When I'm 64

Committee on Aging Frontiers in Social Psychology, Personality, and Adult Developmental Psychology

Laura L. Carstensen and Christine R. Hartel, *Editors*

Board on Behavioral, Cognitive, and Sensory Sciences
Division of Behavioral and Social Sciences and Education

NATIONAL RESEARCH COUNCIL
OF THE NATIONAL ACADEMIES

THE NATIONAL ACADEMIES PRESS
Washington, D.C.
www.nap.edu

THE NATIONAL ACADEMIES PRESS 500 Fifth Street, N.W. Washington, DC 20001

NOTICE: The project that is the subject of this report was approved by the Governing Board of the National Research Council, whose members are drawn from the councils of the National Academy of Sciences, the National Academy of Engineering, and the Institute of Medicine. The members of the committee responsible for the report were chosen for their special competences and with regard for appropriate balance.

This study was supported by Contract No. N01-0D-4-2139 between the National Academy of Sciences and the National Institutes of Health. Any opinions, findings, conclusions, or recommendations expressed in this publication are those of the author(s) and do not necessarily reflect the views of the organizations or agencies that provided support for the project.

Library of Congress Cataloging-in-Publication Data

When I'm 64 / Laura L. Carstensen and Christine R. Hartel, editors.— 1st ed.
p. cm.
Includes bibliographical references.
ISBN 0-309-10064-X (pbk. book) — ISBN 0-309-65508-0 (pdfs) 1. Aging—Psychological aspects. 2. Aging—Social aspects. 3. Older people—United States. I. Title: When I am sixty-four. II. Carstensen, Laura L. III. Hartel, Christine R., 1947-
BF724.55.A35W54 2006
155.67—dc22
2005033689

Additional copies of this report are available from National Academies Press, 500 Fifth Street, N.W., Lockbox 285, Washington, DC 20055; (800) 624-6242 or (202) 334-3313 (in the Washington metropolitan area); Internet, http://www.nap.edu

Printed in the United States of America

Suggested citation: National Research Council. (2006). *When I'm 64*. Committee on Aging Frontiers in Social Psychology, Personality, and Adult Developmental Psychology. Laura L. Carstensen and Christine R. Hartel, Editors. Board on Behavioral, Cognitive, and Sensory Sciences, Division of Behavioral and Social Sciences and Education. Washington, DC: The National Academies Press.

THE NATIONAL ACADEMIES

Advisers to the Nation on Science, Engineering, and Medicine

The **National Academy of Sciences** is a private, nonprofit, self-perpetuating society of distinguished scholars engaged in scientific and engineering research, dedicated to the furtherance of science and technology and to their use for the general welfare. Upon the authority of the charter granted to it by the Congress in 1863, the Academy has a mandate that requires it to advise the federal government on scientific and technical matters. Dr. Ralph J. Cicerone is president of the National Academy of Sciences.

The **National Academy of Engineering** was established in 1964, under the charter of the National Academy of Sciences, as a parallel organization of outstanding engineers. It is autonomous in its administration and in the selection of its members, sharing with the National Academy of Sciences the responsibility for advising the federal government. The National Academy of Engineering also sponsors engineering programs aimed at meeting national needs, encourages education and research, and recognizes the superior achievements of engineers. Dr. Wm. A. Wulf is president of the National Academy of Engineering.

The **Institute of Medicine** was established in 1970 by the National Academy of Sciences to secure the services of eminent members of appropriate professions in the examination of policy matters pertaining to the health of the public. The Institute acts under the responsibility given to the National Academy of Sciences by its congressional charter to be an adviser to the federal government and, upon its own initiative, to identify issues of medical care, research, and education. Dr. Harvey V. Fineberg is president of the Institute of Medicine.

The **National Research Council** was organized by the National Academy of Sciences in 1916 to associate the broad community of science and technology with the Academy's purposes of furthering knowledge and advising the federal government. Functioning in accordance with general policies determined by the Academy, the Council has become the principal operating agency of both the National Academy of Sciences and the National Academy of Engineering in providing services to the government, the public, and the scientific and engineering communities. The Council is administered jointly by both Academies and the Institute of Medicine. Dr. Ralph J. Cicerone and Dr. Wm. A. Wulf are chair and vice chair, respectively, of the National Research Council.

www.national-academies.org

COMMITTEE ON AGING FRONTIERS IN SOCIAL PSYCHOLOGY, PERSONALITY, AND ADULT DEVELOPMENTAL PSYCHOLOGY

LAURA L. CARSTENSEN (*Chair*), Department of Psychology, Stanford University
FREDDA BLANCHARD-FIELDS, School of Psychology, Georgia Institute of Technology
MARGARET GATZ, Department of Psychology, University of Southern California
TODD F. HEATHERTON, Department of Psychological and Brain Sciences, Dartmouth College
GEORGE LOEWENSTEIN, Department of Social and Decision Sciences, Carnegie Mellon University
DENISE C. PARK, Department of Psychology, University of Illinois at Urbana-Champaign
LAWRENCE A. PERVIN, Department of Psychology (emeritus), Rutgers University
RICHARD E. PETTY, Department of Psychology, Ohio State University
ILENE C. SIEGLER, Department of Psychiatry and Behavioral Sciences, Duke University Medical Center
LINDA J. WAITE, Department of Sociology, University of Chicago
KEITH E. WHITFIELD, Department of Behavioral Health, Pennsylvania State University

CHRISTINE R. HARTEL, *Study Director*
TRACY G. MYERS, *Study Director (until March 2004)*
JESSICA G. MARTINEZ, *Senior Program Assistant*

BOARD ON BEHAVIORAL, COGNITIVE, AND SENSORY SCIENCES

Contents

Preface ix

Executive Summary 1

PART ONE: COMMITTEE REPORT

1 Overview 9
2 The Social Side of Human Aging 19
3 Motivation and Behavioral Change 34
4 Socioemotional Influences on Decision Making: The Challenge of Choice 54
5 Social Engagement and Cognition 68
6 Opportunities Lost: The Impact of Stereotypes on Self and Others 80
References 92

PART TWO: BACKGROUND PAPERS

Initiatives to Motivate Change: A Review of Theory and Practice and Their Implications for Older Adults 121
Alexander J. Rothman
A Review of Decision-Making Processes: Weighing the Risks and Benefits of Aging 145
Mara Mather

A Social Psychological Perspective on the Stigmatization of Older Adults 174
Jennifer A. Richeson and J. Nicole Shelton

Measuring Psychological Mechanisms 209
Committee on Aging Frontiers in Social Psychology, Personality, and Adult Developmental Psychology

Measurement: Aging and the Psychology of Self-Report 219
Norbert Schwarz

Optimizing Brief Assessments in Research on the Psychology of Aging: A Pragmatic Approach to Self-Report Measurement 231
Jon A. Krosnick, Allyson L. Holbrook, and Penny S. Visser

Utility of Brain Imaging Methods in Research on Aging 240
Christine R. Hartel and Randy L. Buckner

Research Infrastructure 247
Committee on Aging Frontiers in Social Psychology, Personality, and Adult Developmental Psychology

APPENDIX: Biographical Sketches of Committee Members and Contributors 251

INDEX 259

Preface

Late in 2002 staff of the Behavioral and Social Research Program of the National Institute on Aging (NIA) asked the National Research Council (NRC) to explore research opportunities in social psychology, personality, and adult developmental psychology in order to assist the NIA in developing a long-term research agenda in these areas. The NRC, through the Board on Behavioral, Cognitive, and Sensory Sciences, created the Committee on Aging Frontiers in Social Psychology, Personality, and Adult Developmental Psychology, which I had the honor of chairing, to undertake this task.

Committee members included clinical, personality, social, and life-span developmental psychologists, as well as a sociologist and an economist. Some committee members hold primary expertise in aging; others represent different but related fields. As we educated each other about the broad range of work relevant to our charge it became clear that this was an ideal mix. The committee held four meetings, at which it identified a variety of possible research opportunities and considered the promise of each. As the committee considered priorities, it invited the input of a number of other specialists in vital research areas at a committee-sponsored workshop in September 2003. This made possible an even deeper discussion of the more promising areas of opportunity. Through such consultation and private deliberation, the committee arrived at consensus in giving its recommendations to the NIA. The committee believes it has identified key areas of research in which additional investment may lead to an entirely new understanding about the health and well-being of older people.

On behalf of the committee, I would like to acknowledge the contributions of a number of people who helped us to complete our work. First, we are grateful to Richard Suzman, the sponsor of the project and associate director of the NIA. He posed provocative ideas and questions to the committee and stimulated much thoughtful discussion.

We owe special thanks to several experts from outside the committee whose input was very valuable. Prominent among these are the authors of the six papers prepared for the committee: Mara Mather, University of California at Santa Cruz; Jennifer Richeson, Northwestern University; Nicole Shelton, Princeton University; Norbert Schwarz, University of Michigan; Alexander Rothman, University of Minnesota; Randy Buckner, Howard Hughes Medical Institute and Washington University in St. Louis; Jon Krosnick, Stanford University; Allyson Holbrook, University of Illinois, Chicago; and Penny Visser, University of Chicago.

We also benefited considerably from the presentations and comments at our workshop of Roger Dixon, University of Alberta; John Darley, Princeton University; Annamaria Lusardi, Dartmouth College; Marc Freedman, Civic Ventures; Claude Steele, Stanford University; Charles Carver, University of Miami; Robert Wallace, University of Iowa; William Greenough, University of Illinois at Urbana-Champaign; Dov J. Cohen, University of Illinois at Urbana-Champaign; Michael Feuerstein, Uniformed Services University of the Health Sciences; Marjorie Bowman, University of Pennsylvania School of Medicine; and Lisa Berkman, Harvard University, all of whom contributed to the committee's thinking in important ways.

At the NRC, Christine R. Hartel and Tracy G. Myers served as the study directors for this project. Special thanks are due to Eugenia Grohman, who provided timely counsel and support as well as editing our manuscript with skill and insight; to Kirsten Sampson-Snyder, who managed the review process; to Amy Love Collins and Susan R. McCutchen, who assisted with research for the report; and to Jessica Gonzalez Martinez, our skilled and dedicated project assistant, who was both efficient and considerate.

I would also like to recognize the committee members for their unusually generous contributions of time and expertise and for their professionalism in completing this work. They receive only the compensation of knowing that they have done their best to provide recommendations to the NIA that could advance the field in important ways.

This report has been reviewed in draft form by individuals chosen for their diverse perspectives and technical expertise, in accordance with procedures approved by the Report Review Committee of the NRC. The purpose of this independent review is to provide candid and critical comments that will assist the institution in making the published report as sound as possible and to ensure that the report meets institutional standards for objectivity, evidence, and responsiveness to the study charge. The review comments and draft manuscript remain confidential to protect the integrity of the deliberative process.

We thank the following individuals for their participation in the review of this report: Marilyn S. Albert, Division of Cognitive Neuroscience, Johns Hopkins University; Toni Antonucci, Institute for Social Research Life Course Development Program, University of Michigan; Karlene Ball, Center for Research on Applied Gerontology, University of Alabama at Birmingham; John T. Cacioppo, Department of Psychology, University of Chicago; Medellena (Maria) Glymour, Department of Society, Human Development, and Health, Harvard School of Public Health; Brenda Major, Department of Psychology, University of California at Santa Barbara; Matthew McGue, Department of Psychology, University of Minnesota; and Phyllis Moen, Department of Sociology, University of Minnesota.

Although the reviewers listed above have provided many constructive comments and suggestions, they were not asked to endorse the conclusions or recommendations nor did they see the final draft of the report before its release. The review of this report was overseen by Lisa Berkman, Department of Society, Human Development, and Health, Harvard School of Public Health. Appointed by the NRC, she was responsible for making sure that an independent examination of this report was carried out in accordance with institutional procedures and that all reviewers' comments were considered carefully. Responsibility for the final content of this report, however, rests entirely with the authoring committee and the institution.

Laura L. Carstensen, *Chair*
Committee on Aging Frontiers in Social Psychology,
Personality, and Adult Developmental Psychology

Executive Summary

The "aging of America" has become a familiar part of people's understanding of today's world. This dramatic change in the nation's demography began several decades ago and will continue for many more. By 2030 there will be about 70 million people in the United States who are older than 64, nearly 22 percent of the population. This older population will be quite different from earlier cohorts: it will be more ethnically and racially diverse, with almost 26 percent comprised of ethnic minorities; it will be better educated than any in history; and it will be the first cohort to anticipate old age as a normative stage in life. The "oldest old"—those over 85 years of age—will increase from 4.2 million to 8.9 million by 2030.

The range of late-life outcomes is already dramatic, and it is likely to become more so. Old age is a very different experience for financially secure or well-educated people than it is for poor or uneducated people. Those who are healthy experience old age very differently from those who are ill. Those who are embedded in strong social networks fare much better than those who find themselves alone. Culture, race, and ethnicity, plus the accumulation of individual life experiences, shape the course of people's later years. Understanding individual and social behavior across the life span is key to understanding the diverse outcomes in old age. It is also key to understanding how society can develop the best policies to support longer, healthier lives and to have society benefit from them.

Whether longer life expectancies are good or bad for societies will depend on the nature of old age. To the extent that people come to old age physically and psychologically fit and play integral roles in communities and families, societies will be strengthened. To the extent that older people are infirm, isolated, or dependent, growing numbers of older people will increase the burdens on a relatively smaller younger population. To the extent that older people are healthy and involved, they will likely contribute far more to society than older people in previous generations.

To further advance understanding of how social and individual factors can improve the health and functioning of older adults, the Behavior and Social Research Program at the National Institute on Aging (NIA) requested a study by the National Research Council. The Committee on Aging Frontiers in Social Psychology, Personality, and Adult Developmental Psychology was formed and charged with exploring research opportunities in social, personality, and adult developmental psychology. More specifically, it was charged with identifying research opportunities that have the added benefit of drawing on recent developments in the psychological and social sciences, including behavioral, cognitive, and social neurosciences, that are related to experimental work in social psychology, personality, and adult developmental psychology, and that also cross multiple levels of analysis.

The committee recommends areas of research opportunity that are characterized by recent, provocative findings from psychological science, findings that strongly suggest that additional work will lead to new understanding about the health and well-being of older people. The committee emphasizes areas that have clear applicability to the everyday lives of the nation's older population. Much of this new work will benefit from a life-span perspective that looks not only at older people, but at people who will become old in the coming decades, recognizing that old age outcomes are the product of cumulative effects of behavioral and social processes that occur throughout adulthood.

RECOMMENDATION

On the basis of the needs of the aging population and the benefits to individuals and to society that could be achieved through research, the committee recommends that the National Institute on Aging concentrate its research support in social, personality, and life-span psychology in four substantive areas: motivation and behavioral change; socioemotional influences on decision making; the influence of social engagement on cognition; and the effects of stereotypes on self and others.

Advances in psychological science have brought the field to a critical juncture where—with adequate support—substantial advances are likely in the near future. Of the social sciences, psychology is especially well-equipped to isolate behavioral mechanisms and to understand how to modify them.

Thus, a move away from the description of behavior toward an investigation of its underlying mechanisms and functions would be most productive. Much of the work the committee identified will proceed most effectively in interdisciplinary teams. Psychology brings to interdisciplinary research a number of sophisticated statistical and methodological approaches. Infrastructure support that stimulates the incorporation of these methods into future research will be essential for the greatest progress.

RESEARCH TOPICS

Motivation and Behavioral Change A great deal has been learned in recent years about life-styles that increase or decrease well-being in old age. Information about the value of adequate nutrition, exercise, and preventive health care is widely available throughout the country, but the dissemination of information alone is clearly insufficient to bring about widespread behavioral change. Having knowledge about what to do does not ensure that people live accordingly; getting people to develop and maintain healthy patterns of living involves motivation.

How do you get people to engage in exercises, take their medications, see their doctors, move to assisted living, or even hang up on telemarketers? More broadly, how do you motivate people to maintain goals that are realistic and adaptive while also modifying those goals and developing new ones in response to new challenges and opportunities, such as retirement, relocation, loss, and illness? Research suggests that older people have diminished interest in novelty, which impairs change initiation, but it also supports that the stability of daily routines and contexts will contribute to maintaining changes once they are in place. Research about motivation that addresses the activation and maintenance of behavior change could generate important insights about long-term adherence to healthy life-styles.

Socioemotional Influences on Decision Making The range of choices faced by Americans of all ages has changed significantly in recent years and is likely to increase. Moreover, decisions about many issues, such as financial planning and retirement, have become more complicated, as have choices about health care, while there is also a wider range of options for where and how to live one's later life.

Most current research on decision making at older ages examines the ways in which cognitive decline impairs decision making, yet research also suggests that there is stability or even improvement in automatic, intuitive cognitive processes. For older people, affective heuristics may come to play a more central role in decision making than effortful, deliberative strategies. Such findings have major implications on the processes involved in decision making, particularly on the implications of emotional and social influences.

Significant topics for basic research in this field are the roles of affect, risk aversion, persuasion, self-insight, and regret, in increasing or decreasing the likelihood that older adults make adaptive decisions.

Social Engagement and Cognition Maintaining a "healthy mind" is one of the central concerns of old age, with profound social and economic consequences for older people and for society. Recently, fascinating correlational findings suggest that social relationships and social interactions may affect cognitive functioning at older ages, but these findings have not been examined systematically: they do not establish causal connections nor do they help to identify contributing mechanisms. If there is a causal relationship, it is imperative that researchers identify its properties. Do high levels of social engagement lead to greater intellectual stimulation? Does social engagement mediate depression, which can depress cognitive abilities? Do culture, context, and ethnicity play a role in either minimizing or magnifying the effects of social engagement for cognitive health?

Opportunities Lost: Stereotypes of Self and by Others To the extent that false beliefs influence the ability of societies to use the resources represented in older cohorts, opportunities are lost. Ageism—the attitudes, behaviors, and stereotypes targeted toward older adults because of their perceived age—can affect the opportunities that individuals are afforded during the later years of life. Stereotypes are not just static beliefs: they have both long- and short-term consequences that may function in a pernicious cycle. Stereotyped beliefs about older adults can lead to differential treatment and a loss of access to opportunities. Because people frequently respond to the conscious or unconscious stereotypes held by others (or even by themselves), stereotypes may limit the contributions that older people can make to society.

Aging stereotypes include both positive and negative assessments of older adulthood. In some cases, these beliefs may be particularly difficult to change because they contain some truths. How do negative and positive stereotypes about older adults lead to differential treatment? How do beliefs about aging affect identity and other aspects of self-concept? How can stereotyped beliefs of aging and about older adults be changed? How applicable are the theories and successful intervention strategies in changing race- and gender-based stereotypes for those associated with aging?

DEVELOPING A PSYCHOLOGY OF DIVERSITY

Gender, race, socioeconomic class, culture, and ethnicity are factors that affect virtually all aspects of the health and functioning of older people because of their cumulative effects across the life course. Recognizing this, the NIA has invested significantly in survey research on health disparities between men and women as well as among cultural, racial, and ethnic groups. However, beyond this approach, there has been relatively little investment in understanding how these factors affect fundamental psychological processes and behavioral practices that are associated with aging or even whether the standard measures used in psychological research are reliable and valid across groups. As the U.S. population becomes increasingly diverse across these dimensions, the understanding of subgroups grows in importance. From a scientific perspective, studies of the older population also offer a unique opportunity to study the psychological and behavioral mechanisms that group membership confers and the opportunity to isolate these mechanisms such that behavioral change can occur. The growing diversity of the population means that broad descriptive generalizations about behavior, decisions, social engagement, stereotypes, or any other topic will not characterize large parts of the population accurately.

RECOMMENDATION

The committee recommends that psychological research help to further clarify whether race, culture, ethnicity, gender, and socioeconomic class are associated with fundamental psychological processes represented in each of the committee's recommended research areas.

The study of race, culture, ethnicity, gender, and socioeconomic class should become substantive topics in aging research. The development of psychological theory in these domains will permit important questions about mechanisms to be answered.

RESEARCH INFRASTRUCTURE

The problem-focused nature of our recommendations will require an interdisciplinary approach that focuses on multilevel factors, a research program difficult to carry out with existing funding mechanisms. The research needs to unite the best conceptual and empirical work in personality and developmental and social psychology with work from economics, neuroscience, medicine, demography, engineering, and other fields.

Better research infrastructure is also needed to support and disseminate methods development. Breakthroughs in thought and theory often occur after improvements in measurement techniques and methodology are made.

RECOMMENDATION

In order to carry out the committee's proposed research program, the committee recommends that the National Institute on Aging provide

support for research infrastructure in psychology and methods development in aging research, including interdisciplinary and multilevel approaches, in order to make progress in each of the other recommended areas more likely and more rapid.

New funding mechanisms could encourage interdisciplinary research and build bridges to other branches of government, private foundations, and industry. Infrastructure development could also include extended workshops and topical conferences. Structural changes could also make innovative use of the review process, perhaps by developing special peer review groups.

Part One

Committee Report

1

Overview

Will you still need me,
Will you still feed me,
*When I'm 64?**

Four decades ago the Beatles captured the questions of the baby boomers in their youthful look into the future. If the song were being written today, 74 or 84 might replace 64, but the questions would reflect the same uneasiness about aging. There is great uncertainty about how societies that are top-heavy with older citizens will function. Will people want to work past the traditional retirement age? Will employers hire them? Will people remain healthy and mentally sharp or suffer from increasing infirmities? Will younger people need to provide care for older people, or will older people be self-sufficient and socially engaged?

The answers to these questions have major implications for society because of the sheer numbers of the boomer generation and the changing distribution of the U.S. population by age and gender. In 1970, the age distribution of the population, shown in a population pyramid in Figure 1-1, had the broad base and small top typical of a rather young population, but with a bulge near the bottom for the baby boomers and, above that, an indentation for the older "birth dearth" of the Great Depression. By 2000, the age distribution had narrowed at the base, reflecting the larger number of those in midlife and the smaller number of children and young adults; see Figure 1-2. By 2030, the age distribution of the popula-

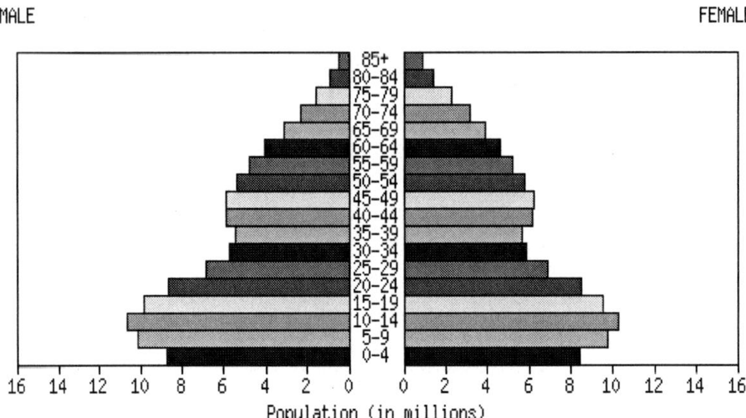

FIGURE 1-1 1970 age distribution by population.
SOURCE: U.S. Census Bureau, International Database. Available: <http://www.census.gov/ipc/www/idbpyr.html (accessed December 2005).

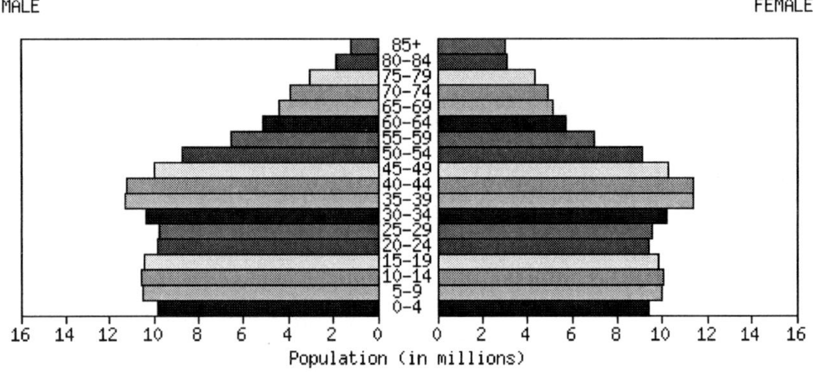

FIGURE 1-2 2000 age distribution by population.
SOURCE: U.S. Census Bureau, International Database. Available: <http://www.census.gov/ipc/www/idbpyr.html (accessed December 2005).

tion will be nearly vertical, with similar numbers of people at every age through midlife and much larger numbers of older adults than at any previous time; see Figure 1-3. By 2030, it is estimated that there will be 12.1 million women and 7.4 million men ages 80 or older, more than twice as many as in the year 2000. In each of the three pyramids, the number of older women is larger than the number of older men.

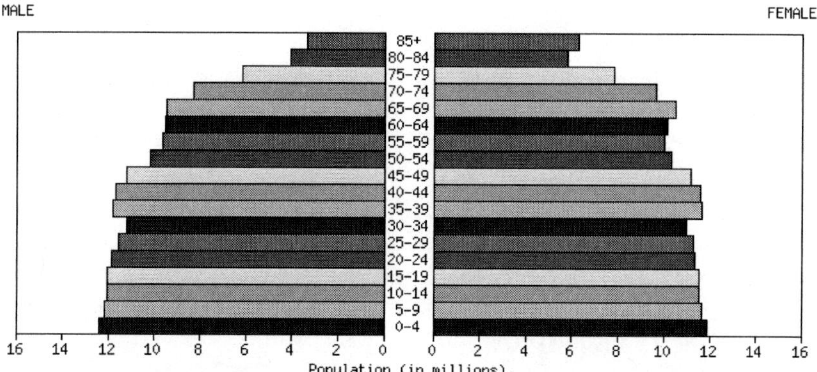

FIGURE 1-3 2030 age distribution by population.
SOURCE: U.S. Census Bureau, International Database. Available: <http://www.census.gov/ipc/www/idbpyr.html (accessed December 2005).

As policy makers and researchers look at the changing U.S. population, they, too, have questions. To date, most of those questions have focused on the societal level—for example, what are the implications for the economy of an aging workforce? What special policy issues will come to the fore because of the extremely large number of women over 80? Increasingly, however, there are questions at the individual level—for example, how will these older people be different from younger adults and, perhaps, different than they were when they were younger? To answer those kinds of questions about the older population, knowledge is needed from a wide variety of disciplines and fields in social and behavioral sciences.[1]

COMMITTEE CHARGE AND APPROACH

To help develop that knowledge, the Committee on Aging Frontiers in Social Psychology, Personality, and Adult Developmental Psychology was formed in response to a request from the Behavior and Social Research Program of the National Institute on Aging (NIA). It was charged to:

> . . . explore research opportunities in social psychology, personality, and adult developmental psychology in order to assist the National Institute on Aging in formulating new directions within its present research portfo-

[1]Throughout this report, "old," "older," and "elderly" are used interchangeably and refer to people ages 65 and older. Subgroups of this population are defined as introduced.

> lios and to develop a long-term research agenda in these areas. The study committee will identify research opportunities that have the added benefit of drawing on recent developments in the behavioral and social sciences, including behavioral, cognitive, and social neurosciences, that are related to social psychology, personality, and adult developmental psychology, and that cross multiple levels of analysis from molecular to macro-levels.

The committee included clinical, personality, and life-span developmental researchers with expertise in aging, as well as researchers whose expertise was highly relevant to aging, but whose research has not focused directly in the field. Considerable time was spent on two initial tasks: to review what has been learned about aging while considering what still needs to be learned, and to consider how to inform the richly descriptive body of research on aging with cutting-edge empirical approaches from several areas in psychology.

The committee's work is fundamentally based on a life-span perspective, on the recognition that people at every stage of life embody everything in their lives, from their initial genetic endowments to their recent experiences, from their individual personality characteristics to the social and cultural milieus in which they have grown up and lived. A life-span perspective not only responds to the committee's charge to consider research from the molecular to the macro level, it also provides a framework in which to begin to bring two disparate areas of research together.

In the field of aging research (gerontology), the corpus of social science research has reflected the efforts—and often the intermingling—of sociology, epidemiology, anthropology, social work, nursing, and psychiatry, as well as psychology. With a handful of important exceptions, experimental social psychology has played a relatively minor role in this research. Because of this history, newcomers to the field sometimes sense a disjuncture between the social science of aging and the mainstream of social psychology, which has been more focused on basic processes and mechanisms involved in attitudes, beliefs, and self-regulation.

In part, the disjuncture reflects the interdisciplinary nature of gerontology and the conceptualization of behavioral science research. In part, it reflects the fact that the early mission of behavioral science research focused on identifying problems of older adults, such as isolation, caregiving, and dementia. However, as life-span psychology emerged and directed attention to normal aging, researchers were increasingly urged to embed individuals in a broad historical, physical, and social context, which involved disciplines and approaches other than those typically considered in the purview of psychology. As cohort differences became increasingly evident, cross-sectional age comparisons, absent broader contextual consideration, became suspect.

The time now is ripe to develop a research agenda that pulls from and crosses the historical disjunctures between the psychology of aging and mainstream psychology and reaches out to other disciplines.

KEY QUESTIONS

Future generations of older Americans may be healthier or more infirm than today's elderly; they may work longer or retire earlier; they may maintain active engagement in communities or pursue lives of leisure. These alternative scenarios will have enormous influence on the future of aging societies, and behavior is key to all of them. The seeking and timing of preventive health care and people's abilities to start—and to sustain—healthy regimens in everyday life are crucial. People who maintain nutritious diets lower their risk of certain diseases. People who get regular exercise and do not smoke experience better outcomes in old age than those who are sedentary and smoke. People who have built strong, lasting social networks are more physically healthy in old age and suffer less cognitive decline than those who have not. Social and economic resources and opportunities form a context in which one may or may not have the power to make any choices at all.

The issue, then, for policy makers, as well as researchers, is how to bring about behavioral changes that will result in optimal outcomes for the majority of the population. That is, one essential societal challenge is to help people arrive at old age as mentally sharp and physically fit as possible and with sufficient economic resources. This challenge entails understanding how people initiate and sustain healthy life-styles. It entails understanding how social influences affect long-range planning. Another equally important challenge is to help people come to old age motivated and engaged. This challenge depends not only on individuals' social and emotional characteristics and expectations, but also on the beliefs, attitudes, and behavior of employers, family members, and health care providers.

The field of research on aging may be on the threshold of its most exciting period. Much of the essential descriptive work has been done. The time for major theory building is ripe, as is the time to apply basic research findings to solving social problems. Aging may be a journey driven in part by biology, but the tremendous variability in aging, even in identical twins, makes it clear that environmental influences—mediated by emotion, cognition, and behavior—significantly affect its course.

RECOMMENDED RESEARCH TOPICS

In order to carry out our charge from the NIA, the committee had to consider a broad array of topics, fields, and disciplines that relate to aging and older people. We set two criteria for our recommended research topics: (1) as specified in the charge, they draw on recent and promising work in the social and behavioral sciences; and (2) they offer promise for assisting in the problems of everyday life for older people. The committee sought to identify research opportunities that illuminate fundamental mechanisms and processes in older people that can, in turn, contribute to practical issues in the lives of the nation's current and future older populations. Our search focused on recent developments in the behavioral and social sciences, including behavioral, cognitive, and social neurosciences, which are related to social, personality, and adult developmental psychology.

The committee did not set criteria about the maturity of a field of research or how active it currently is. Rather the committee identified areas poised to make major advances relatively rapidly given sufficient support.

In addition to the above criteria and a life-span perspective, the committee decided to be highly selective and not to offer the NIA a long list of recommended research topics. Thus, the committee's recommendations are not intended as an exhaustive list of promising areas, nor do the committee's selections mean that other areas are not interesting or important. Rather, the committee selected four topics that we concluded met the charge from NIA, represent fertile and promising fields of research, and can contribute to improving the practical aspects of people's lives.

RECOMMENDATION

On the basis of the needs of the aging population and the benefits to individuals and to society that could be achieved through research, the committee recommends that the National Institute on Aging concentrate its research support in social, personality, and life-span psychology in four substantive areas: motivation and behavioral change; socioemotional influences on decision making; the influence of social engagement on cognition; and the effects of stereotypes on self and others.

The committee recognizes that both interdisciplinary and multilevel approaches are required to address the problems of research on aging. The committee supports the development of integrated interdisciplinary work that will take the best conceptual and measurement work from social, personality, and adult developmental psychology and link it with related concepts and measures from many other disciplines, in order to address important social and health problems of relevance to the mission of the NIA.

For example, the emergence of the new field of social neuroscience, which combines methods and insights from neuroscience, cognition, and social psychology, is transforming our understanding of behavior. This issue is discussed more fully in the topic chapters that follow and the papers "Measuring Psychological Mechanisms" and "Utility of Brain Imaging Methods in Research on Aging" later in this report.

DEVELOPING A PSYCHOLOGY OF DIVERSITY

Future cohorts of the nation's older population will be more racially and ethnically diverse than previous or current cohorts. In 2000, slightly more than 15 percent of people ages 65 and older were black, Hispanic, or Asian or Pacific Islander (the largest racial and ethnic groups in the country); in 2030, almost 26 percent will be minorities. Among the oldest old—those ages 85 and older—the change is from 13 percent minority in 2000 to just over 21 percent in 2030.

But the most important fact about the nation's older population is its heterogeneity. It includes both healthy 75-year-olds who still work and jog every day and frail 75-year-olds in nursing homes. It includes people living with or close to family or friends with whom they are deeply involved and people who live alone, far from family and friends. It includes those born into upper-middle-class families in comfortable suburban neighborhoods, whose lives have followed the expected trajectories through school, work, marriage, and family, and those born into poor families in crowded inner-cities, whose lives have encompassed constant uncertainties and struggles. And it obviously includes men and women of all sexual orientations and of all ethnicities and races, U.S. born or not.

Gender, race, social class, and ethnicity affect opportunities, skills, and liabilities across life, and they significantly relate to old age outcomes. In addition to these characteristics and experiences, attitudes, motivation, and dispositions are also major determinants of people's behavior and, thus, of their decisions and further experiences. Subsequently, given the almost limitless possible combinations of characteristics and experiences that people can have, it is not surprising that the range of late-life outcomes is dramatic. This range of individual life trajectories may be the most important characteristic of the nation's current and future older population.

Although individual-level factors are keys to outcomes in old age, they cannot be considered in isolation from society-level forces. Gender, race, socioeconomic class, culture, and ethnicity provide opportunities to compare outcomes in groups of older people that hold quite different beliefs about aging and display different behavioral and social styles. The NIA has invested significantly in survey research on health disparities between men and women as well as among cultural, racial, and ethnic groups (e.g., Nguyen et al., 2004; Terracciano et al., 2003; Thayer et al., 2003).

RECOMMENDATION

The committee recommends that psychological research help to further clarify whether race, culture, ethnicity, gender, and socioeconomic class are associated with fundamental psychological processes represented in each of the committee's recommended research areas.

Each of the substantive research areas proposed in this report requires the examination of diverse samples. In this way important questions can be answered, such as how group membership(s) may alter types of challenges encountered by older adults or may influence the array of choices made in daily living or how multiple group memberships along with age can affect the extent to which individuals experience and are affected by stereotyping. Existing research on the topics selected by the committee has produced mostly normative findings with very few studies that explore the range of responses that could be expected of the diverse aging population. Of necessity, therefore, the following chapters are limited mostly to normative results; this state of the science is another reason for the recommendation by the committee to make diversity such a significant research consideration.

SUPPORTING THE INFRASTRUCTURE

The research agenda proposed in this report requires strategies for involving excellent psychologists from many specialties in research on aging. It also requires bringing together social, personality, and developmental psychologists with scholars from other social sciences who are actively engaged in research on aging. Moreover, because the problems of aging represent a combination of biological, psychological, and societal influences, both interdisciplinary and multilevel approaches are required. Implementing such interactive research will require innovative funding that creates conditions for collaboration.

RECOMMENDATION

In order to carry out the committee's proposed research program, the committee recommends that the National Institute on Aging provide support for research infrastructure in psychology and methods development in aging research, including interdisciplinary and multilevel approaches, in order to make progress in each of the other recommended areas more likely and more rapid.

Currently, the Behavioral and Social Research Program at NIA recognizes the need for aggressive strategies to encourage researchers at universities work across disciplines, as does the National Institutes of Health (NIH) (see "Roadmap" <http://nihroadmap.nih.gov/> [accessed December 2005]).

We strongly support extending these approaches to encourage new partnerships not only across disciplines within a university and across different universities, but also with government agencies, foundations, and professional societies. In particular, we ask the NIH to consider encouraging nonprofit organizations or even universities to apply for NIA funding to administer small grants programs to promote specific aspects of interdisciplinary work.

In order to facilitate collaboration between disciplines, funding mechanisms need to provide for sustained contact between researchers in different disciplines and mutual education in the approaches of each discipline. This could be done at the level of individual researchers, through paired career awards, or at the level of centers, modeled on the R24 infrastructure grants[2] or on the grants for transdisciplinary centers.[3] In addition, to further encourage developing methods and sharing methods across disciplines, we encourage funding for technical assistance workshops and short courses. (Other ideas for new grant mechanisms are described in the paper "Research Infrastructure" in this volume.)

Methodological and analytical approaches hold special promise for the field of aging research. The measurement of change over time—which is essential to a deep understanding of aging—is also an area in which rapid progress is being made. It is critical that issues of methodology and measurement receive attention and priority: good research depends on the use of appropriate techniques and tools. In the paper "Measuring Psychological Mechanisms" in this volume, the committee offers brief explorations of measurement topics. This paper does not, by any means, cover all the methodological issues that are relevant to research on aging and social psychology, but it highlights some approaches that are particularly relevant to the topics on the committee's recommended research agenda. They are examples of the kind of cross-fertilization of ideas and techniques that can occur between researchers in psychology and other disciplines in research on aging.

The topics we recommend for a focused research program on aging for the NIA can benefit enormously from the kind of support envisioned by the committee's recommendation on infrastructure. Flexibility to cross disciplines, foster small-scale efforts, and encourage the development of innovative methodology for approaching the exciting questions in aging research, will lead to major strides in understanding certain key aspects of aging in a short time.

---

[2]See <http://obssr.od.nih.gov/RFA_PAs/MindBody/MBFY04/Start.htm#infrastructure%20 initiatives> (accessed December 2005).

[3]See <http://grants.nih.gov/grants/guide/rfa-files/RFA-RM-04-004.html> (accessed December 2005).

REPORT STRUCTURE

The next chapter briefly reviews some of the key work and findings from psychology and aging research that provided a foundation for the committee's recommendations and for the rest of the report. With this foundation, Chapters 3 through 6 detail the questions and issues that should be pursued in our four recommended areas: motivating change, decision making, social engagement and cognitive function, and stereotypes. Throughout these chapters we note the roles of gender, socioeconomic status, race, culture, and ethnicity. Our intensive discussions on these topics led to the conclusion that the broad areas of culture and ethnicities can rarely be studied in isolation; rather, they need to be components of most work in aging, including the committee's four recommended areas of research.

The papers in the second part of this volume present background material to complement the committee's report. The first three papers cover topics that relate directly to three of the committee's recommended research topics: motivating change, decision making, and stereotypes. The four shorter papers discuss methodology and measurement, as described above. The final paper presents additional ideas about the kinds of research funding mechanisms that would facilitate carrying out the committee's research recommendations.

2

The Social Side of Human Aging

As people grow older, they are the sum of all that they were born with and have lived through; to a large degree, they are reflections of the social and environmental advantages and disadvantages of the times in which they lived. The life-span approach considers human development embedded in this broader context. It is an approach that has had a profound influence on the study of social aging. A life-span perspective makes it clear that old age cannot be viewed as an insular stage of life—separate from all that comes before—but rather as a stage in the continuum of development.

This chapter presents a brief overview of research from social, personality, and developmental psychology that provided the foundation for the committee's deliberations and illuminated some of the key challenges that are likely to be encountered in carrying out the proposed recommendations. This necessarily brief summary covers the life-span approach; personality and self concept; social relations; emotional well-being; social cognition; and gender, race, and socioeconomic status. In the recommendations we tie these findings about aging to recent advances in mainstream psychology concerning regulatory mechanisms, behavior change, planning, and decision-making—linkages that may lead to progress in areas of economics, health, and well-being.

THE LIFE-SPAN APPROACH

Life-span theory was laid out in a series of edited volumes, which first appeared in the 1970s (Goulet and Baltes, 1970) and continued into the

1990s (Featherman, Lerner, and Perlmutter, 1994). These volumes provided a conceptual framework for the psychological and sociological study of human development across the full life span. As the empirical literature grew and fed back into theory, general conclusions about aging began to crystallize (see Baltes, 1991). One reliable observation is that the balance between gains and losses—albeit weighted increasingly toward loss—continues to include growth in old age (Heckhausen, Dixon, and Baltes, 1989). Of particular relevance to this report, social relations and emotional well-being appear to be areas typified by growth. Indeed, self-knowledge, well-honed skills in self-regulation, and stable social relationships may represent the very resources on which people draw on in order to face the challenges of aging.

One important theme that runs throughout the literature on social aging concerns *selection*. Choices made throughout life to pursue intimate relationships, professions, families, and avocations make people focus increasingly on specific individuals and narrower life domains. Throughout adulthood, people actively construct skills and hone environments to meet selected goals. People become increasingly sure about who they are and more accepting of their strengths and weaknesses. The investment of resources in selected domains of life means that these same resources cannot be allocated elsewhere. In other words, breadth is sacrificed for depth. The meta-model of what is called selective optimization with compensation, developed by Baltes and Baltes (1990; see also Baltes, 1997; Freund and Baltes, 1998), views development as increasingly optimized on expert performance in selected domains. In the context of this model, the relative strength of social ties, satisfaction with relationships, and generally good mental health (as discussed below) very likely represent optimization in selected domains.

Of course, development is not driven purely by choice. Selections are also made by outside forces that place people on particular paths and offer limited opportunities. Sociologists refer to the "Matthew effect" (Merton, 1968) to describe the cumulative advantages and disadvantages associated with the roles assigned to individuals as a function of gender, race, and socioeconomic status (Dannefer, 2003). Furthermore, the longer life expectancy of women compared to men and the significant increases in the culturally and racially diverse populations in the United States speak to the critical importance of understanding how gender, race, culture, and ethnicity affect aging. The number of people ages 80 and over will increase by 2030 to more than 19.5 million—a doubling of the current population, and 63 percent will be female. Current projections also suggest that by 2050 the total number of non-Hispanic whites ages 65 and over will nearly double, the number of blacks ages 65 and over will more than triple, and the number of Hispanics will increase almost ten-fold (U.S. Census Bureau, 2004a).

Gender, race, culture, and ethnicity are important moderators of aging that place people on very different trajectories, which subsequently influence behavioral opportunities, environmental constraints, and frequently very significant differences in life-styles. For example, if a middle-class woman with health insurance reports the same symptom as a poor woman to a health care provider, treatment likely varies. If a black man jogs on city streets for exercise he is more likely to become a target of suspicion by passersby than a white woman. Retirement "decisions" for the socioeconomically disadvantaged are often not decisions at all. The literature in psychological science tends to consider individuals as causal agents. Yet, the physical and social contexts in which people age likely affect myriad aspects of life—including diets, exercise, beliefs, and social concepts—in profound ways that remain relatively unexplored.

Human development is an interactive process that requires consideration of multiple levels of analysis to understand any aging phenomenon, whether of changes in cognition or in emotional well-being (Dixon, 2000). The early findings from the human genome project provide an elegant example. The project promises to grant remarkable insights into the genetic influences on human behavior. Yet, just as surely the human genome project is revealing the limits of purely genetic explanations for behavior.[1] Indeed, some of the most exciting advances address the question of how social factors modify genetic expression. An example comes from Caspi and colleagues (2003), who identified individuals who differed on the 5-HTT (serotonin transporter) gene. People who had one or two copies of the short allele of this polymorphism and who also experienced more stressful life events had an elevated risk of becoming depressed. Another examination of aging phenomena using multiple levels of analysis was recently completed by Epel et al. (2004). They found that women under high levels of perceived chronic stress had much higher levels of cellular senescence, as evidenced by accelerated rates of telomere shortening, than did women under lower levels of stress. A life-span approach points to the need for a developmental diathesis-stress model, in which the developmental trajectories of risk and protective factors are charted to illuminate differential effects as a function of age of exposure (Gatz, Kasl-Godley, and Karel, 1996).

The following sections briefly describe some forces that may be sources of either risk or protection during the life span and their consequences in old age.

---

[1]A summary of genomics and behavior genetics can be found in Plomin and McGuffin (2003), and a discussion of the ethical and social implications of these scientific developments is available from the Hastings Center (Parens, 2004).

PERSONALITY AND SELF-CONCEPT

Stereotypes about older people suggest extremes, ranging from the incompetent fool to the compassionate and wise elder (Cuddy and Fiske, 2002; Hummert, 1990). To believe the stereotypes is to believe that age transforms the very core of who people are. In the realm of personality traits, however, people are more like themselves when they were younger than any old person stereotype. Cross-sectional surveys of men and women ages 18 to 89 show that old people are not necessarily more rigid; if anything, they are less so (Krosnick and Alwin, 1989; Visser and Krosnick, 1998).

Various taxonomies of traits have been offered over the years, but unquestionably the five-factor model (commonly referred to as the "Big Five") is most widely accepted today. Based on factor analyses of self-descriptions, the five traits that reliably emerge across many studies of Europeans and Americans are: (1) openness to experience, (2) conscientiousness, (3) extraversion, (4) agreeableness, and (5) neuroticism. There is some evidence that the core set of traits that differentiates people are genetically based and that they exert their influence throughout the life course: genetic influence is as strong in older age as early adulthood; yet, different genes may change in importance at different ages (Gatz, Pedersen, Plomin, Nesselroade, and McClearn, 1992; Heiman, Stallings, Hofer, and Hewitt, 2003).

As conceptualized by the five-factor model, personality in old age is not radically different from a person's younger years. After the age of about 30, personality traits are highly stable, particularly in terms of rank order. That is, relative extraverts in youth become relative extraverts in old age. There are only very modest mean differences between ages, amounting to less than one standard deviation, in samples drawn from the United States, Germany, Portugal, Israel, China, Korea, and Japan: older adults (up to age 76) score slightly higher than younger adults (age 18 and older) on agreeableness and conscientiousness and slightly lower on neuroticism, extraversion, and openness to experience (McCrae et al., 1999; see also Labouvie-Vief, Diehl, Tarnowski, and Shen, 2000). The big message about personality is about stability (McCrae and Costa, 1994; McCrae et al., 1999; Yang, McCrae, and Costa, 1998).

To be clear, there is no dispute about whether people change in adulthood. They do. Adults are inevitably changed in idiosyncratic ways by the life experiences they encounter, including such major life events as becoming a parent, or less dramatic but persistent experiences associated with, for example, the pursuit of a particular career and the consequent development of a particular type of expertise. Psychologists argue that such changes do not mean that personality changed, however; rather they expect that personality shapes the direction of such changes. The field is only beginning to develop sophisticated models that link and integrate findings from different approaches (Hooker and McAdams, 2003).

Because traits are associated with important aspects of people's functioning, including health behaviors and ways of coping, their consistency allows for reasonable predictions about health and well-being in old age (Bosworth et al., 1999; Caspi and Roberts, 1999; Whitbourne, 1987). Traits predict responses to major life events (Costa, Herbst, McCrae, and Siegler, 2000), such as Alzheimer's disease (Siegler, Dawson, and Welsh, 1994), and the development and even prognosis of coronary heart disease (Hemingway and Marmot, 1999; Williams et al., 2000). McCrae and Costa (1994) argue that certain psychopathologies, specifically major affective disorders, result from a trait-like configuration of personality factors that place individuals at risk to experience chronic periods of negative affect. The dimension of optimism-pessimism represents another important variable related to healthy functioning (Carver and Scheier, 1999). Optimism is related to higher subjective well-being, lower distress, better coping, and faster recovery from illness. Findings from longitudinal study populations have shown that personality traits can be used to predict mortality (Smith and Spiro, 2002).

The idea that stable personality traits such as neuroticism, conscientiousness, and extraversion may affect the trajectory of one's life has been well explored (see, e.g., Costa and McCrae, 1990), but the possibility that traits that are highly adaptive in one group may be less so in another, as a function of racial, ethnic, or cultural membership, is relatively novel and could contribute substantially to the understanding of aging processes. It is also possible that personality measures designed for majority populations do not accurately measure these constructs in members of minority racial, cultural, or ethnic groups and that different constructs may better characterize other groups (Jackson, Antonucci, and Gibson, 1990).

Other personality approaches, such as that proposed by Albert Bandura (1989), consider individual differences to reflect a complex interplay of factors, including temperamental inheritance, that reflect exposure to different types of environments, acquired beliefs and expectations, and the capacity for self-regulation (Bandura, 1989; see also Pervin, 2003). Richard Lazarus's (1991) research on stress and coping also takes an interactional or transactional perspective on personality. In this view, individuals differ both in the external tasks they face and the adaptive resources they possess. This is particularly important during transitional stages in people's lives, for example, when new adaptive tasks are faced by the elderly and the resources needed to master those tasks are limited. In this view, the delicate balance between gains and losses that occurs in the second half of life has important implications for personality. The longer people live, the more likely they will encounter difficult challenges, including the deaths of friends and loved ones, assaults on their own physical health, and threats to social status. At the same time, experience in life accrues, perspectives change, and individual adjustments play a role in the process. Resilience and wisdom have been of particular interest to life-span developmentalists because they involve the use of age-based experience to compensate for losses in circumscribed domains (Staudinger, 1999; Staudinger, Marsiske, and Baltes, 1995).

Because they are rooted in adaptation, life-span developmental approaches naturally lead to consideration of the ways that goals and goal attainment change throughout life (Baltes and Baltes, 1990; Brandtstädter, Wentura, and Rothermund, 1999; Carstensen, Isaacowitz, and Charles, 1999). Carstensen and colleagues, for example, have shown that the perception of time left in life strongly influences goals. Because aging is inextricably and positively associated with limitations on future time, older people and younger people differ in the goals they pursue (Carstensen et al., 1999). Cross-sectional studies with men and women ages 20 to 83 show that older people are more likely to pursue emotionally meaningful goals; younger people are more likely to pursue goals that expand their horizons or generate new social contacts. Brandtstädter and his colleagues (1999) argue that people adjust goal strivings to accommodate external and internal constraints placed on goal achievement at different points in the life cycle. For example, a central finding coming out of this line of work is that older people respond to the loss of resources in advanced age by downgrading the importance of some previously desirable goals.

Self-concept changes with age, but self-esteem—the evaluative aspect of self-concept—tends not to change (Crocker and Wolfe, 2001). Self-concept refers to the beliefs that people have about themselves, including such characteristics as likes, dislikes, values, appearance, and competencies. By and large, cross-sectional research with men and women between ages 18 and 86 shows that older people report less distance between their actual and ideal selves than younger adults, suggesting that they are striving less for personal growth and are more satisfied with who they are (Cross and Markus, 1991; Ryff, 1991). Relatively nuanced beliefs about the aging process also shape self-concept. For instance, McFarland, Ross, and Giltrow (1992) found that older adults' recollections of the past were influenced by their theories of aging. In essence, they found that older adults who believe that memory typically declines with age reported that their memories had been much better earlier in life, and, indeed better than is typically reported by young adults. Thus, views of the self appear to influence the course of aging. Indeed, one recent study by Levy, Slade, Kunkel, and Kasl (2002) provides the tantalizing finding that beliefs about aging, as assessed at ages 50 to 94, predicted longevity: people with strong, positive attitudes lived on average 7.5 years longer than those with negative attitudes.

SOCIAL RELATIONS

In the social realm there is considerable continuity across adulthood. Psychologists Robert Kahn and Toni Antonucci (1980) described a social pattern common across cultures in which people form what they term "social convoys." Social convoys are units or bands of people who accompany individuals through life. The researchers show that although these convoys expand and contract across adulthood, they contain a core set of people, mostly kin, who remain present for decades and whose presence predicts functioning of the individuals embedded in them. In this regard, there is considerable stability in social network composition across adulthood. Some researchers argue that this social stability contributes to the continuity of personality. Caspi and Herbener (1990) found that people tend to choose spouses similar to themselves, and they show that people who have spouses similar to themselves are less likely than people with dissimilar spouses to display personality change in adulthood. Thus, it may be that stability is maintained across the life course because people actively create environments that maintain stability. The strength of social ties as predictors not only of psychological well-being but also of morbidity and mortality was established more than 25 years ago (Berkman and Syme, 1979). More recent longitudinal research shows that emotional solidarity between parents and adult children predicts parental survival (Silverstein and Bengtson, 1991).

Although stable in their core, social networks do become smaller with age (Cumming and Henry, 1961). For many years this narrowing was presumed to be due primarily to morbidity and mortality and to place older people at risk, but a different process has been revealed. Longitudinal studies that have included participants ages from 18 to over 100 suggest that adults engage in a sort of pruning process, beginning long before old age, in which emotionally close social relationships are retained while more peripheral relationships are increasingly excluded (Carstensen, 1992; Lang, 2000). By old age, social networks comprise a relatively larger proportion of emotionally close social partners, a change that appears to have positive consequences for well-being in older people (Lang and Carstensen, 1994; Lansford, Sherman, and Antonucci, 1998).

Older people—both men and women—do spend more time alone (Baltes, Wahl, and Schmid-Furstoss, 1990), but interestingly, until advanced old age, loneliness is less prevalent in older adults than younger adults (Victor, Scambler, Bond, and Bowling, 2000; see also Page and Cole, 1991). In cross-sectional studies of men and women ages 13 to 99, older people are less ambivalent about and more satisfied with relationships than younger people (Fingerman, Hay, and Birditt, 2004). For example, older parents grow more satisfied with their relationships with their children, who have become adults (Fingerman, 2000; Rossi and Rossi, 1990), and the quality of relationships with adult children is strongly associated with parent well-being (Ryff, Lee, Essex, and Schmutte, 1994). Marital satisfaction is also higher in older couples than their younger counterparts (Charles and Carstensen, 2002), and couples (ages 73-93) in a longitudinal study report increasing closeness over time (Field and Weishaus, 1992).

Of course, the positive side of social relations should not be overstated. There can be an important downside to the longevity of family ties, again related to their emotional quality. Although family relationships are, by and large, positive, they are not always so. Close relationships characterized by negative exchanges appear to hold deleterious physical and mental consequences. Over time, negative social exchanges have more potent and deleterious effects than the benefits of positive exchanges (Newsom, Nishishiba, Morgan, and Rook, 2003). Thus, the fact that families last a lifetime can have negative effects, as well as positive ones.

It is also important to keep in mind that even in the strongest relationships, special strains occur in later life, including caregiving and widowhood, and that these strains are different for women and men and experienced quite differently across ethnic groups. Not only does psychological strain accompany caregiving—fully half of all caregivers become clinically depressed (Gallagher, Rose, Rivera, Lovett, and Thompson, 1989)—but the risk of death in the caregiver also increases (Schulz and Beach, 1999). In addition, responsibilities often place severe restrictions on engagement in other activities, ranging from work to social engagement. Otherwise pleasurable activities are forgone so that caregivers can attend to their partners. Interestingly, activity restriction appears to mediate the relationship between caregiver burden and depressed affect even more than the direct physical demands of caregiving (Williamson, Shaffer, and Schulz, 1998). Social norms clearly affect who will become a caregiver and the nature of the caregiving experience. Wives and daughters are far more likely to assume caregiving roles (England, Keigher, Miller, and Linsk, 1991). When husbands do assume the caregiving role, they are more likely to hire professional aides to assist them; moreover, friends and neighbors are more likely to help a husband care for a wife than vice versa (Zarit, Orr, and Zarit, 1985). Among African Americans, beliefs in cultural norms about family care appear to reduce negative physical effects on the caregivers (Dilworth-Anderson, Goodwin, and Wallace, 2004).

The loss of very long-term relationships is common in old age: in 2000, 1.3 million people ages 65 and over had been widowed (representing 32.4 percent of this age group; U.S. Census Bureau, 2004b), and levels of well-being can be reduced for years after the death of a spouse (Lucas, Clark, Georgellis, and Diener, 2003). Women are at much greater risk of being widowed, due to gender differences in life expectancy and the cultural practice of women marrying older men. Among older people, 45 percent of older women are widowed, compared with only 14 percent of men (U.S. Census Bureau, 2004). However, widowhood appears to take a special toll on men. Bereaved husbands are more likely to show distress than wives (Lichtenstein, Gatz, and Berg, 1998). Also, ethnicity matters: almost 40 percent of older white women are married and living with their spouses, compared with only 22 percent of black women (U.S. Census Bureau, 2004b).

Another fundamental aspect of social relations is in the relationship of self to the group. In addition to individual differences, race, culture, and ethnicity exert strong effects. There is compelling evidence that, for example, East Asians' identity is more tightly bound within social groups than for Western cultural groups (Markus and Kitayama, 1991). The effects of aging may actually be different for individuals in cultures with a less individualistic orientation. Moreover, as cultural experiences accrue across the life span, culture-based differences in behavior may become more pronounced in older adults than in younger ones (Park, Nisbett, and Hedden, 1999). There is a growing literature that suggests that social identity and support may play an important protective role against morbidity and mortality. If factors like racism increase stress and affect health, one might expect that social constructs such as identity and family cohesion, at least in healthy families, may be protective against health insults in late life. Similarly, positive aspects of identity and self that are related to racial identity may help to buffer against perceived and actual racism and ageism.

One final point about social networks and aging: although research shows that the overall size of social networks is relatively unimportant for well-being and that the elderly are not particularly vulnerable to isolation, when it does occur, isolation holds notably deleterious consequences for well-being, including an increase in morbidity and mortality (Berkman and Breslow, 1983; Hawkley and Cacioppo, 2003).

EMOTIONAL WELL-BEING

Surveys of men and women ages 20 to over 80 find that older people are as satisfied with life as younger people (Diener and Suh, 1998), which is somewhat intriguing given the loss of social resources noted above. Expectations about satisfaction are guided, in part, by cultural beliefs. In one study of men and women ages 25 to 74, younger people rated their well-being lower than did older people. However, asked about expectations for the future, younger people anticipated a brighter future while older people predicted lower satisfaction in the future (Staudinger, Bluck, and Herzberg, 2003).

Rather than treat well-being as a unidimensional construct, Ryff and her colleagues (1989) have taken a differentiated approach to emotional well-being and identified important nuances to the satisfaction construct. Ryff conceptualizes well-being in terms of self-acceptance, environmental mastery, purpose in life, personal growth, positive relations with others, and autonomy. The dimensions appear to have differential relationships with age, with older adults scoring higher than younger adults on environmental mastery and autonomy, but lower on purpose in life and personal growth. Socioemotional selectivity theory also predicts a motivational shift in later life, away from expanding horizons to finding emotional meaning in life (Carstensen et al., 1999). Consistent with findings that emotional meaning increases in importance with age, older people (men and women up to age 75) seem to perform well on problems that involve emotional matters (Blanchard-Fields, Jahnke, and Camp, 1995).

By their own assessments, older people control their emotions better than younger people (Aldwin, Sutton, Chiara, and Spiro, 1996; Diehl, Coyle, and Labouvie-Vief, 1996; Gross and Levenson, 1997; Lawton, Kleban, Rajagopal, and Dean, 1992; McConatha, Leone, and Armstrong, 1997). Although based mostly on global subjective evaluations, such findings are highly reliable across diverse samples of people from age 10 to 92. Overall, there is compelling evidence that at least some aspects of emotional experience and regulation reliably improve with age. Human emotions are most often experienced in social contexts, and it is likely that there are links between increased selection in social partners and emotional experience. Older people—including men and women up to age 95—choose social partners who fulfill emotional goals (Fredrickson and Carstensen, 1990; Fung, Carstensen, and Lutz, 1999; Fung, Lai, and Ng, 2001) and are happier when their social networks are built to meet these goals (Lang and Carstensen, 2002).

Emotional experience, in contrast to satisfaction (which is a more evaluative construct), speaks to the frequency and intensity of felt emotions and the ability to regulate strong emotions when they occur. Emotion regulation appears to be particularly well preserved in old age. By and large, older people report that they experience relatively fewer negative emotions than younger people (Mroczek, 2001), an observation supported by cross-sectional studies of men and women ages 18 to 95 (Carstensen, Pasupathi, Mayr, and Nesselroade, 2000; Gross et al., 1997; Lawton, Kleban, and Dean, 1993) and by longitudinal studies that followed individuals ages 16 to over 65 at baseline for more than 20 years (Charles, Reynolds, and Gatz, 2001). Even after a traumatic event, older people appear to cope better than their younger counterparts. A study that assessed emotional distress before and after the 1994 Northridge, California, earthquake, for example, found that the oldest old ruminated the least (Knight, Goetz, Heller, and Bengtson, 2000). With the exception of highly arousing or "surgent" emotions, they experience similar (Lawton et al., 1993) or even higher levels of positive emotions than young people well into late life (Mroczek and Kolarz, 1998).

Similar themes resonate in mental health research findings. Rather than a risk factor, age appears to be a protective factor in the etiology of mental health disorders (Gatz et al., 1996; Robins and Regier, 1991). With the exception of the dementias, research shows that older adults suffer relatively low rates of all mental health problems, including depression. Older people (men and women ages 63 to 92) also report fewer fears and anxieties than college undergraduates (Powers, Wisocki, and Whitbourne, 1992). Results of the National Health Interview Survey show that serious psychological distress is least likely to be reported by men and women over the age of 65 (National Center for Health Statistics, 2005). In no way should such findings downplay the seriousness of psychopathology when it occurs; however, such findings do help to place such cases in a context that suggests that aging per se does not increase risk of psychopathology.

SOCIAL COGNITION

Social cognition refers to processing information about social matters and the influence of social context on cognitive processing. Research on cognitive aging documents deterioration in a broad array of basic cognitive processes, including speed of processing, working memory, executive functions, attention, and inhibition. These results are from cross-sectional studies that compared high school or college students and sometimes middle-aged adults to older men and women up to age 92 (Oberauer and Kliegl, 2004; Park et al., 2002; Salthouse, Atkinson, and Berish, 2003; Smith, Park, Earles, Shaw, and Whiting, 1998). Longitudinal studies of men and women ages 70 to 103 at baseline show also that age gradients are more negative over time (Singer, Verhaeghen, Ghisletta, Lindenberger, and Baltes, 2003). Yet the research also suggests that reasoning about emotionally charged matters is well maintained. Older people (largely in their 60s and 70s) solve interpersonal problems more flexibly than younger people (college undergraduates), especially those that are emotionally charged (Blanchard-Fields, 1998; Blanchard-Fields et al., 1995), and they display greater evidence for motivated reasoning about social targets when character traits are emotionally laden (Hess, Waters, and Bolstad, 2000). Even on cognitive tasks known to show age-related decline, like source memory, older people (60-75) perform better when the source concerns emotionally significant characteristics of people (Rahhal, May, and Hasher, 2002). Such findings are in keeping with the idea that older people are motivated to maintain social and emotional harmony in day-to-day life and so direct cognitive resources to those goals.

Support for this finding is also evident in studies of attention (Mather and Carstensen, 2003) and memory, with cross-sectional comparisons of young and middle-aged men and women to older adults ages 56 to 89, including both white and African American participants (Charles, Mather, and Carstensen, 2003; Denburg, Buchanan, Tranel, and Adolphs, 2003; Fung and Carstensen, 2003; Kensinger, Brierley, Medford, Growdon, and Corkin, 2002). Older people attend to and remember emotional images better than neutral images. Most of these studies find that emotionally *positive* information is particularly salient (Charles et al., 2003; Denburg et al., 2003; Mather et al., 2004). For young adults, emotionally negative material is better remembered than emotionally positive material in young adults; age is associated with a shift favoring the positive—a developmental phenomenon referred to as the *positivity effect* (Carstensen and Mikels, 2005).

Another important line of research to emerge from social cognition in recent years concerns stereotype threat (Steele, 1997). It appears that at least part of the documented decline in cognitive functioning can be attributed to beliefs about aging and the social context of the testing. Because there are widespread beliefs in the culture that memory declines with age, tests that explicitly feature memory may invoke performance deficits in older people. In one study, Lynn Hasher and her colleagues (Rahhal, Hasher, and Colcombe, 2001) compared memory performance for young adults (ages 17 to 24) to older adults (ages 60 to 75) under two conditions. In the first condition, experimental instructions stressed that memory was being tested, with the experimenter repeatedly stating that participants should "remember" as many statements from a list as they could. In the second condition, experimental instructions were identical except that emphasis was placed instead on learning, that is, participants were instructed to "learn" as many statements as they could. This study showed rather dramatic effects: there were age differences when memory was emphasized, but there were no differences when learning was emphasized.

Hess and his colleagues (2003) have also documented the effects of stereotype threat with respect to memory and aging. Younger people outperformed older people on a memory task, but the age difference was significantly reduced in the older participants who were primed by a positive account of memory among older people. Apparently, this priming enabled those who read the positive account to use an effective memory strategy, while those who read an account of memory deficits in old age were not as likely to do so.

Findings from experiments that prime age stereotypes map well onto findings about the influence that beliefs about aging have on self-concept and memory performance (Miller and Lachman, 1999). Older people who believe they have control over their memories set different goals for themselves and evaluate their performance differently than those who do not

(West and Yassuda, 2004). Importantly, age-related changes in control beliefs are domain specific: in a large probability sample of people ages 25 to 75, greater control was perceived by older people over some parts of life and less over others (Lachman and Weaver, 1998a).

Another important and different type of question in social cognition research is how racially or culturally bound views of aging might affect the aging process itself. For example, it is widely believed that East Asians, particularly the Chinese, hold more positive views of aging than Westerners (Palmore, 1990) and that these positive views act as a buffer against some aspects of age-related decline, such as decreases in cognitive function. When examining women and men ranging from 60 to 90, this assertion was supported by Levy (1996), but not by Yoon et al. (2000). The study of race, culture, and ethnicity also informs the understanding of cognitive and neural function, providing evidence for aspects of the neurocognitive aging process that are malleable—that is, shaped by race, culture, and ethnicity—or invariant—that is, shaped by biological aging (Park and Gutchess, 2002).

GENDER, RACE, AND SOCIOECONOMIC STATUS

In the United States, gender, race, and socioeconomic status indubitably play important roles in shaping developmental pathways. Arguably, the culmination of these pathways is most striking in old age. The experience of old age for a poor, European American female is very different from the experience of an educated, Asian American male. Women live longer than men. They are also more likely to assume caregiving roles, become widowed, and suffer from chronic diseases. They are more likely to be poor and more likely to be institutionalized at the end of their lives.

Racial differences in health are profound. African Americans are more likely than European Americans to suffer from hypertension; Hispanics, from diabetes (Pleis and Coles, 2002). Level of education predicts the risk of dementia (Gurland et al., 1999; Weintraub et al., 2000). Socioeconomic status predicts longevity (National Research Council, 2004, p. 54). In other words, gender, race, and socioeconomic status are associated with very different health outcomes. Differences arise not purely out of hardship, nor does social privilege inevitably lead to better outcomes (Lachman and Weaver, 1998b).

Some, but not all, research suggests that the effects of socioeconomic class and physical strain appear to be mediated by a subjective sense of mastery such that high degrees of mastery may buffer the effects of economic disadvantage (Lachman and Weaver, 1998b; Singer and Ryff, 1999). Indeed, some of the more intriguing questions about well-being in later life concern the relative resilience of African Americans, who suffer on many objective measures of well-being including health, but show relatively high levels of psychological well-being (Jackson, 1996).

Race, gender, and socioeconomic status are associated with a host of social and behavioral differences, and differences in values, expectations, and behavioral practices. Apparent age and gender differences in family values may be explained, for example, by religious beliefs (Blanchard-Fields, Hertzog, Stein, and Pak, 2001). Elderly African Americans are more likely to want life-prolonging medical care than Asian or European Americans (Lawton, 2000). When African American caregivers hold strong cultural values, their physical health is better preserved than when they do not (Dilworth-Anderson et al., 2004). Also, the difference between the kind of family care considered desirable for older people and the amount of family care actually available can cause strains in Asian American families (Chiu and Yu, 2001). Even widely accepted social psychological principles demand qualification. Research findings from social psychology, for example, have long pointed to a relationship between choice and likability; it is taken as axiomatic that freely chosen options are rated more favorably than options selected by others. A recent study by Snibbe and Markus (2005), however, found that although this relationship is apparent in college students, it is not apparent in people with lower levels of educational attainment.

In order to make significant progress beyond the strong correlations among group status and old age outcomes, it will be important to understand the conditions under which aging experiences are universal, as well as the conditions under which experiences are unique. And it will be essential to identify the mechanisms responsible for those differences. The social science literature leaves no doubt that socioeconomic class, gender, and race play important roles in shaping old age outcomes. However, at the level of mechanisms, understanding of how such group memberships affect psychological processing is only beginning. How race, culture, and ethnicity affect decision-making processes, effective interventions for change, types of social events that affect healthy minds, as well as how they affect stigmatizing experiences and views of aging are just some of the unknown territories related to the country's increasingly diverse older population. Investigation of these factors might also help explain some of the persistent health disparities observed among these groups as well as ways in which individual differences at the psychological level exacerbate or diminish group differences. For example, racial and ethnic differences in appearance and attitudes toward body image could be significant factors that affect the effectiveness of programs to reduce obesity. Moreover, aspects of aging that are universal across cultures can provide insight into aspects of aging that are biologically based in contrast to those that are culturally situated.

The psychological mechanisms that lead to the observed social, behavioral, and physiological differences are not well understood, and there are many important domains in which research offers high yield at both practical and theoretical levels. The study of the slow and steady accumulation of life experiences that characterize development, however, may answer some of the most interesting and important questions we ask about ourselves.

3

Motivation and Behavioral Change

Getting people to develop and maintain healthier patterns of living involves the issue of motivation: How do you get people to perform and maintain behaviors that are in their own best interests but that can be bothersome or difficult to do, such as eating properly, exercising, moderating bad habits, and following through on doctors' directives? More broadly, how do you motivate people to strive for goals that are realistic and adaptive as well as to modify those goals in response to new challenges and opportunities (e.g., for older adults, retirement, relocation, loss, illness)? The need for change is constant throughout life, as people seek new opportunities, try to improve their life-styles, enter new relationships, and control undesirable behaviors. Such behaviors carried out in early and midlife have profound effects on well-being throughout the life span. The committee considered the factors that promote or obstruct attempts at change, as well as the factors that support or interfere with the maintenance of change. At issue are the best ways to motivate efforts to change for the better at all stages of life, and, more specifically, to understand the special needs of older adults in motivating them to change for their own benefit.

Understanding the myriad factors that promote and maintain change is a daunting but crucial enterprise. Even when people say that they want to change, procrastination and acceptance of the status quo are commonplace (Anderson, 2003). More than two-thirds of older patients admitted to emergency rooms, for example, even those with known preexisting medical conditions, do not have advance directives, and a large percentage of those surveyed say that procrastination is the cause (Llovera et al., 1999). Deferral of action has also been well documented in employer-sponsored savings plans and health insurance plans: default "options" are far more likely to be adopted than alternatives, for example (Choi, Laibson, Madrian, and Metrick, 2003). Thus, a great deal of inertia needs to be overcome before change can occur (Baumeister and Heatherton, 1996).

It is currently unknown whether older people are more or less likely than younger ones to initiate change, but it is clear that aging often entails the need to make changes and that the types of changes older people must consider are particularly pressing. For example, many older adults need to watch their diets not only for aesthetic reasons or general physical health, but because of immediate consequences to cardiovascular functioning, blood sugar regulation, or other health problems; failing to take medications may be imprudent and risky when one is in middle age, but downright disastrous in old age because of disease progression. Likewise, exercise can profoundly reduce the likelihood of falls in older people, the consequences of which are far more likely to result in death than in any other age group (Greenhouse, 1994). In short, poor health practices might interact with age to exacerbate negative health outcomes. Thus, behavior change can be an issue of life or death for older people. Understanding how change can be motivated and the ways in which older and younger people may differ in the initiation and maintenance of change is critically important. Large differences between individuals within groups of older and younger adults must also be investigated because broad variations due to chronological age, gender, or level of ability also influence the initiation and maintenance of behavior change.

Older people might have unique motives for change: for example, they might be especially and uniquely family oriented, and thus, wish to be less of a burden to their families, or they might be motivated to maintain an exercise program in order to retain physical functioning. Or they might be uniquely motivated by a behavior change that would promote global good. For instance, older adults might be willing to make a contribution to the needs of one generation in hopes that their contribution might flow through to other generations. Whether these unique age-specific motivators are sufficient to initiate and maintain change remains to be investigated.

The committee sees an important role for psychology in understanding the best strategies for motivating change. This includes a better scientific understanding of the factors that promote change and the factors that maintain change. In the fields of social and personality psychology, the committee viewed two distinct conceptual approaches as being relevant. First, many psychologists focus on self-regulation, which is concerned with personal efforts to initiate and maintain change. This approach is most concerned with internal sources of change, such as how people choose to make changes, their sense of self-efficacy for change, the strategies they undertake to maintain change, and the factors that interfere with their abilities to remain changed. Internal sources of change include the implicit beliefs and values that are associated with different cultures, races, and ethnicity, which shape the lens with which one views the world and result in profound effects on behavior. Research is needed not only to understand the neural, cultural, and psychological processes involved in self-regulation, but also to understand how these processes may change during aging.

The second approach focuses on external sources of change, such as how information can be presented to change attitudes or persuade people to change. From this perspective, research examines social influence and the methods that can be used to change people's behaviors. Research is needed to examine the specific social influence and attitude factors that are relevant to motivating change in older people. The rest of this chapter is divided into two parts, examining the internal and external approaches to self-regulation. Much of the experimental work discussed in this chapter has been carried out in younger or middle-aged people, which is fitting, given the consequences of earlier self-regulation (or its failure) to later life. But the studies must now be carried out in older people, as well.

MOTIVATION AND SELF-REGULATION

Self-regulation is the process by which people control or alter their thoughts, emotions, and behaviors. At its core, self-regulation involves overriding existing habits or contextually triggered impulses and sustaining efforts over time until a specified goal is reached. It involves the capacity to project oneself into the future, form adaptive attitudes, make plans, choose among alternatives, focus attention on pursuit goals, inhibit competing thoughts, and detect discrepancies between one's current states and goal states (Bandura, 1997, 2001; Baumeister and Heatherton, 1996; Carver and Scheier, 1982; Gollwitzer, Fujita, and Oettingen, 2004; Leventhal, Leventhal, and Contrada, 1998; Mischel, 1996; Muraven and Baumeister, 2000). Although humans have the capacity to delay gratification, control appetites and impulses, and persevere in order to attain goals, people of all ages have difficulty with self-regulation. Indeed, failures of self-regulation are among the most important and perplexing problems facing modern society, and, for reasons discussed above, they may pose especially serious difficulties for older people.

Self-regulation is becoming increasingly well understood in social psychology, with an ever-increasing emphasis on how motivational factors may be important for successful self-regulation. For instance, recent models view self-regulation as a limited resource that can be depleted with situational demands (Gross and Levenson, 1997; Muraven and Baumeister,

2000). In contrast is the theory that repeated acts of self-regulation lead to greater self-regulatory capacity, and this may be especially important among older adults. For example, Park et al. (1999) reported that older adults were more adherent in taking medication than middle-aged adults, in part because of lower levels of environmental demands. The increased regularity and predictability of everyday life for older adults may promote habit and self-regulation with age.

The issue of self-regulation must be addressed at multiple levels of analysis: from neurochemistry, neuroanatomy, brain systems, cognition, and emotion; to such familial and societal contexts as socioeconomic status and including gender, race, culture, and ethnicity. At each level, attention is needed to whatever encourages people to inhibit or exhibit certain behaviors, thoughts, or emotions. Research is needed to understand how neural and psychological processes involved in self-regulation may change with age and influence effective change.

A lack of cross-disciplinary interaction and communication among scientists may be one reason that there is still limited understanding of why and when self-regulation succeeds or fails. Social and developmental psychologists have developed complex theories and models of self-regulation, but these theories often fail to consider underlying neurobiological functions or structures. At the same time, neuroscientists have made tremendous gains in understanding the link between brain and behavior, but too often these findings are not informed by the social and cultural contexts that shape and guide human lives. Thus, research is needed that crosses levels of analysis, from molecular genetics to social psychology and sociology.

Moreover, further attention needs to be given to self-regulation outside of the laboratory, such as attempted changes in people's lives (Heatherton and Nichols, 1994). There is consistent evidence that people are able to make important changes in their lives, and many people who do change do so without any form of professional assistance (Prochaska, Velicer, Guadagnoli, Rossi, and DiClemente, 1991). Indeed, Stanley Schachter (1982) observed that clinical studies provide an especially pessimistic assessment of change, in that he found that most individuals who had lost substantial amounts of weight and kept it off or who had quit smoking had done so without formal treatment. Similarly, there is evidence that those who curb problematic drinking do so on their own, without formal treatment of any kind (Peele, 1989). Even those with serious drug dependencies, including alcoholism and heroin addiction, are able to change or alter their problematic behaviors (Klingemann, 1991; Sobell, 1991). Still, there is a surprising paucity of information about the factors that predict change in natural environments, and this may be especially relevant as people become older. Schachter (1982) observed that a greater number of attempts to lose weight or quit smoking predicted greater success, perhaps in part because people develop more successful strategies over time. It is also possible that people develop greater self-regulatory strength through repeated efforts (Muraven and Baumeister, 2000). Researchers must move beyond laboratory and clinical settings to study the way people go about trying to make important changes in their daily lives.

Age Differences in Self-Regulation

Self-regulation is clearly important for people of all ages, although certain aspects of self-regulation may be especially relevant for older adults, such as adherence to medical regimens, following a specified diet to control health problems, and maintaining physical activity (Balkrishnan, 1998; Brown and Park, 2003; Christmas and Andersen, 2000; Diehl, Coyle, and Labouvie-Vief, 1996; Kahana and Kahana, 1975; Schneider, Friend, Whitaker, and Wadhwa, 1991). Social psychologists have long been interested in examining and promoting methods that can be used to encourage people to engage in healthful behaviors (Salovey, Rothman, and Rodin, 1998). This interest is driven both by researchers wanting to test their theories in applied settings outside the laboratory and by a growing awareness in the medical community that people's personal beliefs and actions can have a profound effect on their physical and mental health. Individuals' beliefs and attitudes about aging are also related to outcomes, as are perceptions about the controllability of life. In fact, older people's subjective *perceptions* of their health status predict mortality better than physician-rated health (Idler et al., 2004; Mossey and Shapiro, 1982).

Given that self-regulation is crucial for successful living across the life span, it is surprising that it has received only modest attention in the research on developmental aging. Developmental changes are also scientifically intriguing because successful self-regulation draws on areas in which there are both age-related gains, such as in emotion regulation, and age-related declines, such as in working memory and attention. Because models developed in social psychology allow for the breakdown of these factors, they are likely to be particularly useful in understanding age differences in self-regulation.

Some evidence warrants optimism regarding self-regulatory capacities among older adults (Blanchard-Fields and Chen, 1996; Hess, 1994). Research has found older adults to be better at emotional control and emotional stability (Gross et al., 1997; Lawton, Kleban, Rajagopal, and Dean, 1992; Thayer, Newman, and McClain, 1994) and that they may also be able to delay gratification longer (e.g., Green, Fry, and Myerson, 1994) than younger adults. Similarly, Diehl, Coyle, and Labouvie-Vief (1996) demonstrated that older adults have greater impulse control than children and young adults, primarily because of the use of more efficacious coping strategies (see also Labouvie-Vief, Hakim-Larson, DeVoe, and Schoeberlein, 1989). The evidence indicates that self-regulatory capacity increases over the life course, with children being the least capable and older people being the most capable.

In contrast to the evidence just described, research in cognitive neuroscience suggests that some aspects of self-regulation may degrade with aging. Given declines in executive functions that frequently accompany aging, it is important to examine how these declines affect the capacity and motivation for self-regulation. Self-regulation requires a number of executive functions, such as working memory, allocating attention, inhibiting prepotent behavioral responses, and initiating novel strategies. A variety of evidence indicates that various neural circuits in the prefrontal cortex are involved in executive functions and self-regulation (Banfield et al., 2004; Bechara, 2003). There is currently considerable debate about whether different brain structures are involved in different types of executive functions or whether some structures enable all executive functions and direct other structures to perform subsidiary tasks (e.g., Breiter and Rosen, 1999; Cohen, Botvinick, and Carter, 2000; Gehring and Knight, 2000, 2002; Grafman, 1999; Kerns et al., 2004; Posner and Rothbart, 1998; Raichle, 2000; Richeson et al., 2003; Smith and Jonides, 1999). Understanding the coordination and integration of brain structures that support behavioral and mental self-regulation is one important goal of neuroscience research, especially to the extent that there is reduction of prefrontal cortex functioning with aging (Salat et al., 2004; Tisserand and Jolles, 2003). Basic research must be conducted to examine the neural mechanisms that support self-regulation with a particular emphasis on which, if any, of the mechanisms change with age.

Initiating or Maintaining Change

Among young people, the maintenance of change programs appears to be more difficult than initiation. Young people are eager to start exercise programs, quit smoking, or lose weight, but failure rates in maintenance are very high (Baumeister, Heatherton, and Tice, 1994). Indeed, a sense of hope that permeates people's lives when they decide to make changes is a strong motivator of initial efforts to change, even if it does not itself predict long-term change (Polivy and Herman, 2002). Inherent in this idea is that notion that some degree of negative affect is crucial for initiating change; people do not attempt to fix what they don't believe is broken. Thus, people attempt to diet when they are dissatisfied with how they look, they quit drinking when it causes problems in their lives, and they save money because they are worried about not having enough when they need it. To the extent that older adults experience fewer negative emotional states, it may be that they are less likely to spontaneously initiate life change on their own. At the same time, there is a greater likelihood that they will be encouraged by physicians or family members to make healthy changes to prolong their lives. Thus, research is urgently needed to understand more thoroughly the factors that initially prompt change, especially for older people.

Rothman (in this volume) notes that one factor that prevents initiation of change is that many people are hesitant to accept information that calls their basic health practices into question. People often respond to negative health diagnoses by minimizing the seriousness of the condition or emphasizing its prevalence (Ditto and Croyle, 1995). This reaction is especially a concern during the aging process when people might misinterpret their symptoms as resulting from aging rather than from disease processes.

Social and health psychologists have developed a number of methods that encourage efforts to change in people of all ages. For instance, message tailoring involves presenting information that is personally relevant for specific individuals, and this method is generally more successful than generic messages that are aimed at a broad audience (see Rothman, in this volume). The manner in which the message is framed also matters a great deal. It is generally believed that if the goal is to promote the use of detection measures (such as screening for cancer), then messages that emphasize losses have stronger effects than those that emphasize gains. In contrast, the promotion of preventive behaviors (such as eating a healthy diet) is best accomplished through messages that focus on gains. However, there is evidence that with older adults emphasizing gains may be more effective in both cases (Löckenhoff and Carstensen, 2004).

One hypothesis is that with age it becomes harder to make behavioral changes, but once those changes are initiated, older adults find them easier to maintain. There is reason to infer from the existing aging literature that change in older adults may entail special challenges in the area of initiation. Passivity on the part of institutionalized older adults has been widely documented (Baltes, 1995, 1996), perhaps because of reinforcement processes (Baltes and Wahl, 1991). And some memory decline in normal aging directly affects self-initiated cognitive strategies (Cabeza et al., 2004; Logan et al., 2002). For example, in healthy older adults, self-initiated memory strategies show reliable deficits with age, while strategies that are externally primed show no age decline (Einstein et al., 1995; Wingfield and Kahana, 2002). It is also possible that older adults see fewer opportunities for change or believe that their efforts to change will have less positive outcomes (Leventhal, Leventhal, and Contrada, 1998).

Yet older people are able to change their behavior. Medication adherence is better among older than middle-aged adults, attributed in part to more stable daily routines (Park et al., 1999) and psychotherapy efficacy is as good with adults between the ages of 61 and 90 as with their younger counterparts ages 21 to 59 (e.g., Reynolds et al., 1996). The difficulty of initiating change, as well as the ease of maintenance, may be related to the stability of contextual cues in late adulthood. There is sound evidence that older adults lead more routine and less varied lives than young adults (Martin and Park, 2003). This stability may make initiating change difficult; at the same time, the presence of stable environmental cues may help maintain behavior. Thus, context plays an important role in maintaining behavior.

These findings are in agreement with research demonstrating that imagining a context in which a future behavior is to be performed greatly enhances the probability that the behavior will be completed (Gollwitzer and Schaal, 2001; Gollwitzer et al., 2004). Chasteen, Park, and Schwarz (2001) reported that older adults were much more likely to remember to perform a simple action of writing the data on a paper at the end of a laboratory study if they imagined completing the action, in comparison with simply repeating the planned action. In a recent study, Liu and Park (2004) demonstrated that older adults were much more likely to maintain use of a glucose monitor over a 4-week period if they spent only a few minutes imagining the context in which they would perform the action at the time they received the monitor, in comparison with people who rehearsed trying to remember performing blood glucose monitoring. These researchers hypothesize that it is the stability of older adults' lives and the regularity in which they encounter the same contextual cues (e.g., they eat meals at the same time every day) that resulted in the maintenance of complex behavior for a month, based on only a few minutes of rehearsal. Further investigation of mechanisms for initiating and maintaining changes in health behavior is needed, with an emphasis on the role of contextual stability. The findings with older adults will also provide valuable strategies for younger adults who are trying to maintain change and also have the potential to inform the understanding of self-regulation at a very broad level.

The Avoidance of Novelty

Generally speaking, change involves novelty. It involves learning new information, modifying routines, and very often making new social contacts, whether change agents or simply new people. There is good evidence that older people have less motivation to explore new ways of living. They tend to be lower in the personality trait of sensation seeking (Lawton et al., 1992) and, as shown in cross-cultural studies, also less open to new experiences (McCrae et al., 2000). Instead, they tend to focus attention away from novelty toward familiar, predictable aspects of life. One prominent conceptual model in life-span psychology noted above, selective optimization with compensation, postulates explicitly that a narrowing of breadth coupled with heightened effort and expertise in selected areas of life reflects successful adaptation to old age (Baltes and Baltes, 1990).

For somewhat different reasons, socioemotional selectivity theory makes similar predictions. According to selectivity theory, perceived constraints on time result in motivational changes that favor goals related to regulating emotional states over goals associated with gaining knowledge or otherwise expanding one's horizons. In studies that use social choice paradigms, for example, older participants are reliably more likely to opt for well-known, emotionally significant partners over novel social partners (Fredrickson and Carstensen, 1990; Fung and Carstensen, 2004; Fung, Carstensen, and Lutz, 1999; Fung, Lai, and Ng, 2001). Even basic cognitive processes, like memory and attention, appear to be affected by motivational changes. Empirical tests of selectivity theory demonstrate that memory for advertisements is better when slogans promise emotional rewards than when they promise informational rewards (Fung and Carstensen, 2003). Thus, there is considerable evidence that, with age, people grow more interested in emotional satisfaction and less interested in seeking novelty. This resistance to trying new things has important implications for initiating change, and it is an important priority for research to illuminate how the motivation to avoid change influences self-regulation, as well as basic cognitive and emotional processes.

Emotional Processes and Self-Regulation

It has been widely noted that negative emotional states lead to relapse for a number of addictive behaviors, such as alcoholism and smoking. Distress increases craving for alcohol among those trying to control alcohol intake (Litt et al., 1990), which, in turn, leads to drinking (Hull and Young, 1983; Miller et al., 1974). Similarly, the single most important trigger for smoking urges is a negative emotional state (Marlatt, 1985; Shiffman, 1982): people smoke in order to control stress (Kassel, Stroud, and Paronis, 2003). Emotional distress has also been identified as a major determinant of diet failure and binge eating (Greeno and Wing, 1994; Heatherton and Baumeister, 1996). According to this research, when a person's emotional state conveys negative implications about the self, people are especially motivated to shut out painful self-awareness, either by external means (such as consuming alcohol) or by restricting attentional focus to potent stimuli through cognitive narrowing. The resulting mental state may indeed be less distressing, but it is also likely to lead to disinhibition, and the long-term consequences of these escapist strategies might exacerbate future distress (see Heatherton and Baumeister, 1996). Thus, it is people who feel personally deficient or who experience threats to the self who are most likely to break their diets, spend excessively, or binge drink.

The literature on self-concept and aging suggests that despite objective threats to self, from physical disabilities to ageism, older people are surprisingly satisfied with their self-views (Greve and Wentura, 2003). Discrepancies between ideal and actual selves, for example, are smaller than those observed in younger people, when groups with mean ages of 19.3, 46.0, and 73.4 are compared (Ryff, 1991). Studies of well-being also suggest that aging is associated with less interest in personal growth (Ryff, 1995). In other words, aging is associated with greater satisfaction with the status quo and less interest in improving the self. One experience sampling study also revealed less variability in self-descriptions in everyday life (Charles and Pasupathi, 2003). Thus, because negative affect is an important trigger of self-regulation failure, it may be that older adults succeed at self-regulation more often than younger adults because they do not experience as much dissatisfaction. This hypothesis further reinforces the idea that although initiating change may be more difficult for older adults, maintaining change may be easier.

It is also possible that the relation between negative emotions and self-regulation is due to inadequate coping and the possibility that people use alcohol, drugs, or food as a coping strategy. Accordingly, it may be that older adults are less prone to self-regulation failure because they use strategies that minimize negative affect in their daily lives (Mather, in this volume). It is unclear whether putative self-regulatory differences observed as a function of age are due to changes in cognitive skills or capacities or to changes in the degree of experienced negative affect. Considered together, it is apparent that the more positive emotional experiences of older adults may discourage initial change but serve to enhance any changes that do occur. Research should examine the general role of affect in self-regulation, with an emphasis on how emotional changes that occur during aging may be associated with initiation or maintenance. Moreover, additional research should examine how emotional processes are involved in change that adds new behaviors (such as exercise) as opposed to change that eliminates them (such as poor health habits).

Individual Beliefs and Attitudes

A vast literature demonstrates the role that efficacious beliefs play in instigating and maintaining change in young people (Bandura, 2001), and there is additional evidence that they play a similar role in older adults. Self-efficacy and personal beliefs have long been known to play critical roles in self-regulation (Bandura, 1989, 1997; Mischel, Cantor, and Feldman, 1996;

Mischel, Shoda, and Rodriguez, 1989) and research demonstrates that feelings of control over the environment are important for self-motivation across the life span (Brandtstädter and Rothermund, 1994; Seeman, McAvay, Merrill, Albert, and Rodin, 1996). Racial, cultural, and ethnic group membership confer an identity that is part of the conception of the self and connectedness of the self to others that directs choices and decision behaviors. Such group membership plays a crucial role in the development of self-efficacy and personal beliefs, especially about control over the environment. A comparison among different groups could highlight the mechanisms of most importance and suggest interventions for members of all groups. Studies of individual variability within these groups could provide further information for designing the most useful interventions.

There is considerable evidence that self-efficacy beliefs are related to motivation and health. In terms of the former, self-efficacy beliefs are associated with the selection of goals, effort, and persistence in the face of frustration, emotion (e.g., anxiety and depression), and coping with stress and disappointment. In relation to the latter, self-efficacy beliefs are associated with healthy behaviors, enhanced immunological system functioning, and the avoidance of relapse (Bandura, 1997). Self-efficacy is especially important for encouraging patient compliance with medical regimens (Schneider et al., 1991). Tying the two together, it is clear that motivating people to change involves helping them to set specific health-related goals and influencing their self-efficacy beliefs in relation to these goals and other life tasks. But far more needs to be known about the mechanisms involved, especially in specific individuals, and how to activate them.

Social Facilitation and Barriers to Change

A variety of evidence suggests that social support is an important component of successful life change (Clifford, Tan, and Gorsuch, 1991). For instance, social support has been found to be valuable for achieving and maintaining weight loss in younger and middle-aged people (Perri et al., 1988). Social support may enhance change because it contributes to self-efficacy (Major et al., 1990) and increases general well-being, and it also may buffer against the strain caused by high-stress life events (Cohen and Wills, 1985; Gentry and Kobasa, 1984). In the context of racial, cultural, and ethnic identity, it is also important to recognize the shielding mechanism and social support that may be provided by membership in a specific racial or ethnic group. As discussed above, relapse is commonly associated with perceived emotional distress (Brownell, Marlatt, Lichtenstein, and Wilson, 1986), but significant others may be able to assuage negative emotional experiences by helping people cope with high-risk situations (Marlatt, 1985). Family, friends, coworkers, and health care professionals can provide the emotional and esteem support, feedback, information, reinforcement, and direct assistance that a person involved in change frequently needs (Clifford et al., 1991; Marlatt, 1985). Moreover, making public commitments and having a "buddy" who shares attempted change might also be a useful strategy for change. The social networks of older people typically involve a small circle of close relatives and friends, suggesting that those in their social networks might be potent motivators of change (Lang and Carstensen, 1994).

However, some research has also shown that social support may interfere with motivation or behavioral change (Kelly, Zyzanski, and Alemagno, 1991). This finding may reflect the fact that people tend to associate with others who have similar ideas, personalities, and backgrounds (Caspi and Herbener, 1990), which would tend to promote stability. But when people change, their ties with other people change as well. It is possible that others sometimes will actively hinder change because they feel threatened by the implications of potential changes. For example, spouses who wish to continue smoking may be unlikely to offer support and encouragement to a partner who is contemplating quitting smoking because such advice would be dissonant with their own behavior. Social support is likely to be effective only when the supporter already holds the attitudes and identity that the person is trying to adopt. Again, because the social networks of older people are small and restricted to significant others, it is likely that any negative social effects will be larger for older than for younger adults. It is crucial that researchers examine the role of other people in efforts to initiate and maintain change.

In general terms, it might be that older adults are less likely to be influenced by social forces. Most theories of social influence do not consider adult development. Theoretical and empirical work in life-span developmental psychology, however, suggests that age may reduce susceptibility to social influence. Under certain conditions and relative to their younger counterparts ages 18-35, people between the ages 63 and 85 display lower rates of social conformity (Pasupathi, 1999).

PERSUASION AND ATTITUDE CHANGE

In addition to self-regulation processes, social psychologists have developed a rich literature on the psychological processes underlying attitude formation and change. In fact, the topic of attitudes and persuasion is one of the most well developed in social psychology, with numerous established theories and findings (for reviews, see Eagly and Chaiken, 1993; Petty and Wegener, 1998). Attitudes refer to individual's evaluations of people (including themselves), objects (e.g., one's medication), issues (e.g., changing Social Security), and actions (e.g., moving to a retirement home). Attitudes can be based on a person's values, specific beliefs, emotions, and behaviors (both actual and anticipated). As noted above, forming attitudes is typically necessary before decisions can be made or behaviors enacted. Thus, if older people are going to change their diets or exercise more, they first need to develop favorable attitudes toward these behaviors and toward making these changes.

Indeed, a major premise of research in social psychology is that attitudes are important because they guide people's decisions and actions (e.g., Fishbein and Ajzen, 1975; Sanbonmatsu and Fazio, 1990). Stated simply, people will choose an option they like over one they dislike. When two options are both evaluated positively (or negatively), the option evaluated more positively (or less negatively) typically will be selected. Thus, if a person likes Coke more than Pepsi, Coke is more likely to be purchased. If two options are equivalent in their desirability, then the option toward which one holds the more confident or accessible attitude will be chosen (Petty and Krosnick, 1995). The attitudes of others are also important in influencing actions. For example, if people believe that you are forgetful, they will tend to act in a manner toward you that is consistent with this belief, and this action may in turn elicit the forgetful behavior that is expected (see Snyder, 1992). Thus, both people's own attitudes and the attitudes that others have about them can influence behavior.

Because of the critical role that attitudes have in guiding behavior, understanding how evaluations are formed and changed and whether these judgments are strong or weak (e.g., how confident or accessible they are) is an important undertaking. Considerable research has examined attitude change processes in younger adults and much can be learned from this work. In contrast, relatively little effort has been aimed at understanding how older adults form or change their attitudes.

There are several areas of research that seem ripe for exploration with respect to older people. One area focuses on the underlying mechanisms by which attitudes are formed or changed and what techniques are most effective in persuading older people. These may or may not be dependent on cultural values and racial or minority group membership. Understanding of persuasion can be useful from the standpoint of producing desirable changes (e.g., a physician persuading older patients to take their medications) and protecting people from undesirable agents of influence (e.g., avoiding telephone scams). A second area concerns the unique role that emotional factors might play in the choices that older adults make. This is of particular interest because of evidence that emotional regulation processes become better and more important with age. A third area involves investigating the factors in older people that produce an initial change in possible contrast with those that are responsible for maintaining a change once it has occurred. A fourth area of research concerns the distinction between implicit and explicit attitudes (e.g., Greenwald and Banaji, 1995). Explicit attitudes are those evaluations that a person consciously endorses; implicit attitudes are evaluative tendencies that may be automatically activated without a person's awareness (Fazio and Olson, 2003). Although much attention has been paid to how to change explicit attitudes, researchers are only beginning to examine how to modify implicit attitudes, and very little work in this area has been undertaken with older adults.

Attitude Change Processes: Thoughtful or Automatic

Researchers are just beginning to consider the unique aspects of communicating with and modifying the attitudes and behaviors of older people (e.g., Spotts and Schewe, 1994). Factors that affect their compliance with medical regimens have received particular attention (e.g., Brown and Park, 2003), with some clear findings, especially with respect to such factors as the cost of medication, insurance coverage, complexity of the medical regimen, and certain demographic variables (e.g., Balkrishnan, 1998; Salzman, 1995). Far less attention has been paid to persuasion processes in older people and how they might differ from those of younger adults.

One reason persuasion processes might differ in older and younger adults relates to the effects of aging on the frontal regions of the brain. For example, a reduced working memory capacity may lead older adults to seek less information when making a decision, and older people ages 65-75 may thus form attitudes based on less information and with less thought than adults ages 28-55 (e.g., Streufert et al., 1990). Much research in social psychology suggests that the underlying processes of attitude formation and change can be placed along a continuum, ranging from extensive thought about the merits of objects to evaluations based on relatively simple (even automatic) processes that require little thinking (Petty and Cacioppo, 1986). Specifically, when people are not thinking very much, they rely on their intuitions, gut feelings, and simple heuristics to form attitudes and make choices (e.g., if an expert said it, it must be true), but when people are thinking carefully, their idiosyncratic thoughts in response to the message and their thoughts about their thoughts (e.g., was my thought valid?) become important determinants of attitudes (for reviews, see Chen and Chaiken, 1999; Petty and Wegener, 1999).

Many individual and situational variables have been identified that determine where a person is along the thinking continuum and thus what type of influence technique might be most effective. For example, people engage in greater thinking when the message is perceived as personally relevant or when the person feels accountable for a decision. In terms of personality, some people are prone to rely on deliberative processing (Cacioppo and Petty, 1982) while others tend to be more reliant on heuristics and intuitions (see Epstein, 2003).

The thinking continuum is particularly interesting to examine in light of aging because, as noted above, people tend to rely less on deliberative forms of thinking and more on intuitive modes as they grow older. It is important to note that extensive thinking does not necessarily produce better decisions than does relying on gut feelings or intuition. This is because a person's extensive thinking can be biased in various ways, and intuition can be a proxy for a person's expertise. Nevertheless, if older adults are less motivated or less able to seek and process information than younger adults, attitude modification processes that rely more on heuristics and intuitions might be more effective than strategies that rely on high amounts of information processing and thinking. Thus, older people may be more likely to base evaluations on the first information presented (primacy effect), or on a smaller number of information dimensions, or on simple inferences, shortcuts, and associations (e.g., if it makes me feel good, I like it; Schwarz and Clore, 1983). The strategies that are most effective in modifying the attitudes of older adults should be investigated.

One reason the amount of thinking behind one's attitudes is important is because thoughtful attitudes tend to be more persistent over time, more resistant to change, and more influential on one's behavior. Also, people tend to have more confidence in judgments that are based on large amounts of information, and judgments based on considerable thinking tend to be more accessible (see Petty and Krosnick, 1995). Thus, if the newly developed attitudes of older adults are based on less information processing, these attitudes may be held with little confidence, or one's new attitudes may be low in their accessibility, causing decision making to be more stressful (see Fazio, 1995). If decision making is somewhat stressful because of holding attitudes with low confidence, decision making will be avoided. The committee believes that this is an important topic for exploration.

How to maximize thoughtful decision making and how to tailor or frame information to be maximally effective for older adults are among the many other research issues that could be examined with respect to persuasion and the concerns of the older population (see Rothman, in this volume). From the perspective of contemporary models of persuasion, there are several mechanisms by which framing or tailoring might work. For example, targeting a message for older people (rather than a younger audience) might be effective because tailoring makes the message seem intuitively appealing (e.g., "the message resonates with me, so it must be good") or because tailored messages get people to think carefully about the information because of the heightened perceived self-relevance. Which of these mechanisms is operating is of importance because the latter process is likely to lead to stronger attitudes than is the former. Also of interest is the possibility that for some older message recipients, tailoring may not have the expected effects. For example, if some older adults hold negative implicit or explicit attitudes toward old people generally (Richeson and Shelton, in this volume), the normal positive effects of tailoring would not be expected. This, too, should be explored.

Emotional Factors in Attitudes and Decision Making

Older adults show increased focus on emotional goals, such as avoiding regret and maximizing satisfaction (Mather, in this volume). Considerable research in social psychology has focused on how emotions, in comparison with cognition, affect individuals' attitudes and ultimately their actions. Common models of attitude formation assume that people consider the cognitive (utilitarian) and affective (emotional) consequences of adopting an advocacy position or making a choice (e.g., Abelson et al., 1982). Although some attitudes are based largely on cognition, others are based largely on affect, and still others are based on both (Crites, Fabrigar, and Petty, 1994; Eagly, Mladinic, and Otto, 1994).

As noted in Chapter 4, psychological models hold that two aspects of beliefs are of particular importance for people—the likelihood of the consequences considered and the desirability of those consequences (e.g., Fishbein and Ajzen, 1975). Thus, if a person is deciding whether to move into a new retirement community, she might consider whether the move would be too expensive and whether the move would make her happy. For each of these perceived consequences, the person would then consider how likely it was that the move would be expensive and how likely the move would be to produce happiness. The person would also consider how desirable it would be to spend the anticipated amount of money and how desirable it would be to attain happiness from the move. Furthermore, social psychological research suggests that being in an emotional state can influence the perceived likelihood and desirability of consequences: for example, being in a happy state can make positive consequences seem even more likely than when not happy (DeSteno et al., 2000; Lerner and Keltner, 2001). These likelihood and desirability "forecasts" (Gilbert and Wilson, 2000) about the cognitive and affective consequences of a considered action are important because they can determine the person's attitudes, which would in turn influence the particular choices made and behaviors implemented.

If one wants to modify people's attitudes in a thoughtful way, persuaders can introduce new consequences that people have not considered previously, or they can try to influence the perceived likelihood or desirability of consequences that are already known. Thus, if a person thinks that it is somewhat likely that moving will produce a little happiness, a persuader can attempt to convince a person that moving is very likely to produce a lot of happiness. To the extent that the perceived likelihood or desirability of the consequences change, the overall attitude toward the move will also change.

Within this framework, research might focus on whether older decision makers weigh emotional consequences more than cognitive ones in attitude formation and decision making. In addition, the role that emotional factors or anticipated emotions have in influencing likelihood and desirability forecasts for older individuals could be investigated. Other topics of interest would include understanding why older adults show greater susceptibility to some forms of persuasion (e.g., phone scams). Is this due to cognitive deficits (e.g., inability to counterargue a sales pitch) or enhanced weighting of emotional benefits (e.g., enjoyment of talking to someone)?

As noted above, research suggests that emotion regulation improves with age (Gross et al., 1997). One strategy people use to maintain their positive moods is to avoid negative information (Wegener and Petty, 1994), including avoidance of processing of messages with negative overtones or consequences (Wegener, Petty, and Smith, 1995). Thus, it could be that older adults are more likely than younger ones to avoid threatening or fearful messages as a mood regulation strategy. Because of emotional regulation and lack of ready attitudes (or attitudes lacking in confidence), they may avoid decision making in order to avoid stress. The notion of avoiding distress also suggests that older adults may be more susceptible to the effects of cognitive dissonance (Festinger, 1957) than younger adults. For example, research has shown that decision making can produce dissonance (unpleasant tension) when people must accept some undesirable features of a chosen alternative and forgo some attractive features of a rejected one (Brehm, 1956). As a result, people tend to exaggerate the positive aspects of the chosen alternative and minimize the positive features of the rejected alternative after making their choice. To the extent that older adults have a greater aversion to negative states, they could be more susceptible to this dissonance effect (see Mather, in this volume).

Initiation and Maintenance of Change

Just as research on self-regulation suggests that the processes involved in the initiation of change may differ from those involved in the maintenance of change, so too does the literature on externally initiated change. In particular, as noted above, when people are considering change, they are largely influenced by their expectations, both emotional and cognitive, regarding the outcomes of changing (e.g., Will I be happier? Will it be easier to walk to the store if I move?). However, once change has occurred, research suggests that people are influenced by their assessment of their post-change experiences. Research on post-change processes is especially prominent in the work on consumer behavior. Researchers have studied *expectancies* about product performance as a determinant of initially selecting a brand, but post-trial *satisfaction* with the product as a determinant of whether the brand will continue to be purchased (e.g., Oliver, 1993). That is, once a person has purchased a new product or engaged in some new behavior (e.g., taking high blood pressure medicine), the experience can either match, exceed, or fall short of one's expectations. The higher one's initial expectations for a behavior change, the more likely one is to initiate the change because more positive attitudes will be formed when expectancies of desirable outcomes are high. However, the higher one's positive expectancies for a change, the less likely it is that the experience of the change will actually match the expectancies. The disappointment following failure to meet expectations can lead to behavioral termination (e.g., Westbrook, 1987). One interesting possibility is that if older people are more focused on positive rather than negative emotions (Ybarra and Park, 2002), any disappointments following behavior change are less likely to undermine the new behavior than they are for younger people.

In addition to post-change dissatisfaction, other factors may work against maintenance of change, and these factors with their implications for change in later life are only beginning to receive serious research attention. For example, once a new attitude is formed, the old attitude and the associated behaviors do not just disappear. Rather, long-standing behaviors can re-emerge, and old attitudes can still be potent when people are not thinking about how to behave (e.g., Ouellette and Wood, 1998; Petty, Baker, and Gleicher, 1991; Wilson, Lindsey, and Schooler, 2002), or if antithetical cultural practices engulf the person. Research has yet to explore the consequences of conflict between old and new attitudes and behaviors and how it might be possible to both decrease the effects of old attitudes and associated behaviors as well as reinforce new ones at all stages of life. Since the consequences of attitudes and behaviors formed in early and midlife are so profound in later life, this and related research topics are on the committee's suggested research agenda.

Changing Implicit and Explicit Attitudes

As noted above, social psychologists have recently begun to explore the possibility that individuals may hold not only *explicit attitudes*, those that can be reported on direct self-assessments, but also *implicit attitudes*, automatic evaluative tendencies of which people may not be aware and that can sometimes conflict with the explicit attitude (see Wilson et al., 2002). Implicit attitudes can stem from a variety of sources, such as media portrayals, and they tend to govern behavior when people are not deliberately considering their actions (Dovidio et al., 1997). Social psychologists have developed various procedures to assess people's automatic attitudes, such as the priming measure (Fazio et al., 1995) and the implicit association test (Greenwald, McGhee, and Schwartz, 1998).

Although decades of research studies have examined how to change people's more conscious explicit attitudes, attention has only recently begun to turn to modifying implicit attitudes. Yet, such understanding is of potentially great importance for older people to the extent that automatic processes do not decline with aging as much as deliberative processes. That is, if older adults are more prone to rely on automatically activated evaluations rather than deliberately considered ones, understanding how to produce desirable automatic attitudes in older people can reap considerable benefits.

CONCLUSION

The need for change is constant throughout life, as people strive to live healthful, productive lives. Aging often entails the need to make significant life-style modifications, from taking new medications to relocation to developing new social networks. Unlike younger adults, who may not experience any negative effects from their life-styles for many years, the consequences for older adults of failing to commence or sustain health behaviors are often immediate and potentially life threatening.

The literature on self-regulation among older adults is sparse, focusing primarily on emotional regulation or adherence to specific medical directives. Interestingly, the literature suggests that older adults may be less likely to initiate behavioral changes, but more likely to maintain any changes that do occur. A major factor that prompts efforts to change, but also sabotages those efforts, is emotional distress. Given evidence that older adults are generally satisfied with their lives and that they avoid negative information, it is possible that the factors that prompt and support change are very different for older adults than for younger ones. However, it is as yet unclear whether self-regulatory differences observed as a function of age are due to changes in cognitive skills, functional neurological capacities, degree of experienced negative affect, or some other factors. Understanding self-regulation among older people is not only important for bettering the lives of older adults, but also provides a unique opportunity for psychologists to examine theoretical models.

People live longer in part because of advances in medicine, but also because they have quit smoking, watched their diets, and generally are motivated to look after themselves. Many of the most common causes of mortality are related to behaviors that people should be doing more often (e.g., eating healthfully, exercising) or avoiding (e.g., excess alcohol consumption, smoking). Motivating change often entails the communication of persuasive messages to change people's attitudes about engaging in these behaviors. Very little is known about persuasion processes in older people—and how they might differ from those of younger adults—or about the roles of racial, cultural, or ethnic preferences in those processes over the life course. Given that older adults are motivated to avoid processing negative information and perhaps are more likely to use heuristic processing than younger adults, it is possible that framing or tailoring messages to older audiences might be an especially efficacious means of encouraging long-term change. It is apparent that research that examines the role of socioemotional processes in self-regulation and persuasion holds great promise for developing methods to motivate older adults to make needed changes in their lives.

4

Socioemotional Influences on Decision Making: The Challenge of Choice

The publication of Milton Friedman's *Free to Choose* in 1980 (Friedman and Friedman, 1980) represented a high-water mark in positive public attitudes toward choice. By contrasting the constraints of socialism with the expanse of choices available in the unregulated free-market system he advocated, Friedman's book served as a kind of manifesto for the idea that more choice is always better. Little more than 20 years later, a new arrival on bookstore shelves is giving voice to what seems to be a widespread reappraisal of this faith in the benefits of choice. In *The Paradox of Choice,* Barry Schwartz (2004) argues that Americans are confronted by an ever-increasing proliferation of decisions they wish they didn't have to make, to the point that they have become shackled by what Schwartz calls a "tyranny of choice."

Schwartz provides few details about how the extent or burden of choice differs across age groups, perhaps because he had little research to draw on in reaching any conclusions on the matter. It seems likely, however, that many older Americans would agree with the message of the book. Indeed, although the burden of choice affects Americans of all ages, it likely affects older Americans differently. Today's elderly came of age in a world with fewer choices in their everyday lives. Electricity was provided by a centralized utility source, pensions were selected by employers, and health care plans were fixed. Today, consumers young and old must choose among different providers of electricity, gas, and, in some municipalities, even water. Employers often offer an assortment of health insurance options that differ in terms of out-of-pocket costs, procedures covered, cost caps, and co-payments. There are also new options, and hence greater need for decision making, when it comes to television, Internet, and cellular phone services: all of these can take alternate forms—analog or digital, land lines or satellite—and come in complicated packages differing in cost, speed, coverage, and so on. To the extent that they use such services, but are less savvy than younger people with new technologies, these choices are likely to pose special challenges for older adults.

In addition, many older adults are compromised in the cognitive domains necessary to process new information and make decisions based on that information. Ironically, even programs designed specifically for older people, like Medicare, are becoming increasingly complicated in terms of the decisions required by participants. New proposals for private Medicare substitutes and add-ons, while offering some advantages, undermine the simplicity that was once one of Medicare's strong points. The recent introduction of 73 different versions of Medicare drug cards underscores the problem. And the surprisingly low number of people who have signed up for these cards suggests that the choice problem may be overwhelming (Lind, 2004). Moreover, those who become sick (as, of course, the elderly do disproportionately) may face a whole new set of decisions that patients were previously rarely expected to make—between alternative drugs, procedures, doctors, and hospitals.

Older Americans not only face many new choices themselves, at a time of life when some cognitive abilities may be in decline, but also experience the brunt of the consequences of many choices made earlier in life. In future generations these consequences may be even more significant. Decisions about geographical relocations may influence closeness to family in the decades when family support is critical. Decisions about whether and when to have children will influence financial stability and social status in old age.

Perhaps nowhere, however, are the effects of early decisions more evident than for retirement savings. The most complicated and significant set of new choices results from the widespread shift from defined benefit to defined contribution retirement plans. Defined contribution plans give employees much more control over how much money to put aside and how to invest it, and inevitably result in much greater variability in retirement incomes. Proposed changes in the Social Security system would bring even more choices to workers and additional variability in retirement incomes. More than ever, older Americans' standard of living in retirement will depend on choices they made when they were working—choices that most economists agree are far from optimal and have led to severely suboptimal levels of retirement saving for the population as a whole. Unless significant changes occur, it is very likely that large numbers of older Americans will be facing difficult choices of how much to spend from what is likely to be a much reduced income from retirement savings and Social Security, while at the same time facing potentially catastrophic costs of health care and assisted living.

CAPABILITIES FOR DECIDING

Individuals

The overall burden of choice depends not only on the number and nature of choices one has to make, but also on the capabilities one brings to making those decisions. As Mara Mather summarizes (in this volume), significant declines in mental capabilities are believed to play an essential role in rational decision making. However, very little empirical research has explicitly examined changes in decision-making processes and competencies as a function of age, gender, or level of physical or cognitive ability.

Most of the limited research that has been done focuses on the ways in which cognitive decline impairs decision processes (e.g., Finucane et al., 2002; Peters, Finucane, MacGregor, and Slovic, 2000; Slovic, Finucane, Peters, and MacGregor, 2002). Findings from empirical examinations of older peoples' performance are generally discouraging. For example, Hibbard et al. (2001) presented a sample of Americans with information commonly given to people selecting a health insurance plan and assessed comprehension in terms of respondents' abilities to accurately interpret and report back information about the different plans. Not only were older respondents significantly more likely to make errors than the younger group (25 and 9 percent, respectively), but error rates continued to increase as a function of age within the elderly sample. By age 80, the error rate was 41 percent, and differences in competence as a function of education that were present in the younger subset of the elderly sample had disappeared.

Other research, however, qualifies this rather bleak picture of decision making by the elderly. As noted above, the strategies people use to make judgments and decisions in everyday life draw on an array of mental processes that span a continuum from the intuitive (or emotional) to analytic or deliberative (Hammond et al., 1987; Kahneman, 2003), and aging seems to affect intuitive and deliberative aspects of the decision process quite differently. While active, effortful, information processing declines with age (National Research Council, 2000, pp. 38-39; Park, Nisbett, and Hedden, 1999), automatic, intuitive processing tends to remain stable or even to improve with age (Isaacowitz, Charles, and Carstensen, 2000). Even performance on tests of basic cognitive processes known to decline with age, such as memory and attention, is enhanced when stimuli are emotional (Charles, Mather, and Carstensen, 2003; Denburg, Buchanan, Tranel, and Adolphs, 2003; Mather and Carstensen, 2003; Mather et al., 2004). Positive stimuli are remembered especially well (Charles et al., 2003). And in contrast to studies that ask participants to digest information about health care plans, studies of *social* problem solving, which are more likely to draw on emotional and intuitive processes, find more flexible performance by adults ages 45-75 than by those between 14 and 35 (Blanchard-Fields, Janke, and Camp, 1995). Moreover, whether they are consciously aware of such changes or not, older decision makers do tend to rely on the types of intuitive, emotional processes that they excel at, at least in relative terms. Adaptive decision making in old age seems to involve a shift toward a more intuitive form of decision making that relies less heavily on effortful strategies and instead on affective heuristics (Slovic et al., 2002).

Of course, although attention to emotion may aid decision making in some ways, it can harm decision making in others. For example, there are likely to be times where reliance on "gut" feelings and past experiences may place older people at heightened disadvantage, such as when a decision feels familiar but is actually quite different from decisions made in the past. At first glance, it may appear that older people who are relying on gut feelings may be especially vulnerable to marketers or con artists who are adept at manipulating positive feelings and creating trust when it is unwarranted. Moreover, given evidence that older people are especially motivated to maintain social harmony, they may be more easily persuaded by providers of deceptive information (Chen and Blanchard-Fields, 2000). Yet it is not necessarily the case that older people's increased reliance on emotion puts them at greater risk of being deceived; emotional acumen could lead to greater resistance to persuasion in older adults (see Pasupathi, 1999). One study has shown that older adults' accumulated experience in social interactions enhances their ability to discriminate lies in situations of deception (Bond, Thompson, and Malloy, 2005). Overall, it is clear that there are important age differences in decision making; the nature and the extent of those differences are important topics for research.

It is well established that intense emotion in younger adults can interfere with systematic deliberation and lead to impulsive, myopic, and often self-destructive choices (Baumeister, Stillwell, and Heatherton, 1994; Loewenstein, 1996). The importance of understanding the ways in which decisions are affected by strong emotions in older people is compounded by the fact that old age often presents decisions at times of high emotional strain, such as when a spouse becomes sick or dies or disability demands relocation to new living accommodations. Decisions about health care may be particularly susceptible to the influence of emotions because they often involve emotionally charged tradeoffs (Löckenhoff and Carstensen, 2004). Furthermore, one's perception of self and others and the type of health care decisions to be made, as well as whether an individual is cared for by family or placed in a nursing home, are all affected by a person's gender; socioeconomic status; and racial, cultural, and ethnic identity.

Research on decision making in younger adults highlights the central role of emotion in the decision process, and research on emotion and motivation suggests some intriguing changes with age, yet there has been almost no research examining the implications of such changes for decision making among the elderly. Several aspects of decision-making processes are especially important to understanding potential changes over the life course. Before delving into these specifics, however, a note on methodology is in order.

Some of the most exciting new directions in decision research and in social psychology involve new types of measures (see paper by the committee on "Measuring Psychological Mechanisms"; also Schwarz, Krosnick et al., Hartel and Buckner, all in this volume). For example, measures of implicit attitudes are revealing that people have values and beliefs and automatic tendencies to draw connections between things that they are often unaware of but that can nonetheless exert a powerful influence on decision making (Greenwald and Banaji, 1995; McConnell and Leibold, 2001). Neuroscience methods, most notably functional magnetic resonance imaging (fMRI) have produced a wide range of new insights about both aging and decision making, albeit little on the intersection of these topics (see Adolphs, 2003). Finally, new large-scale field experiments have revolutionized the field of decision making and the closely allied field of behavioral economics, demonstrating that policies inspired by decision research can improve decision making and welfare at the aggregate level (see, e.g., Thaler and Bernartzi, 2004).

Meta-Awareness

In many domains, what one knows about one's own capabilities is as important as the capabilities themselves. The vastly different effects of alcohol and marijuana on driving illustrate the point: although both drugs impair driving and judgment, alcohol makes one feel more competent and aggressive, which encourages one to drive fast, while marijuana makes one feel less competent and causes one to drive more slowly (Hall, Room, and Bondy, 1999). As a result, alcohol is a much larger contributor to accidents and fatalities, even after controlling for differences in use of the two drugs. When studied, metacognition has been viewed as a cognitive process; yet the social and emotional consequences of self-awareness surely play an important role in the views that people hold of their abilities. The case of driving, for example, is directly relevant to the elderly, who often experience impairments in their driving skills. Whether older people continue to drive, and if so, how far and fast they drive, depends not only on their actual driving skills, but also on self-perceptions of their cognitive, sensory, and physical abilities. Because of the link of driving to independence, a decision to stop driving is emotionally charged. Older people may be motivated to minimize their impairments in order to stave off dependence on others. Indeed, there is some evidence that older people show considerable self-awareness about their driving abilities and modify their driving accordingly to reduce risks (Ball, Owsley, Stalvey, Roenker, and Graves, 1998). Clearly, older people with forms of dementia, developmental disabilities, or other types of cognitive impairment may not have such meta-awareness.

There are many other domains in which self-insight might matter for the elderly. For example, working memory has been shown to decline significantly with age. If the elderly are aware of such declines, they may take steps to deal with them, such as using mnemonics or relying more heavily on written information (see, e.g., Schwarz, in this volume). Compliance with drug regimens is another good illustration of the importance of the meta-understanding of one's own cognitive and decision processes. Studies have found that older people actually do better than middle-aged people at adhering to drug regimens (see, e.g., Park et al., 1999). And, while part of the explanation may be motivational, the main cause seems to be the recognition by older people of their own memory limitations, which motivates them to make use of such compliance aids as pill dispensers that signal when it is time to take a pill. In fact, there is a large literature on metacognitive functioning in older adults; it is a valuable basis for research on its implications for changes in decision making with age.

LONG-RANGE PLANNING AND DECISION MAKING

Long-term planning and decision making is an area of research in which there has been a great deal of convergence in findings from psychologists—including social psychologists—and economists. Research coming from both fields documents a common pattern of behavior: a tendency for people to place disproportionate weight on costs and benefits that are immediate, but to treat delayed costs and benefits in a much more evenhanded fashion. For example, someone might choose a $50 dinner immediately over a $70 dinner a week later, but would almost surely state the reverse preference if the delay on both dinners were increased by a year.

However, in apparent contradiction to this common pattern, in many situations people—even those who have trouble with dieting and saving or who procrastinate—express a strong preference for sequences of outcomes that improve over time, as if they care more about later than about earlier outcomes. Putting these two sets of findings together, it appears that people want things to improve over time, but often behave in a fashion that ensures exactly the opposite result. For example, surveys have shown that many people *want* to save more and *plan* to save more, but when faced by temptations, they often incur high levels of debt, including high-interest credit card debt (Angeletos, Laibson, Repetto, Tobacman, and Weinberg, 2003; Bernheim, Skinner, and Weinberg, 2001; Caplin, 2003; Laibson, Repetto, and Tobacman, 1998). As people live longer, long-range planning becomes increasingly important, as does the ability to implement such plans.

Normative models of intertemporal choice (decisions between outcomes occurring at different points in time) assume that there are strong individual differences—that someone who is impulsive in one domain of behavior will also tend to be impulsive in other domains. Yet research shows that people are very inconsistent in their attitude toward the future, in some cases behaving as if present gratifications were all that mattered and in other cases appearing to care more about the future than the present. Indeed, it was research on intertemporal choice by the social psychologist Walter Mischel (1996) that first led him to recognize the importance of situational factors in human behavior, an insight that revolutionized social psychology for decades. Although Mischel emphasized the role played by cognitive self-control strategies in what he termed "delay of gratification"—in a wonderful example, that a child could successfully wait to get a chocolate bar instead of taking an immediately available marshmallow if she cognitively transformed the marshmallow into little white clouds—modern research has revealed a multiplicity of cognitive and motivational mechanisms, any one of which, alone, appears to be capable of producing radical variation in people's weighting of present and future. Different mechanisms, or mixtures of mechanisms, are invoked in different situations, producing striking variability in people's tradeoffs of immediate and delayed costs and benefits.

Different decision contexts, for example, evoke different "choice heuristics"—rules of thumb that people use to help them make decisions (Frederick, Loewenstein, and O'Donoghue, 2003). For example, when presented with a simple choice between two sequences, one improving (e.g., a mediocre restaurant dinner one weekend followed by a superb dinner the following weekend) and the other deteriorating (the same dinners but in reverse order), most people prefer the improving sequence. However, if asked to price the two sequences, most people value the declining sequence more highly, apparently because asking about money evokes considerations of net present value.

Emotions also play an important role in intertemporal decisions. There is considerable support for the idea that intertemporal decisions result from the interaction between two types of neural systems: "hot" affective systems that are inherently short-sighted and "cold" deliberative systems that are more even-handed when it comes to present and future (Loewenstein, 1996; McClure et al., 2004; Metcalfe and Mischel, 1999; Thaler and

Shefrin, 1981). These two systems often reinforce each other, as when the feeling of hunger reminds the deliberative system that it is time to eat. But in some cases they come into conflict, as when the sight of an available snack produces an affective urge to eat but reminds the deliberative system that one is on a diet, producing problems of, and in some cases failures of, self-control. Fluctuations in the intensity of affect can produce erratic, inconsistent patterns of behavior, with short-sighted decisions in situations characterized by intense affect, but much more far-sighted decisions when decision-makers are in affectively neutral states.

MULTIPARTY DECISION MAKING

Although most decision research focuses on individuals, much decision making in fact occurs in social contexts. For example, couples often make decisions jointly (such as where to live), sometimes tacitly coordinate on decision making (as when the husband buys a fancy car and the wife lives extra frugally to compensate), and sometimes provide each other with advice. There is intriguing evidence that for certain tasks, such as retrieving memories about a vacation, older adults benefit more than younger adults from collaboration with their spouses (Dixon and Gould, 1998). However, it is also well documented that couples commonly make decisions about survivor benefits that turn out to be disastrous for the survivor, putting widows especially at a disadvantage (International Longevity Center, 2003). The topic of collaborative decision making remains largely unstudied.

The interpersonal context may be especially important for older people, but the effects of such age-dependent changes remain poorly understood. The smaller social networks of older people may reduce access to potential advisers and advocates, especially for elderly people who are geographically isolated from family members. This is also an area in which culture, race, and ethnicity exert particularly strong effects because of their influence on the relationship of self to the group, particularly the relationship of self to the family. There are references to this topic in the caregiving literature, but it has not been well studied (e.g., Miner, 1995; Smerglia, Deimling, and Schaefer, 2001).

Family cohesion and responsiveness vary significantly on the basis of culture, race, and ethnicity, and the relative effects of these differences in family cohesion are important to understanding decision making and aging. Family cohesion may have quite different effects: with high family cohesion, resources within the family network may be efficiently mobilized to address the care needs; or strong family cohesion may create family discord because of varying opinions about care and responsibility. Because many members of minority cultural, racial, and ethnic populations live longer with physical limitations and have smaller pools of financial resources, reliance on families to provide care in later life is prevalent. Understanding the effects of family cohesion among these groups will become increasingly important as more and more families become responsible for care.

Affective Forecasting

There has been a recent proliferation in research examining affective forecasting—the ability to predict future feelings (Gilbert, Driver-Linn, and Wilson, 2002; Kahneman, 1994; Loewenstein and Frederick, 1997; Loewenstein and Schkade, 1999; Mellers and McGraw, 2001; Wilson and Gilbert, 2003). Most recently, researchers have measured both predicted and experienced affective responses in an effort to identify and explain inaccuracies in affective forecasting. Virtually all of the studies examining different aspects of affective forecasting, however, have involved young or, in some cases, middle-aged adult samples. And with the exception of quite a large body of research on affective forecasting involving changes in health conditions, most studies have focused on the types of events that are especially important to young and middle-aged adults, such as romantic breakups or professional setbacks. Even when it comes to health, however, there has been virtually no systematic research on affective forecasting by older people.

The research on affective forecasting suggests that individuals are generally accurate in making predictions about the valence (positive or negative) of future emotional experiences (Wilson and Gilbert, 2003) and about the specific discrete emotion they will experience (Robinson and Clore, 2001). However, these results must be qualified by other findings that suggest that people have overly simplistic, schema-driven perceptions of the emotional responses to events when thinking about the distant as opposed to near future (Liberman, Sagristano, and Trope, 2002). Furthermore, research suggests that for events that elicit a more complex blend of emotions, individuals may not be as good at predicting the specific mixture of emotions they will experience (Wilson and Gilbert, 2003). Overall, though, people are relatively accurate in identifying specific future emotions.

In contrast, individuals are not accurate at predicting the intensity and duration of their emotional experiences (Baron, 1992; Coughlan and Connoly, 2001; Mellers and McGraw, 2001; Wilson and Gilbert, 2003). Individuals tend to overestimate the enduring effect that future events will have on their emotional well-being. Measurement of this bias has typically used self-report scales and behavioral forecasting measures. This bias is important because evidence suggests that social behaviors and decisions are influenced by affective forecasts.

Recent research has focused on the mechanisms that account for this bias. Sources of affective forecasting errors include misconstruing the nature of the future event; focusing on features of the situation that are of little consequence to a person's emotional experience (Schkade and Kahneman, 1998); memory errors in recalling past emotional experiences (Loewenstein and Frederick, 1997); faulty theories as to what caused an affective state; and failures to correct for unique influences on forecasts. Finally, when they are attempting to forecast their future emotional experiences, people do not account for a variety of processes that ultimately attenuate intense emotional states (e.g., homeostatic processes or defensive processes that diminish the physiological effect) (Gilbert, Lieberman, Morewedge, and Wilson, 2004). Gilbert and colleagues argue that this is the most important source of affective forecasting errors. In other words, people do not take into account the fact that they will ultimately transform events psychologically to regulate their affect. This transformation happens in two different ways. First, individuals underestimate how rapidly they will make sense of a novel and positive event and thus overestimate the duration of positive emotional reactions. Second, when predicting how they will respond to negative events, people fail to anticipate the degree to which their psychological immune systems will speed up their recovery. Both transformational processes seem to be largely automatic and nonconscious. For example, studies show that people who forecasted their emotional reactions underestimated the degree to which they would rationalize a failure to achieve an outcome by blaming an unfair component of the situation or questioning the validity of the feedback (Gilbert, Pinel, Wilson, Blumberg, and Wheatley, 1998). Social psychologists are puzzled by the fact that people do not seem to readily learn from experience that they are equipped with powerful transformational abilities that facilitate recovery from an initial emotional state. A life-span developmental perspective may offer new ways to address this question.

Risk Aversion

Contrary to the stereotype of old people as frightened and risk avoiding, empirical studies have not revealed systematic changes in risk taking with age, beyond those that can be accounted for simply on the basis of changing physical capabilities. And the prevalence of casino gambling among the elderly points to at least one domain in which they contradict the stereotype. How does risk taking relate to age? Are older people generally more or less risk averse than younger people, or are there domain-specific differences?

Not surprisingly, there are reasons to think that risk taking might increase with age and reasons to think otherwise. On one side, as one ages, there are fewer years over which to average or correct mistakes. If one invests in stocks in one's 30s, and the market crashes, you still have several decades to make up your losses prior to retiring. Losing one's "nest egg" in one's later years is likely to be far more consequential. Indeed, many investment advisers recommend a progressive shift toward a safer mix of assets as people age. On the other side, the types of emotional changes that have been shown to occur with age might increase risk taking. There is substantial research supporting the idea that risk aversion is driven by negative emotions, such as fear and anxiety (see, e.g., Loewenstein et al., 2001; Loewenstein and Schkade, 1999). Since negative emotions have been shown to decrease with age, it would be natural to expect risk avoidance to decrease in tandem, especially social risk taking. Older people are notoriously less concerned about how they appear to others. To the extent that social risk aversion is driven by the fear of creating a negative impression, it would be expected to decline with age.

There is relatively little research in this area. Limited findings do suggest that older adults perform well at maximizing gains in gambling tasks (Shiv et al., 2005; Stout, Rodawalt, and Siemers, 2001). However, this research does not address the possibility that different strategies (e.g., loss aversion versus an emphasis on gains) may change as a function of age. Along these lines, other researchers have shown that types of strategy vary as a function of the content of the decision. For example, people use different strategies for socially relevant decisions involving moral issues and personal immediacy (use of social schemas, emotion focus, story construction) than for decisions about stock investments (use of numerical calculations) (Rettinger and Hastie, 2001).

Regrets

The emotion of regret plays a critical role in decision making. It serves as an affective signal, albeit one with a great deal of noise, that previous choices may have been wrong. Not surprisingly, there has been quite a bit of research on the role of regret in decision making. Most of this research focuses on the role of anticipatory regret, shifting one away from choices that have the potential to engender regret (e.g., Bell, 1982, 1985; Larrick and Boles, 1995; Loomes and Sugden, 1982, 1986; Mellers, Schwartz, Ho, and Ritov, 1997; Mellers, Schwartz, and Ritov, 1999). Yet there has been no research on whether the avoidance of regret plays a more or less prominent role in decision making as a function of age. There is some evidence that older people remember their choices more positively than do younger people (Mather and Johnson, 2003). Still, the irreversibility of many decisions made in old age make anticipated regret quite salient.

Gilovich and Medvec (1995) have examined the temporal pattern of regret. Their research shows that, at least in younger adults, when looking back on the recent past there is a general tendency to regret acts of commission (things one wishes one hadn't done); in contrast, when looking back at the distant past there is a tendency to regret acts of omission (things one didn't do that one wishes one had). No research has examined the types of decisions that people regret, or end up feeling good about, late in life. This topic is important, because understanding what types of decisions people do and do not regret in old age might provide a rough guide to the types of mistakes that older people commonly make. Do people who move to assisted living or semi-independent facilities tend to regret the decision? Do people who choose a medical plan or a new physician regret the decision? An investigation of regrets in older age might help to improve decision making not only among the elderly, but also among younger adults who have to make decisions that will affect them later in life.

END-OF-LIFE CARE

Some of the most important practical issues for decision research involve end-of-life care. A very large fraction of total national expenditures on health are incurred in the last 6 months of people's lives. This is not necessarily a mistake: older people tend to be sick and naturally draw on health care resources before they die. However, this fact has raised questions about whether the money is being put to the best use. More importantly, costly health care is often intrusive and degrading and may not be what people want. While the public places great value on "quality of death" (Bryce, Angus, and Loewenstein, 2003)—most people would prefer to die at home, surrounded by family—most people end up dying in hospitals or other sterile environments.

End-of-life decision making often entails great complications, involving many relatives who may hold different opinions and intense and complex emotions, both on the part of the patients and their relatives. Research by Peter Ditto and his colleagues (Fagerlin, Ditto, Danks, and Houts, 2001; Fagerlin, Ditto, Hawkins, Schneider, and Smucker, 2002) shows that patient surrogates often make decisions that are contrary to the wishes of the patient and that advanced directives and living wills barely improve the situation. Moreover, physicians may face financial incentives and fear of malpractice suits that could encourage them to promote tests and services that may not be in the patients' interest. With such a rich mix of complexity, affect, and conflicts of interest, it should come as no surprise that surviving family members often end up feeling deeply dissatisfied with the end-of-life care that their decedent relatives received (Addington-Hall, Lay, Altmann, and McCarthy, 1995; Teno et al., 2004). More research is clearly needed to understand what factors may lead to misguided decisions that result in excessively costly and degrading health interventions for people who are, even with such interventions, almost certain to die.

CONCLUSION

For better or for worse, aging Americans are being faced with more choice in life, from daily purchases to retirement spending to health care. Even decisions about the dying process are being placed increasingly in the hands of individuals. Yet very little is known about decision making by older people and even less about the effects on that decision making of their gender and socioeconomic status or of their life-long identification with a racial, cultural, or ethnic group. The existing literature on decision making and aging is small, and most of it focuses on the ways that cognitive decline may degrade decision competence. Moreover, as in the broader field of decision research, the conceptual approach adapted in most research is one in which decisions are viewed as "rational" processes that entail the weighing of pros and cons about different options and the selection of the option with the most advantages. An emerging approach to decision research, however, suggests that emotional responses to options play a central role in the decision process. Given that emotional functioning appears to be relatively spared from age-related decline, emotional aspects of the decision process are especially important to understand. The area is particularly promising because it may point to aspects of the decision process in which older adults perform relatively well, such as using intuitions in domains in which they are highly experienced.

The research proposed in this chapter promises to shed light not only on the decision-making processes of the elderly, but on decision making more broadly. Multiparty decision making, regret, and risk aversion are aspects of decision making at all ages, and gaining a better understanding of how they operate in the elderly will inevitably shed light on the decision making of younger groups, as well as contributing to more information for today's elderly population. Even end-of-life decisions can be relevant for younger people, who may also face life-threatening health problems.

We know that studying people with brain abnormalities can shed light on decision making. So, studying the relationship between changes in brain physiology and decision making over the life span should provide additional evidence on both decision making and its neural underpinnings. For example, since the time of Phineas Gage, the prefrontal cortex has been thought to be the seat of self-control (Damasio, 1994), yet we know that this area deteriorates with age. Why, then, are older people not generally characterized by a loss of self-control? One possibility is that the subregions of the prefrontal cortex that decline with age are different from those associated with self-control. Another possibility is that the urgency of emotions and physical drives, such as hunger and sex, also decline, perhaps even more rapidly than self-control resources. Understanding why self-control is generally maintained with declining prefrontal cortex function could help us understand the ongoing mystery of self-control.

As the population grows older, the decisions older people make will affect not only their own lives, but also the lives of their families, and public policies and societal functioning as well. Research on social and emotional aspects of decision making and on the intersection of emotional and cognitive processes is particularly promising because the marriage of these areas is likely to yield considerable progress in a relatively short period of time.

5

Social Engagement and Cognition

The ability to maintain mental vitality into late adulthood and function independently are major goals of most older Americans. There is great popular interest in knowing what can be done to preserve good cognitive function and to prevent Alzheimer's disease and other dementias. Although there have been tremendous gains in understanding changes in neurocognitive function with age, there is a surprising dearth of information on social factors that lead to healthy minds in late adulthood. Findings from a few studies suggest that social engagement and absorbing leisure activities may play a role in maintaining cognitive function in late adulthood and even in delaying or preventing dementia. These studies have largely been correlational in nature, so that it is impossible to know whether people who age well have selected engaged life-styles or whether those life-style behaviors themselves promote healthy aging. Caution is also required in assuming that activities that improve cognitive functioning in older adults who do not have dementia will contribute to preventing Alzheimer's disease. However, adopting a more engaged life-style or maintaining participation in the work force might be easier behaviors to adopt than some others that lead to healthy aging, such as changing diet and exercise habits, but are very difficult for most people to do.

Our specific focus is the association between social engagement and cognition. There is a recent report on contextual factors that affect cognitive function in late adulthood (National Research Council, 2000), as well as a burst of research activity that is examining mentally engaging leisure activities as a possible protective factor against dementia (e.g., Verghese et al., 2003). However, the construct of social engagement as a behavioral variable supportive of cognitive health has not been systematically considered in either the cognitive or social psychological literature. Although there is a long history of research on the relationship between social ties and psychological and physical health, less is known about the relationship of social engagement to cognitive health. Thus, because it is a promising yet neglected topic at the intersection of social psychology and adult development and aging, more fully investigating the causal relationships between social engagement and cognition is scientifically—and socially—essential.

AGING AND SOCIAL ENGAGEMENT

It is widely accepted that social engagement is related to many positive outcomes in older adults. People with more social ties have been found to live longer (see reviews by Antonucci, 2001; Bowling and Grundy, 1998), to have better health (see Berkman, 1985; Vaillant, Meyer, Mukamal, and Soldz, 1998), and to be less depressed (Antonucci, Fuhrer, and Dartiques, 1997).

A number of factors occur with older age that may increase the likelihood of decreased participation in meaningful social and intellectual activities in older adulthood. Older adults are retired, not raising children, and have fewer positions of authority than middle-aged and younger adults, so that their lives are not necessarily structured to maintain engagement. In a recent study, older adults (up to age 85) reported being less busy than younger adults (age 35 and older), and older adults described themselves as leading more routine and predictable lives (Martin and Park, 2003). While it would be inaccurate to characterize most older adults as plagued by loneliness, irreplaceable relationships are inevitably lost as people age. The differences in the types of social networks that older adults and younger adults have are well-established: as discussed in Chapter 2, older people have a smaller circle of close relatives and friends, particularly those who are important to them and from whom they derive the most pleasure (Carstensen, Isaacowitz, and Charles, 1999).

Social activities do not inevitably lead to meaningful engagement with others. Moreover, social ties are not always positive, and it is important to recognize that increased engagement may not reliably enhance life satisfaction, as engagement with other people has the potential to be stressful as well as supportive (see Rook, 1992). Thus, it is essential that research on social engagement and cognition simultaneously focus on characterizing the relevant features of social relations that facilitate cognition while testing the effects of social engagement on cognition.

Neurocognitive Function and Cognition

As people age, changes in the brain affect cognitive function. There are significant decreases in many behavioral domains of cognitive function. Although knowledge and verbal skills remain strong, there are measurable decreases in the speed of processing information (Salthouse, 1995), working memory function, and long-term memory processes between people in their 20s and people in their 90s (Park et al., 1996, 2002).

The frontal cortex is a large area important for memory and strategic processing of information while the hippocampus, along with prefrontal cortex, plays a critical role in encoding and long-term retention of information. The frontal cortex shows significant shrinkage with age, as does the hippocampus, although not as much as the frontal areas (Moss and Raz, 2001). There is also evidence that older adults have fewer dopamine receptors than young adults (Volkow et al., 1998). Functional imaging studies present a consistent picture of decreased hippocampal activation and increased frontal recruitment during working memory and long-term memory tasks (Gutchess et al., 2005; Park et al., 2003). The increased frontal activation appears to represent the brain's reorganization to compensate for brain shrinkage, decreased hippocampal function, deterioration in white matter, and loss of dopamine receptors (Cabeza, 2002; Logan et al., 2002; Reuter-Lorenz, 2002). These studies have been cross-sectional and include an age range from college students to those over 85 years old. An important question is what kinds of social and intellectual experiences might support neural function and optimize compensatory activation. Also worth consideration is whether there are any differences in experiences in successive birth cohorts—for example, differences in educational experiences (Castro-Caldas, Petersson, Reis, Stone-Elander, and Ingvar, 1998), exposure to television, and the structure of society—that might contribute to the observed results in brain function.

Evidence indicates that the brain has developed specialized mechanisms for dealing with the social environment. The amygdala appears to be important for using social cues, such as judging whether someone is trustworthy (Adolphs, Tranel, and Damasio, 1998). That is, there are dissociable brain regions that are involved in social and emotional processing. It has further been suggested that aging may have a differential impact on hippocampal as opposed to amygdala function (Denburg, Buchanan, Tranel, and Adolphs, 2003). This finding would help to explain why emotionally significant stimuli—especially positive—are readily remembered by older adults (Charles, Mather, and Carstensen, 2003) and may lead individuals to adopt strategies in which they use relatively more preserved brain regions to support those that are less preserved.

In contrast to normal cognitive aging, dementia is defined as declines in multiple cognitive domains sufficient to interfere with daily functioning. Alzheimer's disease is the most common cause of dementia (Cummings and Cole, 2002). A variety of terms have been applied to intermediate conditions in which there is cognitive decline that is not sufficiently severe to be diagnosed as dementia (e.g., mild cognitive impairment). By age 85, approximately 50 percent of individuals experience significant memory loss (Graham et al., 1997), and 25 percent show dementia that ultimately limits their ability to manage independently (von Strauss et al., 1999). Determining whether heightened social engagement can defer cognitive aging and maintain more years of independent functioning is therefore a critical public health issue.

Mental Stimulation and Cognitive Aging

The relationship between mental stimulation and cognitive aging is currently an active area of investigation. This work has implications both methodological and substantive for the study of social engagement. Engagement is a behavior that involves a high level of both intellectual and social function. There is a growing literature (based on longitudinal data) suggesting that leading an intellectually stimulating life may foster cognitive vitality (Hultsch, Hertzog, Small, and Dixon, 1999; Schooler, Mulatu, and Oates, 1999). Other literature suggests that cognitive stimulation in everyday life can even be an important buffer in delaying onset of Alzheimer's disease or slowing its progression (Wilson, Bennett, Gilley, Beckett, Barnes, and Evans, 2000). It is quite well established that higher education serves a protective effect with respect to dementia. What is not known is the mechanism for this association, although it may be that those with higher education have generally more cognitively stimulating lives (Wilson and Bennett, 2003).

It is important to differentiate the construct of engagement from that of cognitive training. Cognitive training is a manipulation that is a systematic attempt to improve cognitive function through focused training activities. The training literature involves traditional laboratory-based manipulations and resides almost exclusively in the realm of cognitive psychology and is thus considered only briefly here. In contrast, the engagement literature is drawn primarily from social psychology and large epidemiological studies. Overall, the training literature suggests that specific, but not general, increases in cognitive function can be realized with cognitive training. For example, memory training with older adults (who do not have dementia) from their 60s through their 80s can be effective if—in addition to teaching mnemonic techniques—the intervention provides information about memory and aging and includes cognitive restructuring (i.e., altering pessimistic beliefs about memory abilities) and stress reduction, which, if untreated, can reduce scores on memory tests (Lachman et al., 1992; Yesavage, 1984). More recently, Ball and colleagues (2002) completed a major randomized clinical trial with older adults up to age 95 that showed modest effects of training on memory and perceptual speed. The effects of training on cognition tended to be very specific, and there was little evidence for broad improvement in everyday cognitive functioning after specific cognitive tasks were trained (Ball et al., 2002). Notably, this trial included a large African American sample as well as European Americans.

Training designs have also been applied to older adults, ages 70 to over 95, with dementia. For example, Camp and colleagues (Bourgeois et al., 2003; Camp et al., 1997) showed that cognition can be improved in older adults with dementia through training that uses the types of learning that are least affected by aging in the brain and through training in the use of appropriate aids to memory. These interventions sometimes include a social component, such as mentoring of children by adults with dementia, conducting training in group settings where participants are asked to engage in conversational exchanges, and so forth.

EFFECTS OF SOCIAL ENGAGEMENT

Studies that suggest that social engagement and socially absorbing leisure activities play an important role in maintaining cognitive function in late adulthood are not as well developed as those connecting mental activation to cognitive outcomes. The data on engagement and cognitive function are relatively limited and restricted to epidemiologic or longitudinal studies in which engagement is self-selected, and there are few, if any, using clinical trials or random assignment. Greater social engagement—measured in terms of contact with family and friends and participation in social activities—has been shown to reduce risk of cognitive decline over 3, 6, and 12 years (Bassuk, Glass, and Berkman, 1999). Another study suggests that individuals (average age = 65) who engage in many social interactions or who have large social networks show better cognitive function than those who do not (Arbuckle, Gold, Andres, Schwartzman, and Chaikelson, 1992).

Better social connectedness has also been shown to be related to reduced risk of subsequently developing dementia (Fratiglioni, Wang, Ericsson, Maytan, and Winblad, 2000). And individuals who are married and presumably engage in more social interactions than single people are also less susceptible to dementia (Helmer et al., 1999). A number of studies show that more engagement in leisure activities is related to reduced risk of dementia or Alzheimer's disease (Crowe, Andel, Pedersen, Johansson, and Gatz, 2003; Fabrigoule, Letenneur, Dartigues, Zarrouk, Commenges, and Barberger-Gateau, 1995; Scarmeas, Levy, Tang, Manly, and Stern, 2001; Wang, Karp, Winblad, and Fratiglioni, 2002). These studies include international samples, and U.S. samples with African American and Latino participants. In most of these studies, leisure encompasses a range of activities that may have social, intellectual, or physical components, so it is not entirely clear which component is responsible for the protective effect. However, Wang et al. (2002) did demonstrate that engagement in social types of leisure activities (theatre, cards, traveling) was related to reduced risk of dementia. A summary of the literature on social engagement and dementia is available in Fratiglioni, Paillard-Borg, and Winblad (2004).

Other research has examined social and intellectual engagement in occupations rather than leisure. Schooler et al. (1999) reported that individuals who engaged in complex jobs that required decisions and engagement showed better intellectual functioning than adults who had less demanding jobs. In a similar vein, data from the Maastricht Longitudinal Study indicated that individuals with cognitively demanding jobs showed less cognitive decline over a 3-year period than those with less demanding jobs (Bosma et al., 2003). Stern et al. (1995) found lower risk of dementia among those whose occupations had high interpersonal and physical demands. Although randomized clinical trials to test the effect of social engagement on cognition and dementia are not available (see Fratiglioni et al., 2004), interventions whose purpose is to strengthen social ties and improve social support are common in long-term care institutions and senior citizen community settings. Randomization to conditions is unusual. Cognitive tests may be included in the outcomes, and follow-up tests of participants in some of these programs have shown improved memory: for example, Newman, Karip, and Faux (1995) found improved memory in older adults in their 60s and 70s who participated in a volunteer program.

Underlying Mechanisms

The causal mechanisms underlying the cognitive benefits that accrue from social and even intellectual stimulation are unknown. There are many possibilities. One is that social and intellectual stimulation alters neural tissue and pathways. Some evidence for this comes from animal studies in which rats raised in social environments showed greater brain volume than animals raised alone (Bennett, Rosenzweig, and Diamond, 1969). More recently, studies have indicated that older animals in environmentally complex, stimulating environments showed both enhanced learning and increased neural tissue and dendrite growth in old age (Greenough, McDonald, Parnisari, and Camel, 1986; Greenough, West, and DeVoogd, 1978). Other work has suggested that neurogenesis (birth of new neurons) occurs in hippocampal structures and dentate gyrus in old mice that are exposed to an enriched environment (Kempermann, Kuhn, and Gage, 1997, 1998). Finally, there is recent research suggesting that physical exercise in older humans enhances both cognitive function and prevents age-related brain atrophy (Colcombe and Kramer, 2003; Colcombe et al., 2004). These data suggest that neurocognitive function in late adulthood is malleable, and they are consistent with the popular "use it or lose it" argument in American culture (a hypothesis described as the "disuse hypothesis" by Orrel and Sahakian, 1995). In other words, by stimulating neural pathways, the health of the brain is maintained. It is plausible that social engagement could provide sustained neurocognitive stimulation, possibly due to the high degree of comprehension, memory, and problem solving required to manage and sustain social relationships (Byrne and Whiten, 1988). It is also plausible that racial, cultural, and ethnic groups that place a high value on social engagement might provide a cognitive advantage to individuals in those groups over others in more isolated or individualistic groups.

Another plausible interpretation of engagement effects is that highly social individuals in late adulthood are healthier than less engaged individuals. It may be that engagement effects in old age, although real, do not result from a causal relationship, but that individuals with greater physical health also have better cognition and engage in more activities than their frailer counterparts. Because the data collected thus far are largely from studies in which individuals have self-selected whether to be socially active, this interpretation cannot be ruled out until experimental studies of engagement are conducted in which volunteers are randomly assigned to participate in engaging activities (which could include the individual's choosing which social activities to engage in) or in an appropriate control group.

Another related explanation for the observed effect of social engagement on cognition may be long-standing differences in individuals that are responsible both for their greater social engagement and for their being relatively protected from cognitive decline and dementia. Results from the nun study (Danner, Snowdon, and Friesen, 2001; Snowdon, Greiner, and Markesbery, 2000) and from Scottish studies of birth cohorts who received a national survey of mental ability (Whalley, Starr, Athawes, Hunter, Pattie, and Deary, 2000) demonstrated that there are notable differences early in life—in language, emotions, and intelligence—that predict cognitive outcomes in late life. These differences imply that both social engagement and better cognitive function in late life stem from these earlier influences.

Another possible explanation is that social engagement prevents the onset of depression, although some studies have controlled for depressive symptoms and still found protective effects for leisure activities (e.g., Bassuk et al., 1999). An extension of this argument is that social engagement leads to reduced stress. Depression and stress can lead to negative changes in cognitive and neural function, including loss of neurons in the hippocampus through glucocorticoid dysregulation (Sapolsky, Krey, and McEwen,

1986). Thus, the observed effect of social engagement in maintaining cognitive function could be due to the positive effects of social engagement on mental health.

Social engagement effects, particularly those associated with evidence for later onset of Alzheimer's disease, may also be understood in terms of how engagement might foster more assistance with cognitive maintenance. That is, individuals who are engaged may engender a larger network of collaboration and support for tasks for which individual cognitive resources may be insufficient. In line with this thinking, Dixon and colleagues (Dixon, Hopp, Cohen, de Frias, and Bäckman, 2003) have suggested that compensatory mechanisms for declining cognition can operate at the social level. Recruitment or engagement of social partners by older adults to consult or to work together in managing problems of everyday living may compensate for declining cognition and help maintain independence. Dixon and Gould (1998) observed that older couples in their late 60s and 70s, with a history of social interaction, were particularly adept at developing specific compensatory strategies to manage problems of everyday living, while dyads who did not previously know one another were only able to construct mechanisms of general social and emotional support. Here, again, cultural differences in endorsement of communal versus individual values may affect social engagement and, hence, cognitive maintenance.

Finally, the manner in which social engagement may foster cognition could be viewed through the work of social psychologists on the role of social context on performance. Zajonc's (1965) theory of social facilitation and subsequent work identifying conditions under which social facilitation occurs (Bargh and Apsley, 2001) provides a framework for understanding when social engagement might provide cognitive benefits. While learning new skills can be more difficult with an audience, well-practiced skills are performed better in the presence of others. The importance of social context may also be understood in terms of its potential negative effects on cognitive function through the operation of age-related stereotypes (see Chapter 6). Thus, social contexts that emphasize age-related declines while demanding acquisition of new skills could diminish rather than enhance cognitive function.

Technology Training as Engagement

Technology plays an increasingly central role in contemporary lives, and it can be an important tool in maintaining independence in the face of physical frailty, as shopping, banking, and many everyday tasks can be managed with computer technology (Liu and Park, 2003). One provocative and important possibility is that technology training of older adults could have multiple benefits. One obvious benefit is in providing older adults with more tools to help themselves in terms of health information, medication refills, financial management, and shopping (Park, 1997). A second benefit is the potential that technology offers for people to interact easily with friends, family, and special interest groups, providing a particular type of social engagement about which little is known. Older adults report that one of their primary uses of the Internet is maintaining contact with family (Loges and Jung, 2001). One obvious question is whether such remote interactions confer the same benefits that other social interactions offer in terms of both socioemotional and cognitive well-being. A third potential benefit is the possibility that the act of acquiring technology expertise in older adults is socially and cognitively stimulating and enhances cognitive vitality, independent of the effect of using the technology. Although some research has been done on the human factors (Czaja, 2001) and cognitive aspects (Rogers and Fisk, 2001) of technology acquisition (see also National Research Council, 2003), the possibility that technology training results in cognitive gains beyond the acquisition of specific skills because of increasing engagement is worthy of further exploration. Given the multiplicative potential for benefits from learning to use may types of technology, the social and cognitive benefits of technology training and use in older adults is an area in which investigation should be encouraged. In this regard, the gap in access to technology across different communities is a topic that warrants attention.

KEY QUESTIONS

There is a need to sort through the various mechanisms that have been postulated about the effects of engagement. First, it is important to know if social engagement does have a measurable effect on cognition and maintenance of independence in late adulthood, both independently of cognitive stimulation and in concert with it. There have not been any controlled experimental studies examining the effects of sustained social interactions on immediate and longer term changes in cognitive function, although there are sufficient data from epidemiologic studies to suggest strongly that high social function is protective of neurocognitive processes. It is important to assess not only the effects of social interactions on cognitive function, but also the magnitude and duration of such effects and whether these effects have practical value. Controlled investigations on this topic could include development of methodologies that permit characterization and manipulation of social engagement that will lead to concrete recommendations for the types of leisure activities and social interactions that promote healthy intellectual function in late adulthood. Of particular importance is determining the dose-response relationship of sustained social activity for healthy aging, as well as whether there are critical periods across the life span at which social engagement has the greatest effect. The topic of engagement raises several important questions, which are discussed in the rest of this section.

Does engagement augment cognitive function or delay disease onset? Whether any protective effect of social engagement applies chiefly to improved cognition within normal aging or whether it extends to dementia in general or Alzheimer's disease in particular, where it has been argued that social engagement might prevent or delay the onset or affect the course of the disease, must be considered. The question of whether the onset of dementia can be delayed is particularly difficult to investigate, and we do not want to underestimate the profound difficulties in establishing causal direction from engagement to cognition. Because dementia has a long and insidious onset, cognitive changes may begin to occur well before there is clinical recognition of any dementia (Elias et al., 2000). Thus, it is particularly important to be sure that reduced social interaction is not a consequence of the beginning of cognitive decline. Some analytic innovations may be helpful with epidemiological datasets in which risk factors can be both predictors and outcomes of subsequent exposure (Robins, Hernan, and Brumback, 2000; Tilling, Sterne, and Szklo, 2002). Randomized trials will be important in establishing connections between engagement and cognition without the selection effects that plague observational studies. Various strategies can help to optimize these studies, including extended follow up or sampling those most at risk of cognitive impairment.

What types of engagement are most effective? A second major research domain of importance is determining what aspects of social engagement may lead to cognitive health. Social engagement can take many forms, ranging from close familial relationships and interactions, including family caregiving, or other culturally sanctioned social activities, to participation in novel activities that result in acquisition of new behavioral repertoires and ideas. Research that specifically characterizes the types of social engagement that are facilitative of cognitive function is needed. It is also important to understand the role of social networks across the life span in maintaining cognitive function, for example, whether the size of social networks is important, or whether it is the extent of social engagement, regardless of network size, that matters. Due to decreased cognitive function associated with normal aging (Park et al., 2001), older adults may prefer more limited social networks. Alternatively, decreased social networks could hasten normal age-related cognitive decline, in which case efforts to increase social engagement might include increasing social networks.

What is the role of individual differences? A third important question involves the mediating role that individual differences may play in the relationship between cognitive function and social engagement. Individual differences include physical health, which may limit some kinds of social activities but need not preclude meaningful social engagement. Personality differences may also be relevant: for instance, social engagement may have different meanings for those who are more introverted. The effects of social engagement may be most pronounced for people with limited opportunities for social engagement because of the unusual stimulation such engagement would provide. Alternatively, the effects of social interactions may be most salient for those who have a long-standing interest in social engagement and even be unhelpful for others. Demographic variables such as socioeconomic status, education, gender, and marital status might reveal important individual differences, suggesting mechanisms for facilitative effects. These individual differences may point to ways of tailoring activities to achieve social engagement and providing opportunities for engagement in a context in which older people can engage in choice and self-regulation with respect to those activities and relationships.

What is the role of cultural and ethnic factors? Cultural context and ethnicity may play roles in minimizing or magnifying the effects of social engagement on cognitive health. Characterizing cultural differences in social engagement with respect to age will help understanding how different forms and styles of social connectedness interact with cognitive health.

It is a relatively consistent finding that there are differences among cultural, racial, and ethnic groups in cognitive performance in later life. In the United States, cross-racial studies of performance on standardized tests of neuropsychological functioning indicate that European Americans, on average, have a higher level of performance than other groups (typically African Americans) (Escobar et al., 1986; Fillenbaum et al., 1988). Recent research suggests that these mean differences in cognitive performance can be entirely or at least partly accounted for by social factors, such as education, literacy, and health status (e.g., Albert et al., 1995; Manly, Jacobs, Touradji, Small, and Stern, 2002; Whitfield et al., 2000). There may also be differences in familiarity with the types of information presented in the tests, which represent a source of difference in mean performance between groups (Whitfield, 1996; Whitfield et al., 2000; Whitfield and Willis, 1998). These data do not suggest that cognitive functioning differs fundamentally as a function of race or ethnicity; rather, since the cultural contexts in which cognition operates are relatively stable over dozens of years, the hypothesis that culture may affect basic cognitive processes is not implausible. The role of social engagement in various cultural contexts is a question that needs to be answered in order to establish the relationships among cognition, culture, and social engagement in later life.

What types of stimulation alone, or in combination, are effective? Another important question concerns the interrelationship among different types of stimulation—intellectual, social, and physical. There is increasing evidence that physical exercise may improve cognitive function (Colcombe and Kramer, 2003), and it is possible that physical and intellectual stimulation interact with social engagement, conferring maximal neurocognitive protection. Alternatively, perhaps it is the quantity rather than the type of stimulation that makes the difference. This is an entirely unexplored question that is worthy of systematic evaluation.

CONCLUSION

The relationship between social engagement and cognitive health deserves serious research attention because of its potential implications for successful aging in America. There is a broad array of techniques for measuring the interactions between social engagement and cognitive health. Specifically, from the neuroimaging literature there is increasing evidence that older adults may use different neural routes to perform a cognitive task than young adults do (Cabeza, 2002; Park et al., 2001; Reuter-Lorenz, 2002) and that there is more plasticity in neural pathways than was previously understood. The use of neuroimaging tools to understand the effect of engagement manipulations on cognition is important and may reveal other effects as well. Research in both the social and the cognitive psychology of aging has provided rich theoretical models that can be extended to understand the role of social engagement in productive aging. Even more broadly, a full complement of sociological, behavioral, physiological, and neurobiological measures are available to measure both neural and behavioral outcomes of associations between social engagement and cognitive function. Furthermore, the outcome of research on motivation and behavior change and on socioemotional influences on decision making will directly affect the design of any interventions needed to increase social engagement.

Understanding the mechanisms underlying the causes and effects of social engagement, and discovering the types of activities that might maintain and even improve cognitive function is a major issue for public health policy and for the lives of the older population. Identifying culturally appropriate programmatic interventions that would make a contribution to delaying the onset of dementia would have major effects on the number of cases and on the demands on the health care system and on families.

6

Opportunities Lost: The Impact of Stereotypes on Self and Others

There is ample evidence to suggest that negative expectations and stereotypes about the competence of older adults pervade Western culture (e.g., Hummert, 1999; Kite and Wagner, 2002). For example, older adults are characterized as more forgetful and less able to learn new information (e.g., Hummert, Garstka, Shaner, and Strahm, 1994). In addition, young and old people alike believe that there is general memory decline across the latter half of the life span (Lineweaver and Hertzog, 1998; Ryan, 1992; Ryan and Kwong See, 1993). Research corroborates these views: there is abundant evidence that older adults do perform more poorly than younger adults across a wide variety of cognitive tasks (for a review, see Zacks, Hasher, and Li, 2000).

Yet there is also evidence of older adults serving important roles in society. For example, nearly 40 percent of the nation's 1,200 working federal judges have reached senior status and could retire. But, these senior judges are crucial to the justice system and, handling reduced caseloads, carry out nearly 20 percent of the federal judiciary's work (Markon, 2001). This fact is also consistent with the literature on cognitive aging, which shows that reasoning about complex matters relevant to daily life—what some call wisdom–shows no deterioration with age (Baltes and Kunzmann, 2003). Yet pervasive beliefs about age-related decline tend to outweigh beliefs about positive aging in our culture. Most people expect that losses will outnumber gains as they get older (Heckhausen, Dixon, and Baltes, 1989); most people expect their abilities to decline with age (Staudinger, Bluck, and Herzberg, 2003).

Most of the work on stereotyping and aging documents this phenomenon. Far less examines the degree to which negative and positive stereotypes have an effect on the quality of life for older adults. Do negative expectations of older people and ageist beliefs lead people in general, as well as older adults themselves, to underestimate the capacities of older adults? Do positive expectations have the opposite effect?

Negative stereotypes can have harmful consequences for the quality of life of older adults and can also result in a major loss to society. With increases in life expectancy as well as reduced infirmity, many adults are aging well, but negative stereotypes of aging may put society at risk for losing the contributions of these vital and knowledgeable people. The potential individual and social effects underscore the need to understand the content of aging stereotypes in terms of their accuracy and applications. It is especially important to understand how negative stereotypes exacerbate poor performance in areas in which decline is real. That is, beliefs that memory is bad in old age can reduce motivation when increased motivation is needed instead. A framework for predicting and interpreting individuals' behavior is imperative to understand how aging stereotypes drive behavior in both positive and negative ways.

Social psychologists have a long history of studying stereotypes and their effects on judgment and behavior. As outlined in more detail below, stereotypes people have about others can influence how those others are treated and in turn elicit particular behaviors from the others that are consistent with those stereotypes (e.g., Snyder, 1992). In addition, stereotypes can exert a direct influence on the stereotype holder. In particular, activation of a stereotype can cause people to act in a manner consistent with the stereotype (Dijksterhuis and Bargh, 2001), regardless of whether they are members of the stereotyped group or not (Wheeler and Petty, 2001).

EXPLICIT STEREOTYPES

The current literature suggests that both positive and negative stereotypes influence judgments made about older adults in everyday life. There are countless ways in which negative stereotypes can have serious personal consequences on the way older adults are perceived and treated (Pasupathi and Löckenhoff, 2002). For example, Erber and colleagues (2001) find that memory failures are seen as more serious for older adults than younger adults and support the perceiver's negative expectations of aging. Older adults are repeatedly reminded of negative stereotypes associated with aging in a variety of settings, such as media advertising of products and services that focus on such aspects of aging as memory loss, frailty, incontinence, and loss of mobility. Other examples include ageist views of older workers on the job and its harmful effects on employee satisfaction (Gordon et al., 2000; McMullin and Marshall, 2001) and ageist views of patients in a medical setting, who receive less aggressive medical treatment because their physical complaints are dismissed simply as signs of aging. In many settings, patronizing forms of communication are used with older adults despite the fact that it is viewed as debasing and disrespectful (see Hummert, 1999; Kemper, 1994; Ryan, Meredith, and Shantz, 1994). As noted by Richeson and Shelton (in this volume), negative stereotypes of age-related cognitive deficits are far more severe than the actual deficits. Those stereotypes may inhibit older people from attempting and actively participating in new activities or exercising their full potential.

A critical issue that emerges from these findings is the extent to which negative stereotypes affect the behavior of older adults in an everyday context. For example, negative stereotypes may not only affect the attributions of medical personnel regarding an older adult's symptoms (i.e., viewing them as normal aging instead of as treatable conditions), but may also affect the older person's understanding of what normal aging is. Thus, the older adult does not receive enough medical care or doesn't want more medical care because of his or her own stereotypes about normal aging. Do older adults themselves overlook symptoms of disease because they view them as part of normal aging, when they should be taking these symptoms more seriously? Older adults' perceived choices also need to be taken into account. Research should examine knowledge and individual choice on the part of older adults in making medical decisions (see Chapter 4).

Fortunately, positive stereotypes and attitudes toward aging can also affect how older adults are treated. For example, Erber and Szuchman (2002) found that a forgetful older adult is seen as having more desirable traits than a forgetful young adult. Similarly, in legal settings older witnesses are believed to be just as credible as younger witnesses despite older adults' memory failures (Brimacombe, Jung, Garrioch, and Allison, 2003). Thus, despite perceptions of declining memory capacity on the part of older adults, they can still be viewed as credible or desirable. There is even a recent emergence in the mass media of positive stereotypes of aging, with older characters described as powerful, active, and healthy (Pasupathi and Löckenhoff, 2002).

What can be abstracted from these few studies is that the social context moderates perceptions and treatment of older adults. Research is needed to determine the degree to which age-differentiated perceptions of behavior are ageist, where they are prominent, and the extent to which behaviors distance and exclude older adults and the extent to which behaviors are beneficial and protective of older adults. For example, are ageist attitudes less prominent in interpersonal settings? Research is also needed to identify the conditions under which positive or negative stereotypes affect decisions made about older people in everyday life—such as whether an older person should continue to drive or requires assisted living or in communications between older people and health care providers.

IMPLICIT STEREOTYPE ACTIVATION

From a sociocultural perspective, negative age stereotypes are socialized early in life (Kwong and Heller, 2005; Montepare and Zebrowitz, 2002) and become so well ingrained that they may be automatically activated in the mere presence of an older person (Hummert, Gartska, O'Brien, Greenwald, and Mellot, 2002; Perdue and Gurtman, 1990). A social psychological perspective further suggests that stereotypes can be viewed as person perception schemas. By examining the cognitive representation of stereotypes important questions can be addressed: Under what conditions are stereotypes activated? Under what conditions do stereotypes guide social judgments and behavior? Why do behaviors reflect negative stereotypes more so than positive ones?

As reviewed in the paper by Richeson and Shelton (in this volume), there is a wealth of evidence describing positive and negative stereotypes of older adults and a growing literature indicating the conditions under which stereotypes are activated. With respect to stereotype activation in perceivers, the literature identifies physical cues, the subcategory of "old-old" adults, contexts involving physically or mentally demanding tasks, and off-target verbosity as elicitors of negative stereotypes (Bieman-Copland and Ryan, 2001; Hummert, Garstka, and Shaner, 1997). More "youthful" behavior and young-old status are elicitors of positive stereotypes (Hummert et al., 1994). Finally, although both younger and older adults hold negative views associated with aging (Hummert et al., 2002; Nosek et al., 2002; Parr and Siegert, 1993; Ryan, 1992), there is conflicting evidence as to whether older adults themselves have more positive or negative views than younger adults.

Other questions with respect to stereotype activation are the degree to which people are or are not aware of having such evaluative attitudes about the elderly, and the effect that such attitudes have on people's thoughts and actions regarding the elderly. In other words, there is a need to distinguish implicit from explicit activation of stereotypes. For example, with respect to older adults who belong to multiple identity categories (age/gender/race), are the same attitudes activated both consciously (explicitly) and unconsciously (implicitly)?

To examine such implicit constructs and processes, social psychologists have developed a battery of implicit measures that do not call for conscious self-reports of the construct or process. The earliest such measures were in essence disguised self-reports (e.g., thematic apperception tests) or behavioral observations (e.g., how close one sat next to a stranger) from which researchers inferred an underlying attitude or motive. Recently, implicit measures based on reaction times have demonstrated considerable utility in predicting behaviors that could not be predicted by direct self-reports (e.g., Dovidio, Kawakami, and Gaertner, 2002). Furthermore, even when direct self-reports were useful in predicting behavior, implicit measures have been shown to account for additional variance (e.g., Vargas, von Hippel, and Petty, 2004).

Two measures have captured the bulk of recent research attention. One measure is based on priming procedures developed initially by cognitive psychologists. With this measure, participants are presented with different stimuli (e.g., elderly or young faces—the primes) and then asked to indicate the evaluative meaning (i.e., good/bad) of various words (e.g., dirt or flower) as quickly as possible by pressing an appropriate response key on a computer. Reaction times for the classification of the words are assessed. To the extent that elderly faces facilitate responses to negative words or inhibit responses to positive words in comparison to young faces, one can infer that a negative attitude toward the elderly is automatically activated when the face appears (e.g., Fazio, Sanbonmatsu, Powell, and Kardes, 1986).

The second measure is the implicit association test (Greenwald, McGhee, and Schwartz, 1998). It assesses the strength of association between a target concept (e.g., the elderly) and an attribute dimension (e.g., good/bad) by examining the speed with which participants can use two response keys to categorize words (or pictures) when each key is assigned a dual meaning (e.g., elderly/good versus young/bad). If people are classifying young (e.g., spring break) and old (e.g., retirement) terms or positive (e.g., flower) and negative (e.g., dirt) words, the question is whether it is easier to do so when elderly is paired with good or with bad on the response keys. The relative pattern of reaction times to the categorization task is informative with respect to whether the category of elderly is more closely associated with good or bad. Both the priming measure and the implicit association test have been used successfully in research on prejudice toward a wide variety of social groups (see recent reviews by Blair, 2002; Fazio and Olson, 2003).

With respect to aging, Hummert and colleagues (2002), using the implicit association test, found that people of all ages were faster to respond to young-pleasant and old-unpleasant trials than to old-pleasant and young-unpleasant trials. Furthermore, all individuals had implicit age attitudes that strongly favored the young over the old. Again, these experiments and others (Levy, 2003) demonstrate that the activation of negative stereotypes about aging affects people's automatic evaluations without their necessarily being aware of it.

Interestingly, just as activating stereotypes about the elderly can cause elderly individuals to act in a more elderly fashion, so too can activating stereotypes about the elderly cause young people to act in a more elderly manner. Thus, after activating the stereotype of the elderly, young college students walked more slowly down the hall (Bargh et al., 1996) and endorsed more politically conservative attitudes (Kawakami, Dovidio, and Dijksterhuis, 2003). Understanding the mechanisms behind the effect of stereotypes is an area ripe for research. Different explanations have been favored—self-stereotype activation versus other stereotype activation—although the behavioral and judgmental effects of activating these stereotypes are quite similar (Wheeler and Petty, 2002).

MULTIPLE CATEGORIES OF IDENTITY

A few studies have examined categories in addition to age as moderators of age-related stereotypes. Older men are perceived more positively than older women (Kite and Wagner, 2002). A gender-based double standard is applied to typical, but not optimal aging (Canetto, Kaminski, and Felicio, 1995). Simulated juries are more likely to vote for conviction when the victim is an older statesman than an older grandfather (Nunez et al., 1999). Few studies have considered race or ethnicity, with only a handful of studies examining cultural differences.

Researchers in social psychology have recognized the importance of examining the degree to which social context and shifting standards moderate automatically activated stereotypes, such as race and gender (Blair, 2002). They argue that studying a single status category (such as age) from any physical context may exaggerate the importance of global stereotypes and attitudes and obscure the importance of contextual variation. Social judgments typically result from multiple categorizations of the same individual, such as age and role, age and race, or age and gender. There is recent evidence that shows that the automatic evaluations that result from multiple simultaneous categorizations reflect emergent properties of combined categories (e.g., Barden, Maddux, Petty, and Brewer, 2004). For example, whites generally have more negative automatic evaluations of blacks than they do of whites (e.g., Greenwald et al., 1998), but automatic evaluations of "black lawyers" are more positive than automatic evaluation of "white lawyers" (Barden et al., 2004). That is, this particular race and role combination changes the automatic response. This research relies on a social cognitive approach that examines how individuals extract information from multiple sources and combine them in complex ways to produce both controlled and automatic patterns of bias. Research has not yet addressed how automatic evaluations of the elderly are affected by other variables, such as occupational or other roles, gender, or race.

Given the importance of automatic evaluations and stereotypes in affecting behavior, there is a need to further examine the nature of age stereotypes and multiple categories embedded in a social context. As the population of older workers is growing, an important topic is stereotyping in the workforce—the interfaces among employment status and age and occupational roles and stereotypic beliefs. This topic is particularly important in that older adults' alleged incompetence often lies in the eye of the beholder. Since relatively little relationship has been found between age and job performance (Salthouse and Maurer, 1996), it is important to identify social context effects that moderate such perceptions. Other status variables such as health, gender, and ethnicity may interact with age to produce combined categories. How various stereotype categories become activated has implications for hiring practices, training, and retirement.

Another important process that needs to be considered is the context in which the elderly person is being evaluated. According to the *shifting standards* framework, people make judgments about individuals who belong to stereotyped groups on the basis of within-category judgments (Biernat, 2003; Biernat and Manis, 1994). For instance, because men are assumed to be stronger than women, when a women is described as strong there is an implied assumption that she is strong *for a woman*. Thus, the description depends on the context and how the meaning of the word "strong" differs for men and women. Similarly, if one says an elderly person is healthy, it likely reflects a judgment made in comparison to other older adults. And even if there are objective differences in memory performance, an elderly individual may be judged to have a good memory because of the implicit comparison against other older adults.

AGE IDENTITY AND SELF-CONCEPT

Recent research suggests that older adults do not necessarily internalize negative aging stereotypes (Zebrowitz, 2003). It is possible for people to know certain information about themselves, but have contradictory feelings about that information. For instance, although people may be accurate in reporting their objective age and even use terms that are appropriate for their age group, they may subjectively view themselves as being much younger than that age. That is, they may believe certain stereotypes about older adults, but not believe that those stereotypes apply to them because they are not, subjectively, old. On implicit measures of age identity, older adults identify with the category "young" as strongly as do younger adults (Levy and Banaji, 2002). What accounts for individual differences in age identity and what are the effects of those differences on the quality of life for older adults?

It may be possible, paradoxically, that a lifetime of discrimination is protective in old age. There is considerable evidence in the social psychology literature that being the target of discrimination is stressful (Crocker, Major, and Steele, 1998). This stress may be associated with numerous physical health problems, including shortened life expectancy. However, the evidence on mental health is more ambiguous (see Richeson and Shelton, in this volume). For example, decades of research comparing the self-esteem of African Americans to European Americans have found small differences between the groups, with slightly higher self-esteem among African Americans (Porter and Washington, 1979; Rosenberg, 1965). Crocker and Major (1989) argued that recognizing that negative treatment and outcomes are the result of prejudice is protective for self-esteem. That is, African Americans can attribute negative outcomes, such as doing poorly on a task or being treated poorly, to prejudice rather than anything personal. One possibility is that stigmatized group members learn coping strategies for dealing with discrimination (Miller and Major, 2000), perhaps by comparing their outcomes to those who share their stigmatizing condition rather than to the population as a whole. Thus, they might value domains that favor their own group and devalue those that favor other groups (Steele, Spencer, and Aronson, 2002). For those who survive and manage to cope with lifelong prejudice, the experience of aging might be quite different than it is for those who have not faced discrimination. Their coping methods may allow them to deal with ageism in much the same way that was adaptive in the past. Research could examine how the experience of being discriminated against over the life course may prepare elderly members of stigmatized groups to cope with age discrimination.

Attention should be focused on the strategies that older adults use for preserving well-being in the face of age discrimination. For example, they might compare themselves only to people of a similar age and value only those domains in which positive outcomes are associated with aging. Some research suggests that older adults may disidentify with their age group in the face of age discrimination (Zebrowitz and Montepare, 2000) to avoid a stigmatized identity and its harmful effects on well-being. Other studies suggest that identifying with one's older group provides a positive identity in spite of age-related stigmatization (Branscombe et al., 1999; Schmitt et al., 2002). Group identification may enable older adults to avoid negative effects of age discrimination as a form of secondary control (Garstka et al., 2004). In this way older adults could adaptively respond to negative and uncontrollable consequences of age discrimination. It would be important to tease apart and expand the repertoire of control strategies in the context of age discrimination. Furthermore, learning about this repertoire of control strategies may also suggest new ways for people to cope with other stereotypes, including those surrounding the cognitive or physical limitations that frequently occur with aging.

EFFECTS OF INTERNALIZED STEREOTYPES

As noted above, there is emerging evidence that negative stereotypes about aging may affect not only others' perceptions about the abilities of older adults, but also the actual behavior of older adults. In recent years, experimental approaches to social cognition have demonstrated that at least part of the documented decline in cognitive functioning can be attributed to beliefs about aging and the social context of the testing. Because there are widespread beliefs in the culture that memory declines with age, tests that explicitly feature memory may invoke performance deficits in older people. In one study, Tammy Rahhal and her colleagues compared memory performance for adults of different ages (17 to 24 and 60 to 75) under two conditions (Rahhal, Hasher, and Colcombe, 2001). In one, the experimental instructions stressed that memory was being tested, with the experimenter repeatedly stating that participants should "remember" as many statements from a list as they could. In the other condition, the experimental instructions were identical except that emphasis was placed instead on learning, that is, participants were instructed to "learn" as many statements as they could. This study showed rather dramatic effects: there were age differences when memory was emphasized, but there were no age differences when learning was emphasized.

One possible explanation for this finding is "stereotype threat" (Steele, 1997). In a series of studies, Steele and colleagues have shown that when people fear confirming a negative stereotype they may perform badly, possibly due to the anxiety involved (e.g., Steele and Aronson, 1995). Thus, when the task was labeled as a memory task, it might have invoked the forgetful stereotype of the elderly. Alternatively, considerable research also suggests that merely priming stereotypes or specific traits can cause people to act in accordance with the primed concepts even if the stereotypes and traits are not self-relevant. Thus, priming the elderly causes young people to walk more slowly (Bargh et al., 1996), and priming the trait of hostility causes people to cooperate less in a game (Carver et al., 1983). Research is needed to pin down the mechanism by which the elderly and other individuals respond to activated stereotypes and primes.

Thomas Hess and his colleagues have also documented depressed performance when aging decline is emphasized to participants (Hess, Auman, Colcombe, and Rahhal, 2003). In their study, older participants read one of three simulated newspaper articles prior to completing a memory task. One article reaffirmed memory decline and stated that older people should rely on others to help them. The second article described research findings that suggested that memory may improve in some ways with age. The third article was neutral about memory. In this study, younger people outperformed older people in each condition, but the age difference was significantly reduced in participants who read the positive account of memory. Most important, Hess's team identified a potential mediator of these performance differences. Participants had been required to write down as many words as they could remember. Those who had read the positive account about memory were more likely to use an effective memory strategy, called semantic clustering, in which similar words are grouped together. Thus, it appeared that strategic efforts were not recruited as skillfully in those participants who were reminded of age deficits.

Indeed, one recent study by Levy and colleagues (2002) suggests that beliefs about aging, as assessed more than 20 years earlier, predicted longevity: people with strong, positive attitudes lived years longer than those with negative attitudes. Of course, it is possible that those with most negative attitudes were already experiencing more serious declines in health, but this finding raises the important alternative that what people believe about the aging process influences biological aging. Much greater attention needs to be given to how personal beliefs about aging influence psychological abilities (such as memory), as well as physical health.

In sum, the degree to which older adults reach their performance potential may be hindered as a function of stereotype threat. Research can identify the conditions under which stereotype threat effects operate in many everyday situations, especially those that involve relations with others who may hold negative stereotyped beliefs about aging (e.g., work settings). Research can also investigate ways to eliminate stereotype threat, such as exploring socially based remediation strategies for aging-related reductions in basic skills in contrast to more traditional cognitive interventions, such as strategy training or providing a more supportive cognitive environment.

INTERVENTIONS TO CHANGE AGEIST ATTITUDES

There are very few studies that examine ways to change negative beliefs about aging. Changing negative stereotypes is difficult because people encode social information in a stereotype-maintaining way: stereotypes reinforce themselves, and thus are resistant to change (Wigboldus, Dijksterhuis, and Van Knippenberg, 2003). However, social psychological research has investigated ways of changing racist and sexist attitudes, and other forms of in-group and out-group behavior, particularly among youth (Aronson and Bridgeman, 1979; Greenfield, Davis, Suzuki, and Boutakidis, 2002; Jackson et al., 2002; Pettigrew, 1998). This literature has identified some important principles that may have relevance to dealing with ageism in the society. More research connecting the two literatures might lead to more effective means of combating ageism. In turn, such research might benefit social psychological knowledge and theory about preventing and remediating discrimination because of ways that age discrimination may differ from other forms of discrimination.

What has been learned in past research is that contact by itself is generally not enough to change stereotyping and negative attitudes. Yet, those working with ageism often focus on exposing young people to older adults. For example, techniques to change ageist attitudes have included frequent exposure to the elderly, heightening sensitivity to the stereotyping of older people, increasing perspective taking, increasing intergenerational cooperation opportunities, among others (Braithwaite, 2002). However, there is little research that examines the effectiveness of such techniques. Changing communication patterns for younger and older people has been generally ineffective because of the very significant differences in communication style and the content of communication between these groups (Gould and Shaleen, 1999; Harwood et al., 1995; Kemper et al., 1995; Williams, 1996). In fact, these differences result in even more negative perceptions and lessened interest in interaction (Giles et al., 1994; Giles and Coupland, 1991).

Work on challenging automatic biases may prove to be a productive direction for future research. For example, Dasgupta and Greenwald (2001) and Duval et al. (2000) have been more successful in changing negative stereotypes about the elderly by using older exemplars who are associated with fewer automatic biases. However, the mechanisms by which exemplars of admired older adults influence negative stereotypes associated with aging have not been identified. Overall, research on changing negative stereotypes about older age has only begun to illuminate the problem. Research can examine the degree to which paradigms used to change racist and sexist beliefs may apply to ageism and negative stereotypes. Similarly, research can better clarify whether and how greater contact between older and younger people can lead to fewer negative stereotypes.

CONCLUSION

A vast literature documents both positive and negative stereotyping about older people, but little is known about the effects of these stereotypes on their behavior, self-concept, and motivation. Unlike stereotypes that have no basis in fact, aging stereotypes tend to hold a kernel of truth. Yet, since negative stereotypes can undermine optimal performance, it is particularly important to consider the social context that moderates age-related differences in cognitive functioning and others' perception of the elderly. It is important to determine the extent to which the observed declines in older adults' cognitive functioning reflects a cognitive deficiency and the extent to which cognitive impairment is influenced by mechanisms associated with a negative social context.

From a practical perspective, research on stereotypes also suggests that healthy older adults are capable of more effective cognitive functioning when operating within a facilitative social context. Thus, another important topic is identifying those conditions in which positive stereotypes serve a beneficial and protective function that may enhance both the performance of older adults and others' perceptions of the elderly. The complicated roles played by gender; socioeconomic status; and racial, ethnic, and cultural identities in the development, internalization, and rejection of ageist stereotypes also require further investigation. The overall challenge is to develop a more nuanced understanding of the mechanisms underlying both explicit and implicit stereotypes and their effects on society and the functioning of older people.

References

Abelson, R.P., Kinder, D.R., Peters, M.D., and Fiske, S.T. (1982). Affective and semantic components in political person perception. *Journal of Personality and Social Psychology, 42*, 619-630.

Addington-Hall, J., Lay, M., Altmann, D., and McCarthy, M. (1995). Symptom control, communication with health professionals, and hospital care of stroke patients in the last year of life as reported by surviving family, friends, and officials. *Stroke, 26*, 2242-2248.

Adolphs, R. (2003). Cognitive neuroscience of human social behavior. *Nature Reviews Neuroscience, 4*, 165-178.

Adolphs, R., Tranel, D., and Damasio, A.R. (1998). The human amygdala in social judgment. *Nature, 393*, 470-474.

Albert, M.S, Jones, K., Savage, C.R., Berkman, L., Seeman, T., Blazer, D., and Rowe, J.W. (1995). Predicitors of cognitive changes in older persons: MacArthur studies of successful aging. *Psychology and Aging, 10*, 578-589.

Aldwin, C.M., Sutton, K.J., Chiara, G., and Spiro, A. (1996). Age differences in stress, coping, and appraisal: Findings from the normative aging study. *Journals of Gerontology Series B: Psychological Sciences and Social Sciences, 51B*(4), P179-P188.

Anderson, C.J. (2003). The psychology of doing nothing: Forms of decision avoidance result from reason and emotion. *Psychological Bulletin, 129*, 139-167.

Angeletos, G., Laibson, D., Repetto, A., Tobacman, J., and Weinberg, S. (2003). The hyperbolic consumption model: Calibration, simulation, and empirical evaluation. In G. Loewenstein, D. Read, and R.F. Baumeister (Eds.), *Time and decision: Economic and psychological perspectives on intertemporal choice* (pp. 517-543). New York: Russell Sage Foundation.

Antonucci, T.C. (2001). Social relations. In J.E. Birren and K.W. Schaie (Eds.), *Handbook of the psychology of aging* (pp. 427-453). San Diego: Academic Press.

Antonucci, T.C., Fuhrer, R., and Dartigues, J.F. (1997). Social relations and depressive symptomatology in a sample of community-dwelling French older adults. *Psychology and Aging, 12*, 189-195.

Arbuckle, T.Y., Gold, D.P., Andres, D., Schwartzman, A.E., and Chaikelson, J. (1992). The role of psychosocial context, age and intelligence in memory performance of older men. *Psychology and Aging, 7*, 25-36.

Aronson, E., and Bridgeman, D. (1979). Jigsaw groups and the desegregated classroom: In pursuit of common goals. *Personality and Social Psychology Bulletin, 5*, 438-446.

Balkrishnan, R. (1998). Predictors of medication adherence in the elderly. *Clinical Therapeutics, 20*, 764-771.

Ball, K., Berch, D.B., Helmers, K.F., Jobe, J.B., Leveck, M.D., Marsiske, M., Morris, J.N., Rebok, G.W., Smith, D.M., Tennstedt, S.L., Unverzagt, F.W., and Willis, S.L. (2002). Advanced cognitive training for independent and vital elderly study group. Effects of cognitive training interventions with older adults: A randomized controlled trial. *Journal of the American Medical Association, 288*, 2271-2281.

Ball, K., Owsley, C., Stalvey, B., Roenker, D.L., and Graves, M. (1998). Driving avoidance, functional impairment, and crash risk in older drivers. *Accident Analysis and Prevention, 30*, 313-322.

Baltes, M.M. (1995). Dependency in old age: Gains and losses. *Current Directions in Psychological Science, 4*, 1419.

Baltes, M.M. (1996). *The many faces of dependency in old age*. New York: Cambridge University Press.

Baltes, M.M., and Wahl, H.W. (1991). The behavior system of dependency in the elderly: Interaction with the social environment. In M. Ory, R.P. Abeles, and P.D. Lipman (Eds.), *Aging, health and behavior*. Thousand Oaks, CA: Sage.

Baltes, M.M., Wahl, H.W., and Schmid-Furstoss, U. (1990). The daily life of elderly Germans: Activity patterns, personal control, and functional health. *Journals of Gerontology Series B: Psychological Sciences and Social Sciences, 45B*, P173-P179.

Baltes, P.B. (1991). The many faces of human aging: Toward a psychological culture of old age. *Psychological Medicine, 21*, 837-854.

Baltes, P.B. (1997). On the incomplete architecture of human ontogeny: Selection, optimization, and compensation as foundation of developmental theory. *American Psychologist, 52*, 366-380.

Baltes, P.B., and Baltes, M.M. (1990). Psychological perspectives on successful aging: The model of selective optimization with compensation. In P.B. Baltes and M.M. Baltes (Eds.), *Successful aging: Perspectives from the behavioral sciences* (pp. 1-34). New York: Cambridge University Press.

Baltes, P.B., and Kunzmann, U. (2003). Wisdom. *Psychologist, 16*, 131-133.

Bandura, A. (1989). Human agency in social cognitive theory. *American Psychologist, 44*, 1175-1184.

Bandura, A. (1997). *Self-efficacy: The exercise of control*. New York: Freeman.

Bandura, A. (2001). Social cognitive theory: An agentic perspective. *Annual Review of Psychology, 52*, 1-26.

Banfield, J.F., Wyland, C.L., Macrae, C.N., Munte, T.F., and Heatherton, T.F. (2004). The cognitive neuroscience of self-regulation. In R.F. Baumeister and K.D. Vohs (Eds.), *Handbook of self-regulation: Research, theory, and applications* (pp. 62-83). New York: Guilford Press.

Barden, J.A., Maddux, W.W., Petty, R.E., and Brewer, M.B. (2004). Contextual moderation of racial bias: The impact of social roles on controlled and automatically activated attitudes. *Journal of Personality and Social Psychology, 87*(1), 5-22.

Bargh, J.A., and Apsley, D.K. (2001). *Unraveling the complexities of social life: A festschrift in honor of Robert B. Zajonc*. Washington, DC: American Psychological Association.

Bargh, J.A., Chen, M., and Burrows, L. (1996). Automaticity of social behavior: Direct effects of trait construct and stereotype activation on action. *Journal of Personality and Social Psychology, 71*(2), 230-244.

Baron, J. (1992). The effects of normative beliefs on anticipated emotions. *Journal of Personality and Social Psychology, 68*, 320-330.

Bassuk, S.S., Glass, T.A., and Berkman, L.F. (1999). Social disengagement and incident cognitive decline in community-dwelling elderly persons. *Annals of Internal Medicine, 131*, 165-173.

Baumeister, R.F., and Heatherton, T.F. (1996). Self-regulation failure: An overview. *Psychological Inquiry, 7*, 1-15.

Baumeister, R.F., Heatherton, T.F., and Tice, D. (1994). *Losing control: Why and how people fail at self-regulation.* San Diego: Academic Press.

Baumeister, R.F., Stillwell, A.M., and Heatherton, T.F. (1994). Guilt: An interpersonal approach. *Psychological Bulletin, 115*, 243-267.

Bechara, A. (2003). Decisions, uncertainty, and the brain: The science of neuroeconomics. *Journal of Clinical and Experimental Neuropsychology, 25*, 1035-1037.

Bell, D.E. (1982). Regret in decision making under uncertainty. *Operations Research, 30*(5), 961-981.

Bell, D.E. (1985). Disappointment in decision making under uncertainty. *Operations Research, 33*, 1-27.

Bennett, E.L., Rosenzweig, M.R., and Diamond, M.C. (1969). Rat brain: Effects of environmental enrichment on wet and dry weights. *Science, 163*, 825-826.

Berkman, L.F. (1985). The relationship of social network and social support to morbidity and mortality. In S. Cohen and L.S. Syme (Eds.), *Social support and health* (pp. 241-262). New York: Academic Press.

Berkman, L.F., and Breslow, L. (1983). *Health and ways of living: The Alameda County study.* New York: Oxford University Press.

Berkman, L.F., and Syme, S.L. (1979). Social networks, host resistance, and mortality: A nine year follow-up study of Alameda County residents. *American Journal of Epidemiology, 109*, 186-204.

Bernheim, B.D., Skinner, J., and Weinberg, S. (2001). What accounts for the variation in retirement wealth among U.S. households? *American Economic Review, 91*(4), 832-857.

Bieman-Copland, S., and Ryan, E.B. (2001). Social perceptions of failures in memory monitoring. *Psychology and Aging, 16*, 357-361.

Biernat, M. (2003). Toward a broader view of social stereotyping. *American Psychologist, 58*, 1019-1027.

Biernat, M., and Manis, M. (1994). Shifting standards and stereotype-based judgments. *Journal of Personality and Social Psychology, 66*, 5-20.

Blair, I. (2002). The malleability of automatic stereotypes and prejudice. *Personality and Social Psychology Review, 6*, 242-261.

Blanchard-Fields, F. (1998). The role of emotion in social cognition across the adult life span. In K.W. Schaie and M.P. Lawton (Eds.), *Annual review of gerontology and geriatrics* (vol. 17). New York: Springer.

Blanchard-Fields, F., and Chen, Y. (1996). Adaptive cognition and aging. *American Behavioral Scientist, 39*, 231-248.

Blanchard-Fields, F., Hertzog, C., Stein, R., and Pak, R. (2001). Beyond a stereotyped view of older adults' traditional family values. *Psychology and Aging, 16*(3), 483-496.

Blanchard-Fields F., Jahnke, H.C., and Camp, C. (1995). Age differences in problem-solving style: The role of emotional salience. *Psychology and Aging, 10*(2), 173-180.

Bond, G., Thompson, L.A., and Malloy, D.M. (2005). Vulnerability of older adults to deception in prison and non-prison contexts. *Psychology and Aging, 20*(1), 60-70.

Bosma, H., van Boxtel, M.P., Ponds, R.W., Houx, P.J., Burdorf, A., and Jolles, J. (2003). Mental work demands protect against cognitive impairment: MAAS prospective cohort study. *Experimental Aging Research, 29*(1), 33-45.

Bosworth, H.B., Siegler, I.C., Brummett, B.H., Barefoot, J.C., Williams, R.B., Vitaliano, P.P., Clapp-Channing, N., Lytle, B.L., and Mark, D.B. (1999). The relationship between self-rated health and health status among coronary artery patients. *Journal of Aging and Health, 11*(4), 565-584.

Bourgeois, M.S., Camp, C., Rose, M., White, B., Malone, M., Carr, J., and Rovine, M. (2003). A comparison of training strategies to enhance use of external aids by persons with dementia. *Journal of Communication Disorders, 36*, 361-378.

Bowling, A., and Grundy, E. (1998). The association between social networks and mortality in later life. *Reviews in Clinical Gerontology, 8*, 353-361.

Braithwaite, V. (2002). Reducing ageism. In T.D. Nelson (Ed.), *Ageism: Stereotyping and prejudice against older persons* (pp. 311-337). Cambridge, MA: MIT Press.

Brandtstädter, J., and Rothermund, K. (1994). Self-percepts of control in middle and later adulthood: Buffering losses by rescaling goals. *Psychology and Aging, 2*, 265-273.

Brandtstädter, J., Wentura, D., and Rothermund, K. (1999). Intentional self-development through adulthood and later life: Tenacious pursuit and flexible adjustment of goals. In J. Brandtstädter and R.M. Lerner (Eds.), *Action and self-development: Theory and research through the life span* (pp. 373-400). Thousand Oaks, CA: Sage.

Branscombe, N.R., Schmitt, M.T., and Harvey, R.D. (1999). Perceiving pervasive discrimination among African Americans: Implications for group identification and well-being. *Journal of Personality and Social Psychology, 77*(1), 135-149.

Brehm, J.W. (1956). Postdecision changes in the desirability of alternatives. *Journal of Abnormal and Social Psychology, 52*, 384-389.

Breiter, H.C., and Rosen, B.R. (1999). Functional magnetic resonance imaging of brain reward circuitry in the human. In *Annals of the New York Academy of Sciences* (vol. 877, pp. 523-547). New York: New York Academy of Sciences.

Brimacombe, C.A.E., Jung, S., Garrioch, L., and Allison, M. (2003). Perceptions of older adult eyewitnesses: Will you believe me when I'm 64? *Law and Human Behavior, 27*(5), 507-522.

Brown, S.C., and Park, D.C. (2003). Theoretical models of cognitive aging and implications for translational research in medicine. *Gerontologist, 43*, 57-67.

Brownell, K.D., Marlatt, G.A., Lichtenstein, E., and Wilson, G.T. (1986). Understanding and preventing relapse. *American Psychologist, 41*, 765-782.

Bryce, C.L., Angus, D.C., and Loewenstein, G. (2003). Assessing the value of "quality of death." *Society for Medical Decision Making Newsletter, 15*(3), 6.

Byrne, R.W., and Whiten, A. (Eds.). (1988). *Machiavellian intelligence: Social expertise and the evolution of intellect in monkeys, apes, and humans.* New York: Clarendon Press/ Oxford University Press.

Cabeza, R. (2002). Hemispheric asymmetry reduction in older adults: The HAROLD model. *Psychology and Aging, 17*, 85-100.

Cabeza, R., Daselaar, S.M., Dolcos, F., Prince, S.E., Budde, M., and Nyberg, L. (2004). Task-independent and task-specific age effects on brain activity during working memory, visual attention and episodic retrieval. *Cerebral Cortex, 14*, 364-375.

Cacioppo, J.T., and Petty, R.E. (1982). The need for cognition. *Journal of Personality and Social Psychology, 42*, 116-131.

Camp, C.J., Judge, K.S., Bye, C.A., Fox, K.M., Bowden, J., Bell, M., Valencic, K., and Mattern, J.M. (1997). An intergenerational program for persons with dementia using Montessori methods. *Gerontologist, 37*, 688-692.

Canetto, S.S., Kaminski, P.L., and Felicio, D.M. (1995). Typical and optimal aging in women and men: Is there a double standard? *International Journal of Aging and Human Development, 40*(3), 187-207.

Caplin, A. (2003). Fear as a policy instrument. In G. Loewenstein, D. Read, and R.F. Baumeister (Eds.), *Time and decision: Economic and psychological perspectives on intertemporal choice* (pp. 441-458). New York: Russell Sage Foundation.

Carstensen, L.L. (1992). Social and emotional patterns in adulthood: Support for socioemotional selectivity theory. *Psychology and Aging, 7*(3), 331-338.

Carstensen, L.L., Isaacowitz, D.M., and Charles, S.T. (1999). Taking time seriously: A theory of socioemotional selectivity. *American Psychologist, 54*(3), 165-181.

Carstensen, L.L., and Mikels, J.A. (2005). At the intersection of emotion and cognition: Aging and the positivity effect. *Current Directions in Psychological Science, 14*(3), 117-121.

Carstensen, L.L., Pasupathi, M., Mayr, U., and Nesselroade, J.R. (2000). Emotional experience in everyday life across the adult life span. *Journal of Personality and Social Psychology, 79*(4), 644-655.

Carver, C.S., Ganellen, R.J., Froming, W.J., and Chambers, W. (1983). Modeling: An analysis in terms of category accessibility. *Journal of Experimental Social Psychology, 19*, 403-421.

Carver, C.S., and Scheier, M.F. (1982). Control theory: A useful conceptual framework for personality-social, clinical, and health psychology. *Psychological Bulletin, 92*, 111-135.

Carver, C.S., and Scheier, M.F. (1999). Control theory: A useful conceptual framework for personality-social, clinical, and health psychology. In R.F. Baumeister (Ed.), *The self in social psychology. Key readings in social psychology* (pp. 299-316). New York: Taylor and Francis Group.

Caspi, A., and Herbener, E.S. (1990). Continuity and change: Assortative marriage and the consistency of personality in adulthood. *Journal of Personality and Social Psychology, 58*(2), 250-258.

Caspi, A., and Roberts, B.W. (1999). Personality continuity and change across the life course. In L.A. Pervin and O.P. John (Eds.), *Handbook of personality* (2nd ed., pp. 300-326). New York: Guilford Press.

Caspi, A., Sugden, K., Moffitt, T.E., Taylor, A., Craig, I.W., Harrington, H.L., McClay, J., Mill, J., Martin, J., Braithwaite, A., and Poulton, R. (2003). Influence of life stress on depression: Moderation by a polymorphism in the 5-HTT gene. *Science, 301*(5631), 386-389.

Castro-Caldas, A., Petersson, K.M., Reis, A., Stone-Elander, S., and Ingvar M. (1998). The illiterate brain: Learning to read and write during childhood influences the functional organization of the adult brain. *Brain, 121*, 1053-1063.

Charles, S.T., and Carstensen, L.L. (2002). Marriage in old age. In M. Yalom and L.L. Carstensen (Eds.), *Inside the American couple: New insights, new challenges* (pp. 236-254). Berkeley: University of California Press.

Charles, S.T., Mather, M., and Carstensen, L.L. (2003). Aging and emotional memory: The forgettable nature of negative images for older adults. *Journal of Experimental Psychology: General, 132*(2), 310-324.

Charles, S.T., and Pasupathi, M. (2003). Age-related patterns of variability in self-descriptions: Implications for everyday affective experience. *Psychology and Aging, 18*, 524-536.

Charles, S.T., Reynolds, C.A., and Gatz, M. (2001). Age-related differences and change in positive and negative affect over 23 years. *Journal of Personality and Social Psychology, 80*(1), 136-151.

Chasteen, A.L., Park, D.C., and Schwarz, N. (2001). Implementation intentions and facilitation of prospective memory. *Psychological Science, 12*, 457-461.

Chen, S., and Chaiken, S. (1999). The heuristic-systematic model in its broader context. In S. Chaiken and Y. Trope (Eds.), *Dual-process theories in social psychology* (pp. 73-96). New York: Guilford Press.

Chen, Y., and Blanchard-Fields, F. (2000). Unwanted thought: Age differences in the correction of social judgments. *Psychology of Aging, 15*, 475-482.

Chiu, S., and Yu, S. (2001). An excess of culture: The myth of shared care in the Chinese community in Britain. *Ageing and Society, 21*, 681-699.

Choi, J.J., Laibson, D., Madrian, B., and Metrick, A. (2003). Optimal defaults. *American Economic Review, 93*, 180-185.

Christmas, C., and Andersen, R.A. (2000). Exercise and older patients: Guidelines for the clinician. *Journal of American Geriatric Society, 48*, 318-324.

Clifford, P.A., Tan, S., and Gorsuch, R.L. (1991). Efficacy of a self-directed behavioral health change program: Weight, body composition, cardiovascular fitness, blood pressure, health risk, and psychosocial mediating variables. *Journal of Behavioral Medicine, 14*, 303-323.

Cohen, J.D., Botvinick, M., and Carter, C.S. (2000). Anterior cingulate and prefrontal cortex: Who's in control? *Nature Neuroscience, 3*, 421-423.

Cohen, S., and Wills, T.A. (1985). Stress, social support, and the buffering hypothesis. *Psychological Bulletin, 98*, 310-357.

Colcombe, S.J., and Kramer, A.F. (2003). Fitness effects on the cognitive function of older adults: A meta-analytic study. *Psychological Science, 14*, 125-130.

Colcombe, S.J., Kramer, A.F., Erickson, K.I., Scalf, P., McAuley, P., Cohen, N.J., Webb, A., Jerome, G.J., Marquez, D.X., and Elavski, S. (2004). Cardiovascular fitness, cortical plasticity, and aging. *Proceedings of the National Academy of Sciences, 101*, 316-321.

Committee on Aging Frontiers in Social Psychology, Personality, and Adult Developmental Psychology. (2006a). Measuring psychological mechanisms. In National Research Council, *When I'm 64* (pp. 209-218). L.L. Carstensen and C.R. Hartel (Eds.). Division of Behavioral and Social Sciences and Education. Washington, DC: The National Academes Press.

Committee on Aging Frontiers in Social Psychology, Personality, and Adult Developmental Psychology. (2006b). Research infrastructure. In National Research Council, *When I'm 64* (pp. 247-249). L.L. Carstensen and C.R. Hartel (Eds.). Division of Behavioral and Social Sciences and Education. Washington, DC: The National Academes Press

Costa, P.T., and McCrae, R.R. (1990). *Personality in adulthood*. New York: Guilford Press.

Costa, P.T., Jr., Herbst, J.H., McCrae, R.R., and Siegler, I.C. (2000). Personality at midlife: Stability, intrinsic maturation, and response to life events. *Assessment, 7*(4), 365-378.

Coughlan, R., and Connolly, T. (2001). Predicting affective responses to unexpected outcomes. *Organizational Behavior and Human Decision Processes, 85*(2), 211-225.

Crites, S.L., Fabrigar, L.R., and Petty, R.E. (1994). Measuring the affective and cognitive properties of attitudes: Conceptual and methodological issues. *Personality and Social Psychology Bulletin, 20*, 619-634.

Crocker, J., and Major, B. (1989). Social stigma and self-esteem: The self-protective properties of social stigma. *Psychological Review, 96*, 608-630.

Crocker, J., Major, B., and Steele, C.M. (1998). Social stigma. In D. Gilbert, S.T. Fiske, and G. Lindzey (Eds.), *Handbook of social psychology* (4th ed.). Boston: McGraw-Hill.

Crocker, J., and Wolfe, C.T. (2001). Contingencies of self-worth. *Psychological Review, 108*(3), 593-623.

Cross, S., and Markus, H.R. (1991). Possible selves across the life span. *Human Development, 34*, 230-255.

Crowe, M., Andel, R., Pedersen, N.L., Johansson, B., and Gatz, M. (2003). Does participation in leisure activities lead to reduced risk of Alzheimer's disease? A prospective study of Swedish twins. *Journals of Gerontology Series B: Psychological Sciences and Social Sciences, 58B*, P249-P255.

Cuddy, A.J.C., and Fiske, S.T. (2002). Doddering but dear: Process, content, and function in stereotyping of older persons. In T.D. Nelson (Ed.), *Stereotyping and prejudice against older persons* (pp. 3-26). Cambridge, MA: MIT Press.

Cumming, E., and Henry, W. (1961). *Growing old: The process of disengagement.* New York: Basic Books.

Cummings, J.L., and Cole, G. (2002). Alzheimer's disease. *Journal of the American Medical Association, 287*(18), 2335–2338.

Czaja, S.J. (2001). Technological change and the older worker. In J.E. Birren and K.W. Schaie (Eds.), *Handbook of the psychology of aging* (pp. 547-568). San Diego: Academic Press.

Damasio, A.R. (1994). *Descartes' error: Emotion, reason, and the human brain.* New York: G.P. Putnam's Sons.

Dannefer, D. (2003). Cumulative advantage/disadvantage and the life course: Cross-fertilizing age and social science theory. *Journals of Gerontology Series B: Psychological Sciences and Social Sciences, 58B*(6), P327-P337.

Danner, D.D., Snowdon, D.A., and Friesen, W.V. (2001). Positive emotions in early life and longevity: Findings from the nun study. *Journal of Personality and Society Psychology, 80*, 804-813.

Dasgupta, N., and Greenwald, A.G. (2001). On the malleability of automatic attitudes. Combating automatic prejudice with images of admired and disliked individuals. *Journal of Personality and Social Psychology, 81*, 800-814.

Denburg, N.L., Buchanan, T.W., Tranel, D., and Adolphs, R. (2003). Evidence for preserved emotional memory in normal older persons. *Emotion, 3*(3), 239-253.

DeSteno, D., Petty, R.E., Wegener, D.T., and Rucker, D.D. (2000). Beyond valence in the perception of likelihood: The role of emotion specificity. *Journal of Personality and Social Psychology, 78*, 397-416.

Diehl, M., Coyle, N., and Labouvie-Vief, G. (1996). Age and sex differences in strategies of coping and defense across the life span. *Psychology and Aging, 11*(1), 127-139.

Diener, E., and Suh, M.E. (1998). Subjective well-being and age: An international analysis. *Annual Review of Gerontology and Geriatrics, 17*, 304-324.

Dijksterhuis, A., and Bargh, J.A. (2001). The perception-behavior expressway: Automatic effects of social perception on social behavior. In M.P. Zanna (Ed.), *Advances in experimental social psychology* (vol. 33, pp. 1-40). San Diego: Academic Press.

Dilworth-Anderson, P., Goodwin, P.Y., and Wallace, S. (2004). Can culture help explain the physical health effects of caregiving over time among African American caregivers? *Journal of Gerontology: Social Sciences, 59B*(3), S138-S145.

Ditto, P.H., and Croyle, R.T. (1995). Understanding the impact of risk factor test results: Insights from a basic research program. In R.T. Croyle (Ed.), *Psychosocial effects of screening for disease prevention and detection* (pp. 144-181). Oxford, England: Oxford University Press.

Dixon, R.A. (2000). The concept of gains in cognitive aging. In D.C. Park and N. Schwarz (Eds.), *Cognitive aging: A primer*. Philadelphia: Psychology Press.

Dixon, R.A., and Gould, O.N. (1998). Younger and older adults collaborating in retelling everyday stories. *Applied Developmental Science, 2*, 160-171.

Dixon, R.A., Hopp, G.A., Cohen, A-L., de Frias, C.M., and Bäckman, L. (2003). Self-reported memory compensation: Similar patterns in Alzheimer's disease and very old adult samples. *Journal of Clinical and Experimental Neuropsychology, 25*, 382-390.

Dovidio, J.F., Kawakami, K., and Gaertner, S.L. (2002). Implicit and explicit prejudice and interracial interactions. *Journal of Personality and Social Psychology, 82*, 62-68.

Dovidio, J.F., Kawakami, K., Johnson, C., Johnson, B., and Howard, A. (1997). On the nature of prejudice: Automatic and controlled processes. *Journal of Experimental Social Psychology, 33*, 510-540.

Duval, L.L., Ruscher, J.B., Welsh, K., and Catanese, S.P. (2000). Bolstering and undercutting use of the elderly stereotype through communication of exemplars: The role of speaker age and exemplar stereotypicality. *Basic and Applied Social Psychology: The Social Psychology of Aging Special Issue, 22*, 137-146.

Eagly, A.H., and Chaiken, S. (1993). *The psychology of attitudes*. Fort Worth, TX: Harcourt, Brace, Jovanovich.

Eagly, A.H., Mladinic, A., and Otto, S. (1994). Cognitive and affective bases of attitudes toward social groups and social policies. *Journal of Experimental Social Psychology, 30*, 113-137.

Einstein, G.O., McDaniel, M.A., Richardson, S.L., Guynn, M.J., and Cunfer, A.R. (1995). Aging and prospective memory: Examining the influence of self-initiated retrieval processes. *Journal of Experimental Psychology: Learning, Memory, and Cognition, 21*, 996-1007.

Elias, M.F., Beiser, A., Wolf, P.A., Au, R., White, R.F., and D'Agostino, R.B. (2000). The preclinical phase of Alzheimer's disease: A 22-year prospective study of the Framingham cohort. *Archives of Neurology, 57*(6), 808-813.

England, S.F., Keigher, S.M., Miller, B., and Linsk, N.L. (1991). Community care policies and gender justice. In M. Minkler and C.L. Estes (Eds.), *Critical perspectives on aging: The political and moral economy of growing old* (pp. 227-244). Amityville, NY: Baywood.

Epel, E.S., Blackburn, E.H., Lin, J., Dhabhar, F.S., Adler, N.E., Morrow, J.D., and Cawthon, R.M. (2004). Accelerated telomere shortening in response to life stress. *Proceedings of the National Academies, 101*, 17312-17315.

Epstein, S. (2003). Cognitive-experiential self theory of personality. In *Handbook of psychology: Personality and social psychology* (vol. 5). New York: John Wiley and Sons.

Erber, J.T., and Szuchman, L.T. (2002). Age and capability: The role of forgetting and personal traits. *International Journal of Aging and Human Development, 54*(3), 173-189.

Erber, J.T., Szuchman, L.T., and Prager, I.G. (2001). Ain't misbehavin': The effects of age and intentionality on judgments about misconduct. *Psychology and Aging, 16*, 85-95.

Escobar, J.I., Burnam, A., Karno, M., Forsythe, A., Landsverk, J., and Goding, J.M. (1986). Use of the Mini-Mental State Examination (MMSE) in a community population of mixed ethnicity: Cultural and linguistic artifacts. *Journal of Nervous and Mental Disease, 174*, 607-614.

Fabrigoule, C., Letenneur, L., Dartigues, J.F., Zarrouk, M., Commenges, D., and Barberger-Gateau, P. (1995). Social and leisure activities and risk of dementia: A prospective longitudinal study. *Journal of the American Geriatrics Society, 43*, 485-490.

Fagerlin, A., Ditto, P.H., Danks, J.H., and Houts, R.M. (2001). Projection in surrogate decisions about life-sustaining medical treatments. *Health Psychology, 20*, 166-175.

Fagerlin, A., Ditto, P.H., Hawkins, N.A., Schneider, C.E., and Smucker, W.D. (2002). The use of advance directives in end-of-life decision making. *American Behavioral Scientist, 46*, 268-283.

Fazio, R.H. (1995). Attitudes as object-evaluation associations: Determinants, consequences, and correlates of attitude accessibility. In R.E. Petty and J.A. Krosnick (Eds.), *Attitude strength: Antecedents and consequences* (pp. 247-282). Mahwah, NJ: Lawrence Erlbaum.

Fazio, R.H., Jackson, J.R., Dunton, B.C., and Williams, C.J. (1995). Variability in automatic activation as an unobtrusive measure of racial attitudes: A bona fide pipeline? *Journal of Personality and Social Psychology, 69*, 1013-1027.

Fazio, R.H., and Olson, M. (2003). Implicit measures in social cognition research: Their meaning and use. *Annual Review of Psychology, 54*, 297-327.

Fazio, R.H., Sanbonmatsu, D.M., Powell, M.C., and Kardes, F.R. (1986). On the automatic activation of attitudes. *Journal of Personality and Social Psychology, 50*(2), 229-238.

Featherman, D.L., Lerner, R.M., and Perlmutter, M. (1994). *Life-span development and behavior* (vol. 12). Mahwah, NJ: Lawrence Erlbaum.

Festinger, L. (1957). *A theory of cognitive dissonance*. Evanston, IL: Row Peterson.

Field, D., and Weishaus, S. (1992). Marriage over a half century: A longitudinal study. In M. Bloom (Ed.), *Changing lives* (pp. 269-273). Columbia: University of South Carolina Press.

Fillenbaum, G.G., Hughes, D.C., Heyman, A., George, L.K., and Blazer, D.G. (1988). Relationship of health and demographic characteristics to Mini-Mental State Examination score among community residents. *Psychological Medicine, 18*, 719-726.

Fingerman K.L. (2000). "We had a nice little chat." Age and generational differences in mothers' and daughters' descriptions of enjoyable visits. *Journal of Gerontology: Psychological Sciences, 55B*, P95-P106.

Fingerman, K.L., Hay, E.L., and Birditt, K.S. (2004). The best of ties, the worst of ties: Close, problematic, and ambivalent relationships across the lifespan. *Journal of Marriage and Family*, 66, 792-808.

Finucane, M.L., Slovic, P., Hibbard, J.H., Peters, E., Mertz, C.K., and MacGregor, D.G. (2002). Aging and decision-making competence: An analysis of comprehension and consistency skills in older versus younger adults considering health plan options. *Journal of Behavioral Decision Making, 15*, 141-164.

Fishbein, M., and Ajzen, I. (1975). *Belief, attitude, intention, and behavior*. Reading, MA: Addison-Wesley.

Fratiglioni, L., Paillard-Borg, S., and Winblad, B. (2004). An active and socially integrated lifestyle in late life might protect against dementia. *Lancet Neurology, 3*(6), 343-353.

Fratiglioni, L., Wang, H.-X., Ericsson, K., Maytan, M., and Winblad, B. (2000). Influence of social network on occurrence of dementia: A community-based longitudinal study. *The Lancet, 355*, 1315-1319.

Frederick, S., Loewenstein, G., and O'Donoghue, T. (2003). Time discounting and time preference: A critical review. In G. Loewenstein, D. Read, and R.F. Baumeister (Eds.), *Time and decision: Economic and psychological perspectives on intertemporal choice* (pp. 13-86). New York: Russell Sage Foundation.

Fredrickson, B.L., and Carstensen, L.L. (1990). Choosing social partners: How old age and anticipated endings make people more selective. *Psychology and Aging, 5*, 335-347.

Freund, A.M., and Baltes, P.B. (1998). Selection, optimization, compensation as strategies of life management: Correlations with subjective indicators of successful aging. *Psychology and Aging, 13*, 531-543.

Friedman, M., and Friedman, R.D. (1980). *Free to choose: A personal statement.* Harmondsworth, UK: Penguin.

Fung, H.H., and Carstensen, L.L. (2003). Sending memorable messages to the old: Age differences in preferences and memory for advertisements. *Journal of Personality and Social Psychology, 85*(1), 163-178.

Fung, H.H., and Carstensen, L.L. (2004). Motivational changes in response to blocked goals and foreshortened time: Testing alternatives to socioemotional selectivity theory. *Psychology of Aging, 19*, 68-78.

Fung, H.H., Carstensen, L.L., and Lutz, A. (1999). Influence of time on social preferences: Implications for life-span development. *Psychology and Aging, 14*, 595-604.

Fung, H.H., Lai, P., and Ng, R. (2001). Age differences in social preferences among Taiwanese and mainland Chinese: The role of perceived time. *Psychology and Aging, 16*, 351-356.

Gallagher, D., Rose, J., Rivera, P., Lovett, S., and Thompson, L.W. (1989). Prevalence of depression in family caregivers. *The Gerontologist, 29*, 449-456.

Garstka, T.A., Schmitt, M., Branscombe, N.R., and Hummert, M.L. (2004). How young and older adults differ in their responses to perceived age discrimination. *Psychology and Aging, 19*(2), 326-335.

Gatz, M., Kasl-Godley, J.E., and Karel, M.J. (1996). Aging and mental disorders. In J.E. Birren and K.W. Schaie (Eds.), *Handbook of the psychology of aging* (4th ed., pp. 367-382). San Diego: Academic Press.

Gatz, M., Pedersen, N.L., Plomin, R., Nesselroade, J.R., and McClearn, G.E. (1992). Importance of shared genes and shared environments for symptoms of depression in older adults. *Journal of Abnormal Psychology, 101*(4), 701-708.

Gehring, W.J., and Knight, R.T. (2000). Prefrontal-cingulate interactions in action monitoring. *Nature Neuroscience, 3*, 516-520.

Gehring, W.J., and Knight, R.T. (2002). Lateral prefrontal damage affects processing selection but not attention switching. *Cognitive Brain Research, 13*, 267-279.

Gentry, W.D., and Kobasa, S.C.O. (1984). Social and psychological resources mediating stress-illness relationships in humans. In W.D. Gentry (Ed.), *Handbook of behavioral medicine* (pp. 87-116). New York: Guilford Press.

Gilbert, D.T., Driver-Linn, E., and Wilson, T.D. (2002). The trouble with Vronsky: Impact bias in the forecasting of future-affective states. In L. Feldman-Barrett and P. Salovey (Eds.), *The wisdom of feeling* (pp. 114-143). New York: Guilford.

Gilbert, D.T., Lieberman, M.D., Morewedge, C.K., and Wilson, T.D. (2004). The peculiar longevity of things not so bad. *Psychological Science, 15*(1), 14-19.

Gilbert, D.T., Pinel, E.C., Wilson, T.D., Blumberg, S.J., and Wheatley, T.P. (1998). Immune neglect: A source of durability bias in affective forecasting. *Journal of Personality and Social Psychology, 75*, 617-638.

Gilbert, D.T., and Wilson, T.D. (2000). Miswanting: Some problems in the forecasting of future affective states. In J.P. Forgas (Ed.), *Feeling and thinking: The role of affect in social cognition* (pp. 178-197). New York: Cambridge University Press.

Giles, H., and Coupland, N. (1991). *Language: Contexts and consequences*. Belmont, CA: Brooks/Cole.

Giles, H., Fox, S., Harwood, J., and Williams, A. (1994). Talking age and aging talk: Communicating through the life span. In M. Hummert, J. Wiemann, and J. Nussbaum (Eds.), *Interpersonal communication in older adulthood: Interdisciplinary theory and research* (pp. 130-161). New York: Sage.

Gilovich, T., and Medvec, V.H. (1995). The experience of regret: What, when, and why. *Psychological Review, 102*, 379-395.

Gollwitzer, P., Fujita, K., and Oettingen, G. (2004). Planning and implementation of goals. In R.F. Baumeister and K.D. Vohs (Eds.), *Handbook of self-regulation: Research, theory, and applications* (pp. 211-228). New York: Guilford Press.

Gollwitzer, P., and Schaal, B. (2001). How goals and plans affect action. In J.M. Collis and S. Messick (Eds.), *Intelligence and personality: Bridging the gap in theory and measurement* (pp. 139-161). Mahwah, NJ: Lawrence Erlbaum.

Gordon, R.A., Goldstein, S.B., Lips, H.M., Jones, M., Crawford, M., Hebl, M.R., Richard, H.W., Lawrence, S.M., Ford, T.E., Grossman, R.W., and Jordan, E.A. (2000). Examining stereotypes of gender and race. In M.E. Ware and D.E. Johnson, (Eds.), *Handbook of demonstrations and activities in the teaching of psychology, Vol. III: Personality, abnormal, clinical-counseling, and social* (2nd ed., pp. 277-302). Mahwah, NJ: Lawrence Erlbaum.

Gould, O.N., and Shaleen, L. (1999). Collaboration with diverse partners: How older women adapt their speech. *Journal of Language and Social Psychology, 18*, 395-418.

Goulet, L.R., and Baltes, P.B. (1970). *Life-span developmental psychology: Research and theory.* New York: Academic Press.

Grafman, J. (1999). Experimental assessment of adult frontal lobe function. In B.L. Miller (Ed.), *The human frontal lobes: Functions and disorders. The science and practice of neuropsychology series* (pp. 321-344). New York: Guilford Press.

Graham, J.E., Rockwood, K., Beattie, B.L., Eastwood, R., Gauthier, S., Tuokko, H., and McDowell, I. (1997). Prevalence and severity of cognitive impairment with and without dementia in an elderly population. *Lancet, 349*(9068), 1793-1976.

Green, L., Fry, A.F., and Myerson, J. (1994). Discounting of delayed rewards: A life-span comparison. *Psychological Science, 5*, 33-36.

Greenfield, P.M., Davis, H.M., Suzuki, L.K., and Boutakidis, I. (2002). Understanding intercultural relations on multiethnic high school sports teams. In M. Gatz, M. Messner, and S.J. Ball-Rokeach (Eds.), *Paradoxes of youth and sport.* Albany: State University of New York Press.

Greenhouse, A.H. (1994). Falls among the elderly. In M.L. Albert and J.E. Knoefel (Eds.), *Clinical neurology of aging* (2nd ed., pp. 611-626). Oxford, England: Oxford University Press.

Greeno, C.G., and Wing, R.R. (1994). Stress-induced eating. *Psychological Bulletin, 115*, 444-464.

Greenough, W.T., McDonald, J.W., Parnisari, R.M., and Camel, J.E. (1986). Environmental conditions modulate dengeration and new dendrite growth in cerebellum of senescent rats. *Brain Research, 380*, 136-143.

Greenough, W.T., West, R.W., and DeVoogd, T.J. (1978). Sub-synaptic plate performations: Changes with age and experience in the rat. *Science, 202*, 1096-1098.

Greenwald, A.G., and Banaji, M. (1995). Implicit social cognition: Attitudes, self-esteem, and stereotypes. *Psychological Review, 102*, 4-27.

Greenwald, A.G., McGhee, D.E., and Schwartz, J.L.K. (1998). Measuring individual differences in implicit cognition: The implicit association test. *Journal of Personality and Social Psychology, 74*, 1464-1480.

Greve, W., and Wentura, D. (2003). Immunizing the self: Self-concept stabilization through reality-adaptive self-definitions. *Personality and Social Psychology Bulletin, 29*, 39-50.

Gross, J., Carstensen, L.L., Pasupathi, M., Tsai, J., Götestam Skorpen, C., and Hsu, A. (1997). Emotion and aging: Experience, expression and control. *Psychology and Aging, 12*, 590-599.

Gross, J.J., and Levenson, R.W. (1997). Emotional suppression: Physiology, self-report, and expressive behavior. *Journal of Abnormal Psychology, 64*, 970-986.

Gurland, B.J., Wilder, D.E., Lantigua, R., Stern, Y., Chen, J., Killeffer, E.H.P., and Mayeux, R. (1999). Rates of dementia in three ethnoracial groups. *International Journal of Geriatric Psychiatry, 14*, 481-493.

Gutchess, A.H., Welsh, R.C., Hedden, T., Bangert, A., Minear, M., Liu, L.L., and Park, D.C. (2005). Aging and the neural correlates of successful picture encoding: Frontal activations compensate for decreased medial temporal activity. *Journal of Cognitive Neuroscience, 17*, 84-96.

Hall, W., Room, R., and Bondy, S. (1999). Comparing the health and psychological risks of alcohol, cannabis, nicotine and opiate use. In H. Kalant, W. Corrigall, W. Hall, and R. Smart (Eds.), *The health effects of cannabis* (pp. 475-506). Toronto: Centre for Addiction and Mental Health.

Hammond, K.R., Hamm, R.M., Grassia, J., and Pearson, T. (1987). Direct comparison of the efficacy of intuitive and analytical cognition in expert judgment. *IEEE Transactions on Systems, Man, and Cybernetics, 17*, 753-770.

Hartel, C.R., and Buckner, R.L. (2006). Utility of brain imaging methods in research on aging. In National Research Council, *When I'm 64* (pp. 240-246). Committee on Aging Frontiers in Social Psychology, Personality, and Adult Developmental Psychology. L.L. Carstensen and C.R. Hartel (Eds.). Division of Behavioral and Social Sciences and Education. Washington, DC: The National Academies Press.

Harwood, J., Giles, H., and Ryan, E.B. (1995). Aging, communication, and intergroup theory: Social identity and intergenerational communication. In J.F. Nussbaum and J. Coupland (Eds.), *Handbook of communication and aging research* (pp. 133-159). Mahwah, NJ: Lawrence Erlbaum.

Hawkley, L.C., and Cacioppo, J.T. (2003). Loneliness and pathways to disease. *Brain, Behavior, and Immunity, 17*(Supplement 1), S98-S105.

Heatherton, T.F., and Baumeister, R.F. (1996). Self-regulation failure: Past, present, future. *Psychological Inquiry, 7*, 90-98.

Heatherton, T.F., and Nichols, P.A. (1994). Personal accounts of successful versus failed attempts at life change. *Personality and Social Psychology Bulletin, 20*, 664-675.

Heckhausen, J., Dixon, R.A., and Baltes, P.B. (1989). Gains and losses in development throughout adulthood as perceived by different adult age groups. *Developmental Psychology, 25*, 109-121.

Heiman, N., Stallings, M.C., Hofer, S.M., and Hewitt, J.K. (2003). Investigating age differences in the genetic and environmental structure of the tridimensional personality questionnaire in later adulthood. *Behavior Genetics, 33*, 171-180.

Helmer, C., Damon, D., Letenneur, L., Fabrigoule, C., Barberger-Gateu, P., Lafont, S., Fuhrer, R., Antonucci, T., Commenges, D., Orgogozo, J.M., and Dartigues, J.F. (1999). Marital status and risk of Alzheimer's disease: A French population-based cohort study. *Neurol ogy, 53*, 1953-1958.

Hemingway, H., and Marmot, M. (1999). Psychosocial factors in the etiology and prognosis of coronary heart disease: Systematic review of prospective cohort studies. *British Medical Journal, 318*, 1460-1467.

Hess, T.M. (1994). Social cognition in adulthood: Aging-related changes in knowledge and processing mechanisms. *Developmental Review, 14*, 373-412.

Hess, T.M., Auman, C., Colcombe, S., and Rahhal, T.A. (2003). The impact of stereotype threat on age differences in memory performance. *Journals of Gerontology Series B: Psychological Sciences and Social Sciences, 58B*(1), P3-P11.

Hess, T.M., Waters, S.J., and Bolstad, C.A (2000). Motivational and cognitive influences on affective priming in adulthood. *Journals of Gerontology Series B: Psychological Sciences and Social Sciences, 55B*(4), P193-P204.

Hibbard, J.H., Peters, E., Slovic, P., Finucane, M.L., and Tusler, M. (2001). Making health care quality reports easier to use. *Joint Commission Journal on Quality Improvement, 11*, 591-604.

Hooker, K., and McAdams, D.P. (2003). Personality reconsidered: A new agenda for aging research. *Journal of Gerontology: Psychological Sciences, 58B*, P296-P304.

Hull, J.G., and Young, R.D. (1983). Self-consciousness, self-esteem, and success-failure as determinants of alcohol consumption in male social drinkers. *Journal of Personality and Social Psychology, 44*, 1097-1109.

Hultsch, D.F., Hertzog, C., Small, B.J., and Dixon, R.A. (1999). Use it or lose it: Engaged lifestyle as a buffer of cognitive decline in aging? *Psychology and Aging, 14*, 245-263.

Hummert, M.L. (1990). Multiple stereotypes of elderly and young adults: A comparison of structure and evaluations. *Psychology and Aging, 5*, 82-193.

Hummert, M.L. (1999). A social cognitive perspective on age stereotypes. In T.M. Hess and F. Blanchard-Fields (Eds.), *Social cognition and aging* (pp. 175-196). San Diego: Academic Press.

Hummert, M.L., Garstka, T.A., O'Brien, L.T., Greenwald, A.G., and Mellott, D.S. (2002). Using the implicit association test to measure age differences in implicit social cognitions. *Psychology and Aging, 17*(3), 482-495.

Hummert, M.L., Garstka, T.A., and Shaner, J.L. (1997). Stereotyping of older adults: The role of target facial cues and perceiver characteristics. *Psychology and Aging, 12*, 107-114.

Hummert, M.L., Garstka, T.A., Shaner, J.L., and Strahm, S. (1994). Stereotypes of the elderly held by young, middle-aged, and elderly adults. *Journal of Gerontology: Psychological Sciences, 49B*(5), P240-P249.

Idler, E., Leventhal, H., McLaughlin, J., and Leventhal, E. (2004). In sickness but not in health: Self-ratings, identity, and mortality. *Journal of Health and Social Behavior, 45*(3), 336-356.

International Longevity Center. (2003). *Unjust desserts: Financial realities of older women.* New York: Author.

Isaacowitz, D.M., Charles, S., and Carstensen, L.L. (2000). Emotion and cognition. In G. Craik and T. Salthouse (Eds.), *Handbook of aging and cognition* (2nd ed., pp. 593-631). Mahwah, NJ: Lawrence Erlbaum.

Jackson, J.M., Keiper, S., Brown, K.T., Brown, T.N., and Manuel, W.J. (2002). Athletic identity, racial attitudes, and aggression in first year black and white intercollegiate athletes. In M. Gatz, M. Messner, and S.J. Ball-Rokeach (Eds.), *Paradoxes of youth and sport*. Albany: State University of New York Press.

Jackson, J.S. (1996). *New directions: African Americans in the 21st century.* Washington, DC: National Policy Association.

Jackson, J.S., Antonucci, T.C., and Gibson, R.C. (1990). Cultural, racial, and ethnic minority influences on aging. In J.E. Birren and K.W. Schaie (Eds.), *Handbook of the psychology of aging* (3rd ed., pp. 103-123). San Diego: Academic Press.

Kahana, B., and Kahana, E. (1975). The relationship of impulse control to cognition and adjustment among institutionalized aged women. *Journal of Gerontology, 30*, 679-687.

Kahn, R.L., and Antonucci, T.C. (1980). Convoys over the life course: Attachment, roles and social support. In P.B. Baltes and O. Brim (Eds.), *Life-span development and behavior* (vol. 3, pp. 253-286). New York: Academic Press.

Kahneman, D. (1994). New challenges to the rationality assumption. *Journal of Institutional and Theoretical Economics, 150*, 18-36.

Kahneman, D. (2003). A perspective on judgment and choice: Mapping bounded rationality. *American Psychologist, 58*, 697-720.

Kassel, J.D., Stroud, L.R., and Paronis, C.A. (2003). Smoking, stress, and negative affect: Correlation, causation, and context across stages of smoking. *Psychological Bulletin, 129*, 270-304.

Kawakami, K., Dovidio, J.F., and Dijksterhuis, A. (2003). Effect of social category priming on personal attitudes. *Psychological Science, 14*, 315-319.

Kelly, R.B., Zyzanski, S.J., and Alemagno, S.A. (1991). Prediction of motivation and behavior change following health promotion: Role of health beliefs, social support, and self-efficacy. *Social Science and Medicine, 32*, 311-320.

Kemper, S. (1994). "Elderspeak:" Speech accommodations to older adults. *Aging and Cognition, 1*, 17-28.

Kemper, S., Vandeputte, D., Rice, K., Cheung, H., and Gubarchuk, J. (1995). Spontaneous adoption of elderspeak during referential communication tasks. *Journal of Language and Social Psychology, 14*, 40-59.

Kempermann, G., Kuhn, H.G., and Gage, F.H. (1997). Experience-induced neurogenesis in the senescent dentate gyrus. *Journal of Neuroscience, 18*, 3206-3212.

Kempermann, G., Kuhn, H.G., and Gage, F.H. (1998). More hippocampal neurons in adult mice living in an enriched environment. *Nature, 386*, 493-495.

Kensinger, E.A., Brierley, B., Medford, N., Growdon, J.H., and Corkin, S. (2002). Effects of normal aging and Alzheimer's disease on emotional memory. *Emotion, 2*, 118-134.

Kerns, J.G., Cohen, J.D., MacDonald, A.W., Cho, R.Y., Stenger, V.A, and Carter, C.S. (2004). Anterior cingulate conflict monitoring and adjustments in control. *Science, 303*, 1023-1026.

Kite, M.E., and Wagner, L.S. (2002). Attitudes toward older adults. In T.D. Nelson (Ed.), *Ageism: Stereotyping and prejudice against older persons* (pp. 129-161). Cambridge, MA: MIT Press.

Klingemann, H.K. (1991). The motivation for change from problem alcohol and heroin use. *British Journal of Addiction, 86*, 727-744.

Knight, R.G., Gatz, M., Heller, K., and Bengtson, V.L. (2000). Age and emotional response to the Northridge earthquake: A longitudinal analysis. *Psychology and Aging, 15*(4), 627-634.

Krosnick, J.A., and Alwin, D.F. (1989). Aging and susceptibility to attitude change. *Journal of Personality and Social Psychology, 57*(3), 416-425.

Krosnick, J.A., Holbrook, A.L., and Visser, P.S. (2006). Optimizing brief assessments in research on the psychology of aging: A pragmatic approach to self-report measurement. In National Research Council, *When I'm 64* (pp. 231-239). Committee on Aging Frontiers in Social Psychology, Personality, and Adult Developmental Psychology. L.L. Carstensen and C.R. Hartel (Eds.). Division of Behavioral and Social Sciences and Education. Washington, DC: The National Academies Press.

Kwong, S.S.T., and Heller, R. (2005). Measuring ageism in children. In E. Palmore, L. Branch, and D. Harris (Eds.), *The concise encyclopedia of ageism*. Binghamton, NY: Haworth Press.

Labouvie-Vief, G., Diehl, M., Tarnowski, A., and Shen, J. (2000). Age differences in adult personality: Findings from the United States and China. *Journals of Gerontology Series B: Psychological Sciences and Social Sciences, 55B*(1), P4-P17.

Labouvie-Vief, G., Hakim-Larson, J., DeVoe, M., and Schoeberlein, S. (1989). Emotions and self-regulation: A life span view. *Human Development, 32*, 279-299.

Lachman, M.E., and Weaver, S.L. (1998a). Sociodemographic variations in the sense of control by domain: Findings from the MacArthur studies of midlife. *Psychology and Aging, 13*(4), 553-562.

Lachman, M.E., and Weaver, S.L. (1998b). The sense of control as a moderator of social class differences in health and well-being. *Journal of Personality and Social Psychology, 74*(3), 763-773.

Lachman, M.E., Weaver, S.L., Bandura, M., Elliot, E., and Lewkowicz, C. (1992). Improving memory and control beliefs through cognitive restructuring and self-generated strategies. *Journal of Gerontology: Psychological Sciences, 47*(5), P293-P299.

Laibson, D., Repetto, A., and Tobacman, J. (1998). Self-control and saving for retirement. *Brookings Papers on Economic Activity, 1*, 91-172.

Lang, F.R. (2000). Endings and continuity of social relationships: Maximizing intrinsic benefits within personal networks when feeling near to death. *Journal of Social and Personal Relationships, 17*(2), 155-182.

Lang, F.R., and Carstensen, L.L. (1994). Close emotional relationships in late life: How personality and social context do (and do not) make a difference. *Psychology and Aging,* 9, 315-324.

Lang, F.R., and Carstensen, L.L. (2002). Time counts: Future time perspective, goals, and social relationships. *Psychology and Aging, 17*(1), 125-139.

Lansford, J.E., Sherman, A.M., and Antonucci, T.C. (1998). Satisfaction with social networks: An examination of socioemotional selectivity theory across cohorts. *Psychology and Aging, 13*(4), 544-552.

Larrick, R.P., and Boles, T.L. (1995). Avoiding regret in decisions with feedback: A negotiation example. *Organizational Behavior and Human Decision Processes, 63*, 87-97.

Lawton, M.P. (2000). Quality of life, depression, and end-of-life attitudes and behaviors. In G.M. Williamson, D.R. Shaffer, and P.A. Parmalee (Eds.), *Physical illness and depression in older adults: A handbook of theory, research, and practice* (pp. 147-171). Dordrecht, Netherlands: Kluwer Academic.

Lawton, M.P., Kleban, M.H., and Dean, J. (1993). Affect and age: Cross-sectional comparisons of structure and prevalence. *Psychology and Aging, 8*, 165-175.

Lawton, M.P., Kleban, M.H., Rajagopal, D., and Dean, J. (1992). Dimensions of affective experience in three age groups. *Psychology and Aging, 7*, 171-184.

Lazarus, R.S. (1991). Psychological stress in the workplace. *Journal of Social Behavior and Personality, 6*(7), 1-13.

Lerner, J.S., and Keltner, D. (2001). Fear, anger, and risk. *Journal of Personality and Social Psychology, 81*, 146-159.

Leventhal, H., Leventhal, E.A., and Contrada, R.J. (1998). Self-regulation, health, and behavior: A perceptual-cognitive approach. *Psychology and Health, 13*(4), 717-733.

Levy, B.R. (1996). Improving memory in old age through implicit self-stereotyping. *Journal of Personality and Social Psychology, 71*, 1092-1107.

Levy, B.R. (2003). Mind matters: Cognitive and physical effects of aging self-stereotypes. *Journal of Gerontology: Psychological Sciences, 58B*, P203-P211.

Levy, B.R., and Banaji, M.R. (2002). Implicit ageism. In T.D. Nelson (Ed.), *Ageism: Stereotyping and prejudice against older persons* (pp. 49-75). Cambridge, MA: MIT Press.

Levy, B.R., Slade, M.D., Kunkel, S.R., and Kasl, S.V. (2002). Longevity increased by positive self-perceptions of aging. *Journal of Personality and Social Psychology, 83*, 261-270.

Liberman, N., Sagristano, M., and Trope, Y. (2002). The effect of temporal distance on level of mental construal. *Journal of Experimental Social Psychology, 38*, 523-534.

Lichtenstein, P., Gatz, M., and Berg, S. (1998). A twin study of mortality after spousal bereavement. *Psychological Medicine, 28*, 635-643.

Lind, K.D. (2004). *Medicare drug discount card program: How much does card choice affect price paid?* (Pub ID# 2004-16.) Washington, DC: AARP Public Policy Institute. Available: http://assets.aarp.org/rgcenter/post-import/2004_16_discount.pdf (accessed December 2005).

Lineweaver, T.T., and Hertzog, C. (1998). Adults' efficacy and control beliefs regarding memory and aging: Separating general from personal beliefs. *Aging, Neuropsychology, and Cognition, 5*(4), 264-296.

Litt, M.D., Cooney, N.L., Kadden, R.M., and Gaupp, L. (1990). Reactivity to alcohol cues and induced moods in alcoholics. *Addictive Behaviors, 15*, 137-146.

Liu, L.L., and Park, D.C. (2003). Technology and the promise of independent living for older adults: A cognitive perspective. In W. Schaie and N. Charness (Eds.), *Impact of technology on successful aging* (pp. 262-289). New York: Springer.

Liu, L.L., and Park, D.C. (2004). Aging and medical adherence: The use of automatic processes to achieve effortful things. *Psychology and Aging, 19*(2), 318-325.

Llovera, I., Ward, M.F., Ryan, J.G., Lesser, M., Sama, A.E., Crough, D., Mansfield, M., and Lesser, L.I. (1999). Why don't emergency department patients have advance directives? *Academic Emergency Medicine, 6*, 1054-1060.

Löckenhoff, C.E., and Carstensen, L.L. (2004). Socioemotional selectivity theory, aging, and health: The increasingly delicate balance between regulating emotions and making tough choices. *Journal of Personality, 72*, 1395-1424.

Loewenstein, G. (1996). Out of control: Visceral influences on behavior. *Organizational Behavior and Human Decision Processes, 65*(3), 272-292.

Loewenstein, G., and Frederick, S. (1997). Predicting reactions to environmental change. In M.H. Bazerman, D.M. Messick, A.E. Tenbrusel, and K.A. Wade-Benzoni (Eds.), *Environment, ethics, and behavior* (pp. 52-72). San Francisco: New Lexington Press.

Loewenstein, G., and Schkade, D. (1999). Wouldn't it be nice?: Predicting future feelings. In D. Kahneman, E. Diener, and N. Schwartz (Eds.), *Well-being: The foundations of hedonic psychology* (pp. 85-105). New York: Russell Sage Foundation.

Loewenstein, G.F., Weber, E.U., Hsee, C.K., and Welch, N. (2001). Risk as feelings. *Psychological Bulletin, 127*(2), 267-286.

Logan, J.M., Sanders, A.L., Snyder, A.Z., Morris, J.C., and Buckner, R.L. (2002). Underrecruitment and non-selective recruitment: Dissociable neural mechanisms associated with aging. *Neuron, 33*, 827-840.

Loges, W.E., and Jung, J.-Y. (2001). Exploring the digital divide. *Communication Research, 28*, 536-562.

Loomes, G., and Sugden, R. (1982). Regret theory: An alternative theory of rational choice under uncertainty. *Economic Journal, 92*, 805-824.

Loomes, G., and Sugden, R. (1986). Disappointment and dynamic consistency in choice under uncertainty. *Review of Economic Studies, 53*, 271-282.

Lucas, R.E., Clark, A.E., Georgellis, Y., and Diener, E. (2003). Re-examining adaptation and the setpoint model of happiness: Reactions to changes in marital status. *Journal of Personality and Social Psychology, 84*, 527-539.

Madeau, A., and McArdle, J.J. (Eds.). (in press). *Contemporary advances in psychometrics.* Mahwah, NJ: Lawrence Erlbaum.

Major, B., Cozzarelli, C., Sciacchitano, A.M., Cooper, M.L., Testa, M., and Mueller, P.M. (1990). Perceived social support, self-efficacy, and adjustment to abortion. *Journal of Personality and Social Psychology, 59*, 452-463.

Manly, J.J., Jacobs, D.M., Touradji, P., Small, S.A., and Stern, Y. (2002). Reading level attenuates differences in neuropsychological test performance between African American and white elders. *Journal of the International Neuropsychological Society, 8*(3), 341-348.

Markon, J. (2001). Elderly judges handle 20 percent of U.S. caseload. *Wall Street Journal,* October 8.

Markus, H.R., and Kitayama, S. (1991). Culture and the self: Implications for cognition, emotion, and motivation. *Psychological Review, 98*(2), 224-253.

Marlatt, G.A. (1985). Relapse prevention: Theoretical rationale and overview of the model. In G.A. Marlatt and J.R. Gordon (Eds.), *Relapse prevention* (pp. 3-70). New York: Guilford Press.

Martin, M., and Park, D.C. (2003). The Martin and Park Environmental Demands (MPED) questionnaire: Psychometric properties of a brief instrument to measure self-reported environmental demands. *Aging, Clinical and Experimental Research, 15*(1), 77-82.

Mather, M. (2006). A review of decision-making processes: Weighing the risks and benefits of aging. In National Research Council, *When I'm 64* (pp. 145-173). Committee on Aging Frontiers in Social Psychology, Personality, and Adult Developmental Psychology. L.L. Carstensen and C.R. Hartel (Eds.). Division of Behavioral and Social Sciences and Education. Washington, DC: The National Academies Press.

Mather, M., Canli, T., English, T., Whitfield, S., Wais, P., Ochsner, K., Gabrieli, J.D., and Carstensen, L.L. (2004). Amygdala responses to emotionally valenced stimuli in older and younger adults. *Psychological Science, 15*(4), 259-263.

Mather, M., and Carstensen, L.L. (2003). Aging and attentional biases for emotional faces. *Psychological Science, 14*(5), 409-415.

Mather, M., and Johnson, M.K. (2003). Affective review and schema reliance in memory in older and younger adults. *American Journal of Psychology, 116*, 169-189.

McClure, S.M., Laibson, D.I., Loewenstein, G., and Cohen, J.D. (2004). Separate neural systems value immediate and delayed monetary rewards. *Science, 306*, 503-507.

McConatha, J.T., Leone, F.M., and Armstrong, J.M. (1997). Emotional control in adulthood. *Psychological Reports, 80*(2), 499-507.

McConnell, A.R., and Leibold, J.M. (2001). Relations among the Implicit Association Test, discriminatory behavior, and explicit measures of racial attitudes. *Journal of Experimental Social Psychology, 37*, 435-442.

McCrae, R.R., and Costa, P.T. (1994). The stability of personality: Observation and evaluations. *Current Directions in Psychological Science, 3*(6), 173-175.

McCrae, R.R., Costa, P.T., Jr., Ostendorf, F., Angleitner, A., Hrebícková, M., Avia, M.D., Sanz, J., Sánchez-Bernardos, M.L., Kusdil, M.E., Woodfield, R., Saunders, P.R., and Smith, P.B. (2000). Nature over nurture: Temperament, personality, and life span development. *Journal of Personality and Social Psychology, 78*, 173-186.

McCrae, R.R., Costa, P.T., Pedroso de Lima, M., Simoes, A., Ostendorf, F., Angleitner, A., Marusic, I., Bratko, D., Caprara, G.V., Barbaranelli, C., Chae, J.H., and Piedmont, R.L. (1999). Age differences in personality across the adult life span: Parallels in five cultures. *Developmental Psychology, 35*(2), 466-477.

McFarland, C., Ross, M., and Giltrow, M. (1992). Biased recollections in older adults: The role of implicit theories of aging. *Journal of Personality and Social Psychology, 62*, 837-850.

McMullin, J.A., and Marshall, V.W. (2001). Ageism, age relations, and garment industry work in Montreal. *Gerontologist, 41*(1), 111-122.

Mellers, B.A., and McGraw, A.P. (2001). Anticipated emotions as guides to choice. *Currrent Directions in Psychological Science, 10*, 210-214.

Mellers, B.A., Schwartz, A., Ho, K., and Ritov, I. (1997). Decision affect theory: Emotional reactions to the outcomes of risky options. *Psychological Science, 8*, 423-429.

Mellers, B.A., Schwartz, A., and Ritov, I. (1999). Emotion-based choice. *Journal of Experimental Psychology, 128*, 332-345.

Metcalfe, J., and Mischel, W. (1999). A hot/cool-system analysis of delay of gratification: Dynamics of willpower. *Psychological Review, 106*(1), 3-19.

Merton, R.K. (1968). The Matthew effect in science. *Science, 15*(3810), 56-63.

Miller, C.T., and Major, B. (2000). Coping with stigma and prejudice. In T. Heatherton, R. Kleck, M. Hebl, and J. Hull (Eds.), *The social psychology of stigma* (pp. 243-272). New York: Guilford Press.

Miller, L.M.S., and Lachman, M.E. (1999). The sense of control and cognitive aging: Toward a model of mediational processes. In T.M. Hess and F. Blanchard-Fields (Eds.), *Social cognition and aging* (pp. 17-41). New York: Academic Press.

Miller, P.M., Hersen, M., Eisler, R.M., and Hilsman, G. (1974). Effects of social stress on operant drinking of alcoholics and social drinkers. *Behavioral Research Therapy, 12,* 67-72.

Miner, S. (1995). Racial differences in family support and formal service utilization among older persons: A nonrecursive model. *Journals of Gerontology Series B: Psychological Sciences and Social Sciences, 50B,* S143-S153.

Mischel, W. (1996). From good intentions to willpower. In P. Gollwitzer and J.A. Bargh (Eds.), *The psychology of action: Linking cognition and motivation to behavior* (pp. 197-218). New York: Guilford Press.

Mischel, W., Cantor, N., and Feldman, S. (1996). Principles of self-regulation: The nature of willpower and self-control. In E.T. Higgins and A.W. Kruglanski (Eds.), *Social psychology: Handbook of basic principles* (pp. 329–360). New York: Guilford Press.

Mischel, W., Shoda, Y., and Rodriguez, M.L. (1989). Delay of gratification in children. *Science, 244,* 933-938.

Montepare, J.M., and Zebrowitz, L.A. (2002). A social-developmental view of ageism. In T.D. Nelson (Ed.), *Ageism: Stereotyping and prejudice against older persons* (pp. 77-125). Cambridge, MA: MIT Press.

Moss, E., and Raz, A. (2001). The ones left behind: A siblings' bereavement group. *Group Analysis, 34,* 395-407.

Mossey, J.M., and Shapiro, E. (1982). Self-rated health: A predictor of mortality among the elderly. *American Journal of Public Health,* 72, 800-808.

Mroczek, D.K. (2001). Age and emotion in adulthood. *Current Directions in Psychological Science, 10,* 87-90.

Mroczek, D.K., and Kolarz, C.M. (1998). The effect of age on positive and negative affect: A developmental perspective on happiness. *Journal of Personality and Social Psychology, 75,* 1333-1349.

Muraven, M., and Baumeister, R.F. (2000). Self-regulation and depletion of limited resources: Does self-control resemble a muscle? *Psychological Bulletin, 126,* 247-259.

National Center for Health Statistics. (2005). *Health, United States, 2005. With chartbook on trends in the health of Americans.* (Table 61.) Hyattsville, MD. Available: http://www.cdc.gov/nchs/data/hus/hus05.pdf (accessed December 2005).

National Research Council. (2000). *The aging mind: Opportunities in cognitive research.* Committee on Future Directions for Cognitive Research on Aging. P.C. Stern and L.L. Carstensen (Eds.), Board on Behavioral, Cognitive, and Sensory Sciences, Commission on Behavioral and Social Sciences and Education. Washington, DC: National Academy Press.

National Research Council. (2003). *Technology for adaptive aging.* Steering Committee for the Workshop on Technology for Adaptive Aging. R.C. Pew and S.B. Van Hemel (Eds.), Board on Behavioral, Cognitive, and Sensory Sciences, Division of Behavioral and Social Sciences and Education. Washington, DC: The National Academies Press.

National Research Council. (2004). *Critical perspectives on racial and ethnic differences in health in late life.* Panel on Race, Ethnicity, and Health in Later Life. N.B. Anderson, R.A. Bulatao, and B. Cohen (Eds.), Committee on Population, Division of Behavioral and Social Sciences and Education. Washington, DC: The National Academies Press.

Newman, S., Karip, E., and Faux, R.B. (1995). Everyday memory function of older adults: The impact of intergenerational school volunteer programs. *Educational Gerontology, 21,* 569-580.

Newsom, J.T., Nishishiba, M., Morgan, D.L., and Rook, K.S. (2003). The relative importance of three domains of positive and negative social exchanges: A longitudinal model with comparable measures. *Psychology and Aging, 18*(4), 746-754.

Nguyen, H.T., Kitner-Triolo, M., Evans, M.K., and Zonderman, A.B. (2004). Factorial invariance of the CES-D in low socioeconomic status African Americans compared with a nationally representative sample. *Psychiatry Research, 126*, 177-187.

Nosek, B.A., Banaji, M.R., and Greenwald, A.G. (2002). Harvesting implicit group attitudes and beliefs from a demonstration website. *Group Dynamics: Theory, Research, and Practice, 6*(1), 101-115.

Nunez, N., McCoy, M.L., Clark, H.L., and Shaw, L.A. (1999). The testimony of elderly victim/witnesses and their impact on juror decisions: The importance of examining multiple stereotypes. *Law and Human Behavior, 23*, 413-423.

Oberauer, K., and Kliegl, R. (2004). Simultaneous cognitive operations in working memory after dual-task practice. *Journal of Experimental Psychology: Human Perception and Performance, 30*(4), 689-706.

Oliver, R.L. (1993). Cognitive, affective and attribute bases of the satisfaction response. *Journal of Consumer Research, 30*, 418-430.

Orrel, M., and Sahakian, B. (1995). Education and dementia. *British Medical Journal, 310*, 951-952.

Ouellette, J.A., and Wood, W. (1998). Habit and intention in everyday life: The multiple processes by which past behavior predicts future behavior. *Psychological Bulletin, 124*, 54-74.

Page, R.M., and Cole, G.E. (1991). Demographic predictors of self-reported loneliness in adults. *Psychological Reports, 68*, 939-945.

Palmore, E.B. (1990). *Ageism: Negative and positive*. New York: Springer.

Parens, E. (2004). Genetic differences and human identities: Why talking about behavioral genetics is important and difficult. *Hastings Center Report, 341*, S1-S36.

Park, D.C. (1997). Psychological issues related to competence: Cognitive aging and instrumental activities of daily living. In W. Schaie and S. Willis (Eds.), *Social structures and aging* (pp. 66-82). Mahwah, NJ: Lawrence Erlbaum.

Park, D.C., and Gutchess, A. (2002). Aging, cognition, and culture: A neuroscientific perspective. *Neurosciences and Biobehavioral Reviews, 26*, 859-867.

Park, D.C., Hertzog, C., Leventhal, H., Morrell, R.W., Leventhal, E., Birchmore, D., Martin, M., and Bennett, J. (1999). Medication adherence in rheumatoid arthritis patients: Older is wiser. *Journal of the American Geriatrics Society, 47*(2), 172-183.

Park, D.C., Lautenschlager, G., Hedden, T., Davidson, N.S., Smith, A.D., and Smith, P. (2002). Models of visuospatial and verbal memory across the adult life span. *Psychology and Aging, 17*, 299-320.

Park, D.C., Nisbett, R., and Hedden, T. (1999). Aging, culture, and cognition. *Journals of Gerontology Series B: Psychological Sciences and Social Sciences, 54B*, P75-P84.

Park, D.C., Polk, T.A., Mikels, J.A., Taylor, S.F., and Marshuetz, C. (2001). Cerebral aging: Integration of brain and behavioral models of cognitive function. *Dialogues in Clinical Neuroscience: Cerebral Aging, 3*, 151-165.

Park, D.C., Welsh, R.C., Marshuetz, C., Gutchess, A.H., Mikels, J., Polk, T.A., Noll, D.C., and Taylor, S.F. (2003). Working memory for complex scenes: Age differences in frontal and hippocampal activations. *Journal of Cognitive Neuroscience, 15*(8), 1122-1134.

Parr, W.V., and Siegert, R. (1993). Adults' conceptions of everyday memory failures in others: Factors that mediate the effects of target age. *Psychology and Aging, 8*, 599-605.

Pasupathi, M. (1999). Age differences in response to conformity pressure for emotional and nonemotional material. *Psychology of Aging, 14*(1), 170-174.

Pasupathi, M., and Löckenhoff, C.E. (2002). Ageist behavior. In T.D. Nelson (Ed.), *Ageism: Stereotyping and prejudice against older persons* (pp. 201-246). Cambridge, MA: MIT Press.

Peele, S. (1989). *The diseasing of America: Addiction treatment out of control.* Lexington, MA: Lexington Books.

Perdue, C.W., and Gurtman, M.B. (1990). Evidence for the automaticity of ageism. *Journal of Experimental Social Psychology, 26*(3), 199-216.

Perri, M.G., McAllister, D.A., Gange, J.J., Jordan, R.C., McAdoo, W.G., and Nazu, A.M. (1988). Effects of four maintenance programs on the long-term management of obesity. *Journal of Consulting and Clinical Psychology, 56*, 529-534.

Pervin, L.A. (2003). *The science of personality.* New York: Oxford University Press.

Peters, E., Finucane, M., MacGregor, D., and Slovic, P. (2000). The bearable lightness of aging: Judgment and decision processes in older adults (pp. 144-165). In National Research Council, *The aging mind: Opportunities in cognitive research.* Committee on Future Directions for Cognitive Research on Aging. P.C. Stern and L.L. Carstensen (Eds.). Board on Behavioral, Cognitive, and Sensory Sciences, Commission on Behavioral and Social Sciences and Education. Washington, DC: National Academy Press.

Pettigrew, T.F. (1998). Intergroup contact theory. *Annual Review of Psychology, 49*, 63-85.

Petty, R.E., Baker, S., and Gleicher, F. (1991). Attitudes and drug abuse prevention: Implications of the elaboration likelihood model of persuasion. In L. Donohew, H.E. Sypher, and W.J. Bukoski (Eds.), *Persuasive communication and drug abuse prevention* (pp. 71-90). Mahwah, NJ: Lawrence Erlbaum.

Petty, R.E., and Cacioppo, J.T. (1986). The elaboration likelihood model of persuasion. In L. Berkowitz (Ed.), *Advances in experimental social psychology* (vol. 19, pp. 123-205). New York: Academic Press.

Petty, R.E., and Krosnick, J.A. (1995). *Attitude strength: Antecedents and consequences.* Mahwah, NJ: Lawrence Erlbaum.

Petty, R.E., and Wegener, D.T. (1998). Attitude change: Multiple roles for persuasion variables. In D. Gilbert, S. Fiske, and G. Lindzey (Eds.), *The handbook of social psychology* (4th ed., vol. 1, pp. 323-390). New York: McGraw-Hill.

Petty, R.E., and Wegener, D.T. (1999). The elaboration likelihood model: Current status and controversies. In S. Chaiken and Y. Trope (Eds.), *Dual process theories in social psychology* (pp. 41-72). New York: Guilford Press.

Pleis, J.R., and Coles, R. (2002). Summary health statistics for U.S. adults: National Health Interview Survey, 1998. *Vital Health Statistics, 10*(209).

Plomin, R., and McGuffin, P. (2003). Psychopathology in the postgenomic era. *Annual Review of Psychology, 54*, 205-228.

Polivy, J., and Herman, C.P. (2002). If at first you don't succeed: False hopes of self-change. *American Psychologist, 57*, 677-689.

Porter, J.R., and Washington, R.E. (1979). Black identity and self-esteem: A review of studies of black self-concept, 1968-1978. *Annual Review of Sociology, 5*, 53-74.

Posner, M.I., and Rothbart, M.K. (1998). Summary and commentary: Developing attentional skills. In J.E. Richards (Ed.), *Cognitive neuroscience of attention: A developmental perspective* (pp. 317-323). Mahwah, NJ: Lawrence Erlbaum.

Powers, C.B., Wisocki, P.A., and Whitbourne, S.K. (1992). Age differences and correlates of worrying in young and elderly adults. *Gerontologist, 32*(1), 82-88.

Prochaska, J.O., Velicer, W.F., Guadagnoli, E., Rossi, J.S., and DiClemente, C.C. (1991). Patterns of change: Dynamic typology applied to smoking cessation. *Multivariate Behavioral Research, 26*, 83-107.

Rahhal, T.A., Hasher, L., and Colcombe, S.J. (2001). Instructional manipulations and age differences in memory: Now you see them, now you don't. *Psychology and Aging, 16*(4), 697-706.

Rahhal, T.A., May, C.P., and Hasher, L. (2002). Truth and character: Sources that adults can remember. *Psychological Science. 13*, 101-105.

Raichle, M.E. (2000). Functional imaging in cognitive neuroscience. In M.J.F. Farah and E. Todd (Eds.), *Patient-based approaches to cognitive neuroscience: Issues in clinical and cognitive neuropsychology* (pp. 35-52). Cambridge, MA: MIT Press.

Rettinger, D.A., and Hastie, R. (2001). Content effects on decision making. *Organizational Behavior and Human Decision Processes, 85*(2), 336-359.

Reuter-Lorenz, P.A. (2002). New visions of the aging mind and brain. *Trends in Cognitive Sciences, 6*, 394-400.

Reynolds, C.F., III, Frank, E., Kupfer, D.J., Thase, M.E., Perel, J.M., Mazumdar, S., and Houck, P.R. (1996). Treatment outcome in recurrent major depression: A post hoc comparison of elderly ("young old") and midlife patients. *American Journal of Psychiatry, 153*(10), 1288-1292.

Richeson, J.A., Baird, A.A., Gordon, H.L., Heatherton, T.F., Wyland, C.L., Trawalter S., and Shelton, J.N. (2003). An fMRI investigation of the impact of interracial contact on executive function. *Nature Neuroscience, 6*, 1323-1328.

Richeson, J., and Shelton, N. (2006). A social psychological perspective on the stigmatization of older adults. In National Research Council, *When I'm 64* (pp. 174-208). Committee on Aging Frontiers in Social Psychology, Personality, and Adult Developmental Psychology. L.L. Carstensen and C.R. Hartel (Eds.). Division of Behavioral and Social Sciences and Education. Washington, DC: The National Academies Press.

Robins, J.M., Hernan, M.A., and Brumback, B. (2000). Marginal structural models and causal inference in epidemiology. *Epidemiology, 11*, 550-560.

Robins, L.N., and Regier, D.A. (1991). *Psychiatric disorders in America: The Epidemiologic Catchment Area Study*. New York: Free Press.

Robinson, M.D., and Clore, G.L. (2001). Simulation scenarios and emotional appraisal: Testing the convergence of real and imagined reactions to emotional stimuli. *Personality and Social Psychology Bulletin, 128*, 934-960.

Rogers, W.A., and Fisk, A.D. (2001). Understanding the role of attention in cognitive aging research. In J.E. Birren and K.W. Schaie (Eds.), *Handbook of the psychology of aging* (pp. 267-287). San Diego: Academic Press.

Rook, K.S. (1992). Detrimental aspects of social relationships: Taking stock of an emerging literature. In H.O.F. Veiel and U. Baumann (Eds.), *The meaning and measurement of social support* (pp. 157-169). New York: Hemisphere.

Rosenberg, M. (1965). *Society and the adolescent self-image*. Princeton, NJ: Princeton University Press.

Rossi, A., and Rossi, P. (1990). *Of human bonding: Parent child-relationships across the life course*. Hawthorne, NY: Aldine and Gruyter.

Rothman, A. (2006). Initiatives to motivate change: A review of theory and practice and their implications for older adults. In National Research Council, *When I'm 64* (pp. 121-144). Committee on Aging Frontiers in Social Psychology, Personality, and Adult Developmental Psychology. L.L. Carstensen and C.R. Hartel (Eds.). Division of Behavioral and Social Sciences and Education. Washington, DC: The National Academies Press.

Ryan, E.B. (1992). Beliefs about memory changes across the lifespan. *Journal of Gerontology: Psychological Sciences, 47*, P96-P101.

Ryan, E.B., Meredith, S.D., and Shantz, G.B. (1994). Evaluative perceptions of patronizing speech addressed to institutionalized elders in contrasting conversational contexts. *Canadian Journal on Aging, 13*(2), 236-248.

Ryan, E.B., and See, S.K. (1993). Age-based beliefs about memory changes for self and others across adulthood. *Journals of Gerontology Series B: Psychological Sciences and Social Sciences, 48B*(4), P199-P201.

Ryff, C.D. (1989). Happiness is everything, or is it? Explorations on the meaning of psychological well-being. *Journal of Personality and Social Psychology, 57*(6), 1069-1081.

Ryff, C.D. (1991). Possible selves in adulthood and old age: A tale of shifting horizons. *Psychology and Aging, 6*(2), 286-295.

Ryff, C.D. (1995). Psychological well-being in adult life. *Current Directions in Psychological Science, 4*, 99-104.

Ryff, C.D., Lee, Y.H., Essex, M.J., and Schmutte, P.S. (1994). My children and me: Midlife evaluations of grown children and of self. *Psychology and Aging, 9*(2), 195-205.

Salat, D.H., Buckner, R.L., Snyder, A.Z., Greve, D.N., Desikan, R.S, Busa, E., Morris, J.C., Dale, A.M., and Fischl, B. (2004). Thinning of the cerebral cortex in aging. *Cerebral Cortex, 14*, 721-730.

Salovey, P., Rothman, A.J., and Rodin, J. (1998). Health behavior. In D. Gilbert, S. Fiske, and G. Lindzey (Eds.), *Handbook of social psychology* (4th ed., vol. 2, pp. 633-683). New York: McGraw-Hill.

Salthouse, T.A. (1995). Refining the concept of psychological compensation. In R.A. Dixon and L. Bäckman (Eds.), *Compensating for psychological deficits and declines: Managing losses and promoting gains* (pp. 21-34). Mahwah, NJ: Lawrence Erlbaum.

Salthouse, T.A., Atkinson, T.M., and Berish, D.E. (2003). Executive functioning as a potential mediator of age-related cognitive decline in normal adults. *Journal of Experimental Psychology: General, 132*(4), 566-594.

Salthouse, T.A., and Maurer, T.J. (1996). Aging, job performance, and career development. In J.E. Birren and K.W. Schaie (Eds.), *Handbook of the psychology of aging* (4th ed., pp. 353-364). San Diego: Academic Press.

Salzman, C. (1995). Medication compliance in the elderly. *Journal of Clinical Psychiatry, 56*, 18-23.

Sanbonmatsu, D., and Fazio, R.H. (1990). The role of attitudes in memory based decision-making. *Journal of Personality and Social Psychology, 59*, 614-622.

Sapolsky, R.M., Krey, L.C., and McEwen, B.S. (1986). The neuroendocrinology of stress and aging: The glucocorticoid cascade hypothesis. *Endocrine Reviews, 7*, 284.

Scarmeas, N., Levy, G., Tang, M.-X., Manly, J., and Stern, Y. (2001). Influence of leisure activity on the incidence of Alzheimer's disease. *Neurology, 57*, 2236-2242.

Schachter, S. (1982). Recidivism and self-cure of smoking and obesity. *American Psychologist, 37*, 436-444.

Schkade, D., and Kahneman, D. (1998). Does living in California make people happy? A focusing illusion in judgments of life satisfaction. *Psychological Science, 9*, 340-346.

Schmitt, M.T., Branscombe, N.R., Kobrynowicz, D., and Owen, S. (2002). Perceiving discrimination against one's gender group has different implications for well-being in women and men. *Personality and Social Psychology Bulletin, 28*(2), 197-210.

Schneider, M.S., Friend, R., Whitaker, P., and Wadhwa, N. (1991). Fluid noncompliance and symptomatology in end-stage renal disease: Cognitive and emotional variables. *Health Psychology, 10*, 209-215.

Schooler, C., Mulatu, M.S., and Oates, G. (1999). The continuing effects of substantively complex work on the intellectual functioning of older workers. *Psychology and Aging, 14*, 483-506.

Schulz, R., and Beach, S. (1999). Caregiving as a risk factor for mortality. The caregiver health effects study. *Journal of the American Medical Association, 282*(23), 2215-2219.

Schwartz, B. (2004). *The paradox of choice: Why more is less.* New York: HarperCollins Publishers.

Schwarz, N. (2006). Aging and the psychology of self-report. In National Research Council, *When I'm 64* (pp. 219-230). Committee on Aging Frontiers in Social Psychology, Personality, and Adult Developmental Psychology. L.L. Carstensen and C.R. Hartel (Eds.). Division of Behavioral and Social Sciences and Education. Washington, DC: The National Academies Press.

Schwarz, N., and Clore, G. (1983). Mood, misattribution, and judgments of well-being: Informative and directive functions of affective states. *Journal of Personality and Social Psychology, 45*, 513-523.

Seeman, T., McAvay, G., Merrill, S., Albert, M., and Rodin, J. (1996). Self-efficacy beliefs and change in cognitive performance: MacArthur Studies of Successful Aging. *Psychology and Aging, 11*, 538-551.

Shiffman, S.M. (1982). Relapse following smoking cessation: A situational analysis. *Journal of Consulting and Clinical Psychology, 50*, 71-86.

Shiv, B., Loewenstein, G., Bechara, A., Damasio, H., and Damasio, A.R. (2005). Investment behavior and the dark side of emotion. *Psychological Science, 16*(6), 435-439.

Siegler, I.C., Dawson, D.V., and Welsh, K.A. (1994). Caregiver ratings of personality change in Alzheimer's disease patients: A replication. *Psychology and Aging, 9*, 464-466.

Silverstein, M., and Bengtson, V.L. (1991). Do close parent-child relations reduce the mortality risk of older parents? *Journal of Health and Social Behavior, 32*(4), 382-395.

Singer, B., and Ryff, C.D. (1999). Hierarchies of life histories and associated health risks. *Annals of the New York Academy of Sciences, 896*, 96-115.

Singer, T., Verhaeghen, P., Ghisletta, P., Lindenberger, U., and Baltes, P.B. (2003). The fate of cognition in very old age: Six-year longitudinal findings in the Berlin aging study (BASE). *Psychology and Aging, 18*(2), 318-331.

Slovic, P., Finucane, M., Peters, E., and MacGregor, D.(2002). The affect heuristic. In T. Gilovich, D. Griffin, and D. Kahneman (Eds.), *Heuristics and biases: The psychology of intuitive judgment* (pp. 397-420). New York: Cambridge University Press.

Smerglia, V., Deimling, G.T., and Schaefer, M.L. (2001). The impact of race on decision-making satisfaction and caregiver depression: A path analytic model. *Journal of Mental Health and Aging, 7*, 301-316.

Smith, A.D., Park, D.C., Earles, J.L.K., Shaw, R.J., and Whiting, W.L. (1998). Age differences in context integration in memory. *Psychology and Aging, 13*(1), 21-28.

Smith, E.E., and Jonides, J. (1999). Storage and executive processes in the frontal lobes. *Science, 283*, 1657-1661.

Smith, T.W., and Spiro, A. (2002). Personality, health and aging: Prolegomenon for the next generation. *Journal of Research in Personality, 36*, 363-394.

Snibbe, A.C., and Markus, H.R. (2005). You can't always get what you want: Educational attainment, agency, and choice. *Journal of Personality and Social Psychology, 88*(4), 703-720.

Snowdon, D.A., Greiner, L.H., and Markesbery, W.R. (2000). Linguistic ability in early life and the neuropathology of Alzheimer's disease and cerebrovascular disease: Findings from the nun study. *Annals of the New York Academy of Sciences, 903*, 34-38.

Snyder, M. (1992). Motivational foundations of behavioral confirmation. In M.P. Zanna (Ed.), *Advances in experimental social psychology* (vol. 25). San Diego: Academic Press.

Sobell, L.C. (1991). Natural recovery from alcohol problems. In N. Heather, W.R. Miller, and J. Greeley (Eds.), *Self-control and the addictive behaviors.* Sydney, Australia: Pergamon Press.

Spotts, H.E., and Schewe, C.D. (1994). Communicating with the elderly consumer: The growing health care challenge. In P.D. Cooper (Ed.), *Health care marketing: A foundation for managed quality* (3rd ed., pp. 242-255). Gaithersburg, MD: Aspen.

Staudinger, U.M. (1999). Social cognition and a psychological approach to the art of life. In T.M. Hess and F. Blanchard-Fields (Eds.), *Social cognition and aging* (pp. 343-375). New York: Academic Press.

Staudinger, U.M., Bluck, S., and Herzberg, P.Y. (2003). Looking back and looking ahead: Adult age differences in consistency of diachronous ratings of subjective well-being. *Psychology and Aging, 18*(1), 13-24.

Staudinger, U.M., Marsiske, M., and Baltes, P.B. (1995). Resilience and reserve capacity in later adulthood: Potentials and limits of development across the life span. In D. Cicchetti and D.J. Cohen (Eds.), *Developmental psychopathology: Risk, disorder, and adaptation* (vol. 2, pp. 801-847). Oxford, England: John Wiley and Sons.

Steele, C.M. (1997). A threat in the air: How stereotypes shape intellectual identity and performance. *American Psychologist, 52*(6), 613-629.

Steele, C.M., and Aronson, J. (1995). Stereotype threat and the intellectual test performance of African Americans. *Journal of Personality and Social Psychology, 69*, 797-811.

Steele, C.M., Spencer, S., and Aronson, J. (2002). Contending with group image: The psychology of stereotype and social identity threat. In M.P. Zanna (Ed.), *Advances in experimental social psychology* (vol. 34, pp. 379-440). San Diego: Academic Press.

Stern, Y., Alexander, G.E., Prohovnik, I., Stricks, L., Link, B., Lennon, M.C., and Mayeux, R. (1995). Relationship between lifetime occupation and parietal flow: Implications for a reserve against Alzheimer's disease pathology. *Neurology, 45*, 55-60.

Stout, J.C., Rodawalt, W.C., and Siemers, E.R. (2001). Risky decisionmaking in Huntington's disease. *Journal of the International Neuropsychological Society, 7*, 92-101.

Streufert, S., Pogash, R., Piasecki, M., and Post, G.M. (1990). Age and management team performance. *Psychology and Aging, 5*, 551-559.

Terracciano, A., Merritt, M.M., Zonderman, A.B., and Evans, M.K. (2003). Personality traits and sex differences in emotion recognition among African-Americans and Caucasians. *Annals of the New York Academy of Sciences, 1000*, 309-312.

Thaler, R.H., and Benartzi, S. (2004). Save more tomorrow: Using behavioral economics to increase employee savings. *Journal of Political Economy, 112*(1), Part 2, S164-S187.

Thaler, R.H., and Shefrin, H.M. (1981). An economic theory of self-control. *Journal of Political Economy, 89*(2), 392-406.

Thayer, J.F., Merritt, M.M., Sollers, J.J., III, et al. (2003). Effect of angiotensin-converting enzyme insertion/deletion polymorphism DD genotype on high-frequency heart rate variability in African Americans. *American Journal of Cardiology, 92*, 1487-1490.

Thayer, R.E., Newman, R., and McClain, T.M. (1994). Self-regulation of mood: Strategies for changing a bad mood, raising energy, and reducing tension. *Journal of Personality and Social Psychology, 67*, 910-925.

Tilling, K., Sterne, J.A., and Szklo, M. (2002). Estimating the effect of cardiovascular risk factors on all-cause mortality and incidence of coronary heart disease using G-estimation: The Atherosclerosis Risk in Communities Study. *American Journal of Epidemiology, 155*, 710-718.

Tisserand, D.J., and Jolles, J. (2003). On the involvement of prefrontal networks in cognitive aging. *Cortex, 39*, 1107-1128.

U.S. Census Bureau. (2004a). *U.S. interim projections by age, sex, race, and Hispanic origin.* Available: http://www.census.gov/ipc/www/usinterimproj/natprojtab01a.pdf (accessed December 2005).

U.S. Census Bureau. (2004b). *We the people: Aging in the United States.* Available: http://www.census.gov/prod/2004pubs/censr-19.pdf (accessed December 2005).

Vaillant, G.E., Meyer, S.E., Mukamal, K., and Soldz, S. (1998). Are social supports in late midlife a cause or a result of successful ageing? *Psychological Medicine, 28*, 1159-1168.

Vargas, P.T., von Hippel, W., and Petty, R.E. (2004). Using partially structured attitude measures to enhance the attitude-behavior relationship. *Personality and Social Psychology Bulletin, 30*, 197-211.

Verghese, J., Lipton, R.B., Katz, M.J., Hall, C.B., Derby, C.A., Kuslansky, G., Ambrose, A.F., Sliwinski, M., and Buschke, H. (2003). Leisure activities and the risk of dementia in the elderly. *New England Journal of Medicine, 348*, 2508-2516.

Victor, C., Scambler, S., Bond, J., and Bowling, A. (2000). Being alone in later life: Loneliness, social isolation and living alone. *Reviews in Clinical Gerontology 10*(4), 401-417.

Visser, P.S., and Krosnick, J.A. (1998). Development of attitude strength over the life cycle: Surge and decline. *Journal of Personality and Social Psychology, 75*(6), 1389-1410.

Volkow, N.D., Gur, R.C., Wang, G.J., Gowler, J.S., Moberg, P.J., Ding, Y.S., Hitzemann, R., Smith, G., and Logan, J. (1998). Association between decline in brain dopamine activity with age and cognitive and motor impairment in healthy individuals. *American Journal of Psychiatry, 155*, 344-349.

von Strauss, E., Viitanen, M., DeRonchi, D., Winblad, W., and Fratiglioni, L. (1999). Aging and the occurrence of dementia. *Archives of Neurology, 56*, 587-592.

Wang, H.-X., Karp, A., Winblad, B., and Fratiglioni, L. (2002). Late-life engagement in social and leisure activities is associated with a decreased risk of dementia: A longitudinal study from the Kungsholmen project. *American Journal of Epidemiology, 155*, 1081-1087.

Wegener, D.T., and Petty, R.E. (1994). Mood management across affective states: The hedonic contingency hypothesis. *Journal of Personality and Social Psychology, 66*, 1034-1048.

Wegener, D.T., Petty, R.E., and Smith, S. (1995). Positive mood can increase or decrease message scrutiny: The hedonic contingency view of mood and message processing. *Journal of Personality and Social Psychology, 69*, 5-15.

Weintraub, D., Raskin, A., Ruskin, P.E., Gruber-Baldini, A.L., Zimmerman, S.I., Hebel, J.R., German, P., and Magaziner, J. (2000). Racial differences in the prevalence of dementia among patients admitted to nursing homes. *Psychiatric Services, 51*, 1259-1264.

West, R.L., and Yassuda, M.S. (2004). Aging and memory control beliefs: Performance in relation to goal setting and memory self-evaluation. *Journal of Gerontology: Psychological Sciences, 59*, P56-P65.

Westbrook, R.A. (1987). Product/consumption-based affective responses and post-purchase processes. *Journal of Marketing Research, 24*, 258-270.

Whalley, L.J., Starr, J.M., Athawes, R., Hunter, D., Pattie, A., and Deary, I.J. (2000). Childhood mental ability and dementia. *Neurology, 55*, 1455-1459.

Wheeler, S.C., and Petty, R.E. (2001). The effects of stereotype activation on behavior: A review of possible mechanisms. *Psychological Bulletin, 127*, 797-826.

Whitbourne, S.K. (1987). Personality development in adulthood and old age: Relationships among identity style, health, and well-being. In K.W. Schaie (Ed.), *Annual review of gerontology and geriatrics* (vol. 7, pp. 189-216). New York: Springer.

Whitfield, K.E. (1996). Studying cognition in older African Americans: Some conceptual considerations. *Journal of Aging and Ethnicity, 1*(1), 35-45.

Whitfield, K.E., Fillenbaum, G., Pieper, C., Seeman, T.E., Albert, M.S., Berkman, L.F., Blazer, D.G., and Rowe, J.W. (2000). The effect of race and health related factors on naming and memory: The MacArthur Studies of Successful Aging. *Journal of Aging and Health, 12*(1), 69-89.

Whitfield, K.E., and Willis, S. (1998). Conceptual issues and analytic strategies for studying cognition in older African Americans. *African-American Research Perspectives, 4*(1), 115-125.

Wigboldus, D.H.J., Dijksterhuis, A., and Van Knippenberg, A. (2003). When stereotypes get in the way: Stereotypes obstruct stereotype-inconsistent trait inferences. *Journal of Personality and Social Psychology, 84*(3), 470-484.

Williams, A. (1996). Young people's evaluations of intergenerational versus peer underaccommodation: Sometimes older is better? *Journal of Language and Social Psychology, 15*, 291-311.

Williams, J.E., Paton, C.C., Siegler, I.C., Eigenbrodt, M., Nieto, J., and Tyroler, H.A. (2000). Anger proneness predicts CHD risk: A prospective analysis from the Atherosclerosis Risk in Communities Study. *Circulation, 101*, 2034-2039.

Williamson, G.M., Shaffer, D.R., and Schulz, R. (1998). Activity restriction and prior relationship history as contributors to mental health outcomes among middle-aged and older spousal caregivers. *Health Psychology, 17*(2), 152-162.

Wilson, R.S., and Bennett, D.A. (2003). Cognitive activity and risk of Alzheimer's disease. *Current Directions in Psychological Science, 12*, 87-91.

Wilson, R.S., Bennett, D.A., Gilley, D.W., Beckett, L.A., Barnes, L.L., and Evans, D.A. (2000). Premorbid reading activity and patterns of cognitive decline in Alzheimer disease. *Archives of Neurology, 57*, 1718-1723.

Wilson, T.D., and Gilbert, D.T. (2003). Affective forecasting. In M. Zanna (Ed.), *Advances in experimental social psychology*. New York: Elsevier.

Wilson, T.D., Lindsey, S., and Schooler, T.Y. (2002) A model of dual attitudes. *Psychological Review, 107*, 101-126.

Wingfield, A., and Kahana, M.J. (2002). The dynamics of memory retrieval in older adults. *Canadian Journal of Experimental Psychology, 5*, 197-199.

Yang, J., McCrae, R.R., and Costa, P.T., Jr. (1998). Adult age differences in personality traits in the United States and the People's Republic of China. *Journals of Gerontology Series B: Psychological Sciences and Social Sciences, 53B*(6), P375-P383.

Ybarra, O., and Park, D. (2002). Disconfirmation of person expectations by older and younger adults: Implications for social vigilance. *Journals of Gerontology Series B: Psychological Sciences and Social Sciences, 57*(5), P435-P443.

Yesavage, J. (1984). Relaxation and memory training in 39 elderly patients. *American Journal of Psychiatry, 141*, 778-781.

Yoon, C., Hasher, L., Feinberg, F., Rahhal, T.A., and Winocur, G. (2000). Cross-cultural differences in memory: The role of culture-based stereotypes about aging. *Psychology and Aging, 15*, 694-704.

Zacks, R.T., Hasher, L., and Li, K.Z.H. (2000). Human memory. In F.I.M. Craik and T.A. Salthouse (Eds.), *The handbook of aging and cognition* (2nd ed., pp. 293-357). Mahwah, NJ: Lawrence Erlbaum.

Zajonc, R.B. (1965). Social facilitation. *Science, 149*(3681), 269-274.

Zarit, S.H., Orr, N.K., and Zarit, J.M. (1985). *The hidden victims of Alzheimer's disease: Families under stress.* New York: New York University Press.

Zebrowitz, L.A. (2003). Aging stereotypes—Internalization or inoculation? A commentary. *Journals of Gerontology Series B: Psychological Sciences and Social Sciences, 58B*(4), P216.

Zebrowitz, L.A., and Montepare, J.M. (2000). Too young, too old: Stigmatizing adolescents and elders. In T.F. Heatherton, R.E. Kleck, M.R. Hebl, and J.G. Hull (Eds.), *The social psychology of stigma* (pp. 334-373). New York: Guilford Press.

Part Two

Background Papers

Initiatives to Motivate Change: A Review of Theory and Practice and Their Implications for Older Adults

Alexander J. Rothman
University of Minnesota

INTRODUCTION

Unhealthy behaviors and the disorders they cause pervade modern life. As even a cursory review of *Healthy People 2010* (U.S. Department of Health and Human Services, 2001) makes perfectly clear, significant improvements in physical and mental health critically depend on changes in human behavior. The reductions in disease morbidity and premature mortality that would come from increased rates of physical activity; improved compliance with medical recommendations; reduced rates of obesity; and reduced rates of utilization of tobacco, alcohol, and other controlled substances are tantalizing. Moreover, these changes would result in meaningful improvements in quality of life and also increase the potential for dramatic reductions in health care costs.

Yet even though the benefits of these behavioral changes are clear, eliciting consistent changes in people's behavior has proven to be a formidable problem (Baumeister, Heatherton, and Tice, 1994; Rothman, 2000). For example, even though people recognize the health costs posed by smoking, the impact of those costs on behavioral decision making has proven to be quite complex—people downplay the importance of health concerns (Gerrard, Gibbons, Benthin, and Hessling, 1996), underestimate their own personal risk (Weinstein, 1998), or believe their fate is sealed and that cessation will make little difference. Moreover, behavioral decisions unfold in environments that too often hinder people's ability or opportunity to act in a healthy manner.

Although across the life span there are significant shifts in the types of behavioral decisions that people must grapple with, there remains a consistent need for people to recognize and adopt healthy patterns of behavior (Leventhal, Rabin, Leventhal, and Burns, 2001). Given the difficulty people have initiating and maintaining changes in their behavior, there is continued demand for intervention strategies that effectively motivate healthy behavior. To date, efforts to specify and test these strategies have tended not to focus on the behavioral decisions facing older adults. In a similar manner, the theoretical models that have guided these intervention efforts do not address, directly or indirectly, whether the underlying processes generalize to older adults.

In order to stimulate both theoretical and practical initiatives directed at the behavioral practices of older adults, this paper provides an overview of current models of how people decide to initiate and maintain healthy patterns of behavior and the implications of these models for intervention design and implementation. The review is divided into four sections. First, I consider whether people are ready to make changes in their behavior. Second, I examine what can be done to motivate people to initiate changes in their behavior, with a particular focus on communication strategies that have been shown to be effective. Third, I consider whether the factors that guide efforts to initiate a new pattern of behavior are distinct from those that determine whether those actions are sustained over time. Finally, because the development of initiatives to promote healthy behavioral decisions depends on communication between investigators who are working to advance theory and those working to advance practice (Rothman, 2004), I consider what can be done to facilitate this type of collaborative activity. In each section, consideration is given to the implications of the current state of basic and applied science for motivating change in older adults.

IS EVERYONE READY TO CHANGE THEIR BEHAVIOR?

Modern society is replete with opportunities for people to make changes in their behavior. Yet the proportion of adults who act on these opportunities has been modest at best (e.g., Schmid, Jeffery, and Hellerstedt, 1989). In response to this observation, investigators have asserted that people differ in their readiness to change and that it is overly simplistic (and optimistic) to expect that most or all people are prepared to avail themselves of the opportunity to modify their behavior (Prochaska, DiClemente, and Norcross, 1992). Thus, initiatives that provide people with effective methods to modify their behavior must be complemented with initiatives that persuade people that it is both important and possible for them to change their behavior.

A rich array of factors has been invoked to explain why people differ in their readiness to make changes in their behavior (Salovey, Rothman, and

Rodin, 1998). In some cases, especially those involving new hazards, it may be that people are unaware of the dangers posed by their actions. Alternatively, people's understanding of the health problem may lead them to believe (inaccurately) that their current actions are appropriate (Leventhal, Nerenz, and Steele, 1984). Even if people are reasonably well informed, they may choose not to modify their behavior because they perceive the value of the new pattern of behavior to be insufficient to justify a change in their behavior, or because they may not have confidence in their ability to perform the new pattern of behavior (Bandura, 1997). Structural factors may also constrain people's behavioral options, acting either directly on behavior (e.g., the absence of low-fat snack foods at one's workplace may hamper one from taking action) or indirectly by influencing people's beliefs about the behavior (e.g., the absence of low-fat snacks may lead people to perceive them as unpopular or undesirable).

Given the myriad of factors that determine people's behaviors, investigators have worked to formulate systematic accounts of the factors that regulate people's behavioral decisions with respect to health issues (e.g., health belief model [Rosenstock, Strecher, and Becker, 1988]; precaution adoption process model [Weinstein, 1988]; social cognitive theory [Bandura, 1997]; theory of planned behavior [Ajzen, 1991]; theory of reasoned action [Ajzen and Fishbein, 1980]; transtheoretical model of behavior change [Prochaska et al., 1992]).[1] Although these models are remarkably similar in many respects, two general approaches can be identified (see Salovey et al., 1998, for a description of the specific features of each model). Some investigators have proposed that the process by which people decide to make changes in their behavior is best conceptualized as a series of stages and that unique factors determine whether people are able to transition from one stage to the next (e.g., transtheoretical model; precaution adoption process model). The critical implication of the stage-based approach is that intervention strategies are effective only if they target the specific needs of individuals at each stage and therefore interventions need to be stage matched. This approach can be contrasted with the conceptual framework that underlies continuum-based models such as the theory of reasoned action (Ajzen and Fishbein, 1980) or social cognitive theory (Bandura, 1997). In this framework, a single set of factors is identified that affects people's behavioral decisions and, regardless of their readiness to change, people will benefit from information highlighting any or all of these factors

[1]These models strive to specify the psychological factors that direct behavior, but provide limited information about the processes by which these factors (i.e., attitudes and beliefs) are formed or altered. Contemporary models of attitude formation and change (Petty and Wegener, 1998) delineate these processes and are considered in the next section of the paper.

(for a detailed discussion of the relative features of stage- and continuum-based models, see Weinstein, Rothman, and Sutton, 1998).

There is little doubt that a continuum-based framework is more parsimonious than a stage-based framework. Stage models require not only a detailed articulation of the determinants of each stage transition, but also empirical evidence of the predicted dissociations among stage predictors. To date, nearly all of the empirical work that has been conducted cannot distinguish between predictions derived from the two frameworks and thus it is difficult to formulate strong arguments for one perspective over the other (Rothman, Baldwin, and Hertel, 2004; Weinstein et al., 1998).[2] However, it is critical that investigators recognize explicitly which approach is guiding their efforts to motivate people to change their behavior (e.g., is the intervention expected to work consistently across people or will its impact be contingent on where people are in the behavior change process?).

The observation that most people are not ready to implement changes in their behavior does not appear to be less true for older people (Leventhal et al., 2001). In fact, if anything, it has been suggested that older adults are somewhat less interested in opportunities for new experiences (e.g., Fredrickson and Carstensen, 1990), which would suggest an even lower level of readiness to change. Of the two approaches identified above, a stage-based approach may provide some interesting insights into the behavioral practices of older adults as it more readily affords investigators the opportunity to respond to the practical and psychological demands posed by the situations in which people find themselves. The psychological needs and prior experiences that older adults bring to a decision are likely to have a significant effect on where they are most likely to be in the behavior change process. When younger adults express limited interest in modifying their behavior, it is typically thought to reflect a failure to attend to or think through the behavioral decision. However, among older adults, limited interest in modifying, for example, one's diet may indicate that a decision has been made to not make a change, as opposed to simply failing to consider the behavioral alternative (see Weinstein, 1988). This may be particularly true when examining behavioral decisions that involve issues that have been addressed repeatedly throughout the life span. If true, this has implications for initiatives to encourage behavior change. In this case, the failure to act would represent an active choice and thus initiatives would be needed to persuade people to reconsider their decision. Because a

---

[2]Even if subsequent empirical work reveals that a stage-based approach provides a more complete account of behavioral decision making, its impact on intervention efforts may be constrained by the logistical and financial costs associated with its implementation.

decision to not take action may lead people to reaffirm the set of beliefs that guided that decision, persuading people to alter the decision is likely to be more difficult than persuading them to consider a new behavioral alternative.

Asking for Change: Communication Strategies that Motivate Behavior Change

A primary strategy for motivating people to change their behavior has been to provide them with information that will persuade them to alter their behavior (Eagly and Chaiken, 1993).[3] Although in some cases this may involve providing new information about an issue, messages are typically designed to help people recognize or confront issues that are familiar but not seen as important enough to motivate a change in behavior. Thus, the primary challenge in efforts to communicate information is getting people to not only attend to the message but also process it in a manner that maximizes its impact on how they think and feel about the issue (Petty and Wegener, 1998). A critical step in this process is to create a context in which people recognize an issue to be personally relevant. Heightened personal relevance motivates people to not only seek out new information but also process the information in a systematic manner (Petty and Cacioppo, 1990).

There is considerable empirical evidence that people strive to interpret information about themselves in a favorable light (Kunda, 1990). In the health domain, people readily accept information that indicates they are healthy, but are critical of and adopt higher standards of evidence for information that indicates a health problem (e.g., Ditto and Lopez, 1992; Liberman and Chaiken, 1992; see Rothman and Kiviniemi, 1999, for a review). For example, in an elegant series of experiments, Ditto and Croyle (1995) have shown that when people are provided with diagnostic information indicating a health problem, they respond to this information by minimizing its seriousness ("Oh, it's not such a big deal") and increasing perceptions of its prevalence ("Oh, everyone gets it"). Although these processes have not been studied systematically in populations of older adults, there is evidence that older adults misattribute symptoms to aging and that this tendency both reduces emotional distress about the symptoms and delays

[3]Interventions targeted at structural or environmental factors (e.g., access to care, availability of facilities) can also afford significant changes in people's behavior but, aside from brief consideration in the final section of this paper, they fall outside the purview of this paper, which focuses on the psychology of change.

interest in seeking care (Prochaska, Keller, Leventhal, and Leventhal, 1987). It is plausible that this tendency reflects a similar underlying interest in construing health information in a self-protective manner.

Despite evidence that people may resist unfavorable information about their health, it must be recognized that people respond to health information in a myriad of ways. As suggested by Leventhal and colleagues (1984), people may adjust their beliefs to alleviate the sense of threat and anxiety posed by a health concern but still choose to act to reduce the danger posed by the health concern. If investigators assess only people's beliefs about the seriousness of the health problem or how worried they are about the problem, they may develop an incomplete description of how people respond to health information. In fact, Croyle, Sun, and Louie (1993) found that even though people who were informed they had a health problem (high cholesterol) minimized the seriousness of the problem, they nonetheless expressed a heightened interest in information about how to treat the problem. It may be that people's efforts to reduce the perceived seriousness of the problem allows them to manage their affective reaction to the threat to a sufficient degree that they have the psychological resources they need to focus on taking action to reduce their risks (e.g., Aspinwall and Brunhart, 1996). However, if people are too quick or too good at minimizing the problem and the appropriate behavioral response to the problem requires sustained action, over time people may find themselves with insufficient motivation to continue in the necessary action. The observation by Carstensen and her colleagues (Carstensen, Isaacowitz, and Charles, 1999) that older adults prioritize actions that address their emotional needs could indicate that older adults will be particularly interested in regulating their affective reactions to the health information. Such an approach might attenuate any behavioral response to the problem. On the other hand, if older adults are able to maintain a positive emotional state, they may find that they have the psychological resources to deal with challenges to their health in an optimal manner (Salovey, Rothman, Detweiler, and Steward, 2000; Taylor, Kemeny, Reed, Bower, and Gruenewald, 2000). Any strong conclusion about the processes that guide how adults (young and old) respond to health information must wait until investigators assess a sufficiently broad set of indicators to provide a complete description of people's psychological and behavioral response.

Given the challenges associated with providing people with information about their health, are there communication strategies that have been shown to be effective ways to motivate behavior change? Message tailoring and message framing represent two conceptual approaches that not only have been shown to alter people's behavior systematically but also have received sufficient empirical scrutiny that investigators have begun to formulate an understanding of the factors that underlie their effectiveness. The state of the science for each of these approaches and their implications for efforts to motivate behavior change in older adults are examined in turn.

Message Tailoring

Message tailoring is guided by the premise that people will pay more attention to and be more persuaded by information that speaks directly to their own personal concerns.[4] For example, a smoker who is concerned about the social stigma of smoking would be sent a message focusing on that topic, whereas a smoker who is concerned about how smoking is harming the health of his wife would be sent a message focusing on that topic. There is a growing body of empirical evidence indicating that tailored health messages are more effective than generic messages that provide all individuals with the same information (Brug, Glanz, van Assema, Kok, and van Breukelen, 1998; Dijkstra, De Vries, and Roijackers, 1998a, 1998b; Kreuter and Strecher, 1996; Kreuter, Oswald, Bull, and Clark, 2000; see Skinner, Campbell, Rimer, Curry, and Prochaska, 1999, for review).

Why might tailoring messages be more effective? Contemporary models of attitude change and persuasion may provide a rich conceptual framework for understanding how and when tailored messages are maximally effective (Petty, Barden, and Wheeler, 2002). In particular, to the extent that tailored messages are perceived to be personally relevant, recipients of the message will process the information more extensively, which, in turn, should increase its influence on people's thoughts and feelings about the health issue. All else being equal, greater elaboration of a strong health message is desirable as well-reasoned attitudes are more stable over time and better predictors of behavior (Petty and Wegener, 1998).

Tailoring information has been shown to increase the attention people pay to a message. Tailored messages are more likely to be read and remembered than are nontailored messages (e.g., Skinner, Strecher, and Hospers, 1994), are more likely to be discussed with others (e.g., Brug, Steenhuis, van Assema, and De Vries, 1996), and are perceived as more interesting and engaging (e.g., Brug et al., 1996; Kreuter, Bull, Clark, and Oswald, 1999). To the extent that the information addresses an individual's concerns (i.e., the perception that "it speaks to me"), it may be less likely to elicit feelings of reactance and it may be more difficult for people to assert that the

[4]It should be noted that tailored messages are distinct from targeted messages. Message tailoring focuses on matching information to individual-level characteristics (e.g., why Alex resists exercising), whereas message targeting focuses on matching information to group-level characteristics (e.g., why men resist exercising).

message doesn't apply to them (see Gump and Kulik, 1995). In many ways, tailored messages invoke some of the strengths of a self-persuasion strategy, which puts people in situations in which they themselves bring to mind the relevant arguments or reasons for modifying their behavior (Aronson, 1999; McGuire and McGuire, 1991). As with self-persuasion, people who receive tailored messages may be more likely to construe their motivation to modify their behavior as reflecting intrinsic concerns, which have been shown to be predictive of behavior change (e.g., Williams, Ryan, Rodin, Grolnick, and Deci, 1998).

Advances in technology have made the prospect of tailoring messages to a person's unique set of personal concerns feasible, but it is not yet clear how investigators are to determine or prioritize which information should be tailored. For instance, is it more important that people's understanding of the determinants of a health problem are well matched so that they readily infer that they either suffer from or are at risk for a health problem, or should the recommended response to the problem be well matched so that people more easily infer that they can perform the new pattern of behavior? Although stage-based models of behavior change could provide a theoretical framework for selecting the dimensions on which to tailor a message, to date investigators have only compared tailored messages to generic messages. Any conclusions regarding the value of tailoring messages along specific dimensions (e.g., self-efficacy vs. perceived risk) or to a person's stage of change must wait until investigators systematically compare the impact of differentially tailored messages (see Weinstein et al., 1998, for a general discussion of these issues).

Although message tailoring has not been tested systematically with older adults, it provides a framework that can capitalize on the observation that as people age their primary concerns and goals shift. According to socioemotional selectivity theory, older adults prioritize goals that address emotional as opposed to informational needs and thus are more likely to focus on people and opportunities that can address those needs (Carstensen et al., 1999). This would suggest that tailored messages might prove to be particularly persuasive with older adults if they address how modifying one's behavior can satisfy one's emotional needs. However, research on the interplay between emotion and persuasion has found that people's emotional goals (e.g., desire to maintain a positive mood) affect the manner in which they process a message (Wegener and Petty, 1994; Wegener, Petty, and Smith, 1996). To the extent that older adults prioritize their ability to regulate and optimize their current emotional needs and, in particular, strive to construct a world that both heightens the opportunity for positive emotional experiences and constrains the opportunity for negative emotional experiences (i.e., antecedent emotional regulation; Charles and

Carstensen, 1999; Gross, 1998), they may be particularly skilled at minimizing contact with messages about health problems.

A critical assumption implicit in tailoring messages to an individual's set of unique concerns is that the different ways in which people think about a health problem do not differentially predict behavior. For example, when asked to consider cessation, some smokers may focus on the good things they would like to get if they were not smokers (e.g., the extra time and money that they would have available for other interests), whereas other smokers may focus on the unpleasant things about smoking they want to avoid (e.g., the hassle and expenses associated with buying cigarettes and finding a place to smoke). Is it correct to assume that both of these construals are equally likely to motivate behavior?

Andrew Elliot and his colleagues have argued that all goals are not equally motivating and that, in particular, approach goals (i.e., goals that are characterized by a desire to reach a favorable goal state) are more strongly associated with favorable outcomes than are avoidance goals (i.e., goals that are characterized by a desire to stay away from an unfavorable goal state; Elliot and Church, 1997; Elliot and McGregor, 1999). This conclusion rests primarily on data from academic settings that have consistently revealed that the more avoidance goals students report (e.g., desire to not do poorly in the class), the poorer their subsequent academic performance. In a similar vein, contemporary statements of social comparison theory have emphasized that upward social comparisons (i.e., comparing one's performance or condition to that of someone who is doing better) are more likely to elicit improvements in performance than are downward social comparisons (i.e., comparing one's performance or condition to that of someone who is doing worse; Taylor and Lobel, 1989).

Translated into the health domain, this perspective suggests that people who focus on approach goals or upward comparison standards for the behavior (e.g., an interest in dieting predicated on a desire to be thin) will be more successful than those who focus on avoidance goals or downward comparison standards for the behavior (e.g., an interest in dieting predicated on a desire not to be fat), and that tailoring messages to approach goals will be more effective than tailoring them to avoidance goals. Although this prediction follows clearly from empirical findings obtained in academic settings, the extent to which it will be confirmed in the health area is uncertain. In prior studies, avoidance goals have almost always involved the desire to prevent an unpleasant future outcome (e.g., not failing a class). Although similar health goals exist (e.g., not wanting to develop cancer), avoidance goals in the health domain can also involve eliminating the risk of or curing an existing unpleasant state (e.g., shortness of breath). In an initial study of smokers enrolled in a cessation program, my colleagues and I found that smokers whose cessation efforts were motivated by avoidance goals—and, in particular, goals that involved eliminating a current problem—were subsequently more likely to quit smoking (Worth, Sullivan, Hertel, Rothman, and Jeffery, 2005). Specifying the impact of avoidance goals on health behavior change may be particularly important given the observation that older adults frequently possess health-related images of themselves that they want to avoid (Hooker, 1999).

Message Framing

Messages designed to promote a health behavior can be constructed to focus on the benefits of performing the behavior (a gain-framed appeal) or the costs of failing to perform the behavior (a loss-framed appeal). For example, a gain-framed brochure designed to promote prostate cancer screening would emphasize the health benefits afforded by screening, whereas a loss-framed brochure would emphasize the health costs of failing to be screened. According to the framing postulate of prospect theory (Tversky and Kahneman, 1981), how information is framed alters people's preferences. Specifically, people act to avoid risks when considering the potential gains afforded by their decision (they are risk averse in their preferences), but are more willing to take risks when considering the potential losses that may result from their decision (they are risk seeking in their preferences).

What impact might gain- and loss-framed health messages have on people's behavioral practices? In order to specify the relative impact of gain- and loss-framed health appeals, investigators must be able to determine the risk people ascribe to performing the targeted behavior (Rothman and Salovey, 1997). According to prospect theory, the likelihood that a particular frame will effectively motivate behavior is contingent on whether the option under consideration is perceived to reflect a risk-averse or risk-seeking course of action. If a behavior is perceived to involve some risk or uncertainty, loss-framed appeals are more persuasive, but if a behavior is perceived to afford a relatively certain outcome, gain-framed appeals are more persuasive.

In an attempt to apply this framework, Rothman and Salovey (1997; see also Rothman, Kelly, Hertel, and Salovey, 2002) proposed that the function served by a health behavior can operate as a reliable heuristic to predict whether people perceive engaging in a behavior to be risky. Specifically, detection behaviors serve to detect the presence of a health problem, and because they can inform people that they may be sick, initiating the behavior may be considered a risky decision. Although detection behaviors such as mammography provide critical long-term benefits, characterizing them as risky accurately captures people's subjective assessment of these behaviors (e.g., Lerman and Rimer, 1995; Meyerowitz and Chaiken, 1987).

In contrast, prevention behaviors such as the regular use of sunscreen or condoms can forestall the onset of a health problem and maintain a person's current health status. In fact, these behaviors are risky only to the extent that one chooses *not* to engage in them. This distinction in risk perception suggests that loss-framed appeals would be more effective in promoting the use of detection behaviors and gain-framed appeals more effective in promoting the use of prevention behaviors.

The empirical evidence that has been obtained across both laboratory and field studies has provided strong support for the framework set forth by Rothman and Salovey (1997). Efforts to promote the use of detection behaviors have consistently found that loss-framed messages elicit greater interest in or use of behaviors such as breast self-examination (Meyerowitz and Chaiken, 1987; but also see Lalor and Hailey, 1990), mammography (Banks et al., 1995; Cox and Cox, 2001; Schneider et al., 2001; but also see Lerman et al., 1992), HIV testing (Kalichman and Coley, 1995), skin cancer examinations (Block and Keller, 1995; Rothman, Pronin, and Salovey, 1996), and blood-cholesterol screening (Maheswaran and Meyers-Levy, 1990).[5]

Because prevention behaviors typically afford people the opportunity to maintain their health and minimize the risk of illness, gain-framed messages are predicted to elicit greater interest in and use of prevention behaviors. Although only a few studies have tested the impact of gain- and loss-framed appeals on prevention behaviors, the empirical findings have revealed a consistent advantage for gain-framed appeals (e.g., for the use of condoms [Linville, Fischer, and Fischhoff, 1993] and sunscreen [Detweiler, Bedell, Salovey, Pronin, and Rothman, 1999; Rothman, Salovey, Antone, Keough, and Martin, 1993]). Although the pattern of empirical findings from studies that have targeted prevention or detection behaviors is consistent with the framework outlined by Rothman and Salovey (1997), clear evidence that the function of the behavior determines the relative influence of gain- and loss-framed appeals did not come until my colleagues and I systematically studied whether a given health behavior prevented or detected a health problem (Rothman, Martino, Bedell, Detweiler, and Salovey, 1999).

A compelling body of evidence supports the thesis that gain-framed messages are more effective when promoting a prevention behavior while loss-framed messages are more effective when promoting a detection be-

[5]Loss-framed information about a blood-cholesterol test was effective only when college undergraduates were informed that coronary heart disease was a problem for people less than 25 years old (see Rothman and Salovey, 1997, for a broader analysis of this finding).

havior. However, it must not be forgotten that the distinction between prevention and detection behaviors rests on the premise that people perceive engaging in detection behaviors as posing some risk and engaging in prevention behaviors as posing little to no risk. To the extent that there is systematic variability in how people construe a detection or a prevention behavior, the relative influence of gain- and loss-framed appeals becomes more complex (Rothman et al., 2002). Specifically, people who construe engaging in the behavior to be risky (regardless of its function) will be more responsive to loss-framed information, whereas those who do not perceive it to be risky will be more responsive to gain-framed information. Only a few studies have tested whether people's perceptions of a behavior moderate the influence of framed appeals, and all have focused on perceptions of screening behaviors. However, the pattern of results has tended to provide support for the premise that people's response to framed information is contingent on their beliefs about the behavior (Apanovitch, McCarthy, and Salovey, 2003; Meyerowitz, Wilson, and Chaiken, 1991; Rothman et al., 1996).

To date, investigators have not systematically examined the impact of framed messages on the behavioral decisions of older adults, although some studies such as those targeting mammography have included samples of older participants. In light of the thesis that how people construe a behavior determines their response to gain- and loss-framed information, any efforts to use message framing to motivate older adults must be grounded in a clear understanding of how they perceive the targeted behavior. As people get older, their perceptions of screening behaviors may very likely change and this may be particularly true of those behaviors that have to be performed repeatedly. For example, the experience of having had a series of mammograms, all of which were negative, is likely to influence how women perceive the procedure. My colleagues and I (Rothman et al., 2002) have suggested that there may be two distinct types of reactions. Given the repeated experience that the mammogram did not detect a health problem, some women may begin to view the screening as less risky and even anticipate that subsequent screens will prove to be fine as well. This growing sense of reassurance would suggest that over time these women would become more responsive to a gain-framed appeal. However, other women may conclude based on the same series of events that being screened is at least as risky as not being screened, or even more so, if they believe that the string of favorable outcomes must come to an end. In this case, loss-framed appeals should continue to prove more effective.

People's perceptions of screening procedures are also likely to be affected by the fact that, as they age, they will know more and more people who have had an illness detected. Although it is possible that these experiences heighten concern that one's own procedure might find a problem, it is also quite plausible that the increased rate of health problems renders them more normative, which, according to research by Ditto and Croyle (1995), might work to alleviate people's concern about the problem. The notion that health problems are more normative may also enable older adults to shift their focus from the short-term consequences of screening procedures to the longer-term benefits afforded by the early detection of the disease. Alleviating the distress invoked by the health issue may also serve to increase the attention people will pay to the message (Wegener and Petty, 1994) and allow them to focus their efforts on addressing the danger posed by the health threat (Leventhal et al., 1984).

A critical, unresolved issue in the application of message framing with older adults is the impact that gain- and loss-framed information has on decisions regarding treatments for a health problem. Research on message framing and treatment decisions has almost always been limited to responses to hypothetical scenarios (Rothman and Salovey, 1997). The prototypical finding in these studies is that participants have a more favorable reaction to the proposed treatment when it is described in terms of its benefits (e.g., percentage of people who survive the procedure) than in terms of its costs (e.g., percentage of people who die from the procedure). One study examined the use of framed information in actual doctor-patient interactions regarding treatment for breast cancer (Siminoff and Fettig, 1989). Although doctors were found to have a systematic preference for using either gain- or loss-framed language when describing treatments to their patients, there was no report of the effect of the information frame on treatment decisions. Clearly, more research in this area is needed.

Finally, it may be useful to examine how people's general expectations about their health affect their response to framed appeals. Hooker and her colleagues have shown that as people get older, health concerns become increasingly incorporated into how they think of themselves and of who they might become (Hooker, 1999). To the extent that older adults are chronically concerned about the possibility of a health problem, loss-framed appeals might prove to be particularly persuasive. On the other hand, to the extent that they are focused on sustaining a positive view of themselves as healthy and active, gain-framed appeals might prove to be more persuasive. These perspectives converge with the more general observation that individual differences in how people think about goals and goal pursuits can affect the impact of different message strategies (Cesario, Grant, and Higgins, 2004; Lee and Aacker, 2004).

Although considerable progress has been made in delineating the conditions under which gain- and loss-framed appeals are most effective, the processes that underlie these effects are not sufficiently specified. Research on the influence of message framing on older adults should help to enrich our current understanding of the phenomenon.

Moving from Initiation to Maintenance: Why Do People Sustain Behavior Change?

Even when efforts to motivate people to modify their behavior prove successful, the changes that are elicited more often than not prove transient (e.g., diet and exercise to produce weight loss [Jeffery et al., 2000], smoking cessation [Ockene et al., 2000], recovery from substance abuse [Marlatt and Gordon, 1985]). Although some health behaviors need only be done once, the overwhelming majority of behaviors that people are urged to adopt (such as those identified in *Healthy People 2010*) require sustained action and their benefits are contingent on maintenance. Why is it that people who are able to successfully initiate changes in their behavior are more often than not unable to sustain those changes over time? One possibility from dual process models of persuasion is that some behavioral changes are ephemeral because the underlying attitudes that support the changes are weak (e.g., based on little cognitive elaboration) and thus unlikely to persist (Petty and Wegener, 1998). In addition, there may be meaningful differences in the processes that underlie the decision to initiate and the decision to maintain a pattern of behavior.

Current models of health behavior, cited above, have focused on elucidating how people determine whether to adopt a given behavior and have assumed, either implicitly or explicitly, that the factors underlying the decision to maintain a pattern of behavior are no different from those that govern its initiation. For example, the health belief model (Rosenstock et al., 1988), theory of reasoned action (Ajzen and Fishbein, 1980), and theory of planned behavior (Ajzen, 1991) make no direct reference to issues regarding behavioral maintenance other than to define it as a course of action sustained over a specified period of time.[6] By comparison, stage models have identified maintenance as a distinct stage in the behavior change process. However, the primary focus of these theoretical approaches has been to delineate the processes through which people become ready to initiate a change in their behavior (Prochaska et al., 1992; Weinstein, 1988). The distinction between people in the action and maintenance stages is predicated solely on the length of time the behavior has been adopted, and thus the set of cognitive and behavioral strategies predicted to facilitate initial

[6]To the extent that investigators have actively focused on time, it has been to determine how to increase the likelihood that people act on their intentions (Gollwitzer, 1999). Although instructing people to articulate how they will implement their behavioral intention has been shown to increase the likelihood that people will take action, these approaches do not address whether a change in behavior, once enacted, will be maintained.

action are similarly predicted to help sustain that action over time (Prochaska and Velicer, 1997).

Social cognitive theory (Bandura, 1997) does explicitly consider how people regulate their behavior over time and identifies self-efficacy beliefs as a critical determinant of both the initiation and the maintenance of a change in behavior. Confidence in one's ability to take action serves to sustain effort and perseverance in the face of obstacles. The successful implementation of changes in behavior bolsters people's confidence, which, in turn, facilitates further action, whereas failure experiences serve to undermine personal feelings of efficacy. Although the reciprocal relation between perceived self-efficacy and behavior is well documented, this relation needs to be reconciled with the observation that successfully enacted changes in behavior are not always maintained.

I have recently proposed that there are important differences in the decision criteria that guide the initiation and maintenance of behavior change and that these differences may serve to explain why people who are able to make changes in their behavior may subsequently choose not to sustain those changes (Rothman, 2000; Rothman et al., 2004). Behavioral decisions by definition involve a choice between behavioral alternatives. What differentiates decisions concerning initiation from those concerning maintenance are the criteria on which the decision is based. Decisions regarding behavioral initiation involve a consideration of whether the potential benefits afforded by a new pattern of behavior compare favorably to one's current situation, and thus the decision to initiate a new behavior depends both on people holding favorable expectations regarding future outcomes and on their ability to obtain those outcomes. This premise is well grounded by a broad tradition of research (for reviews, see Bandura, 1997; Salovey et al., 1998).

Whereas decisions regarding behavioral initiation are based on expected outcomes, decisions regarding behavioral maintenance involve a consideration of the experiences people have had engaging in the new pattern of behavior and a determination of whether those experiences are sufficiently desirable to warrant continued action. Consistent with Leventhal's Self-Regulatory Model of Illness Behavior (Leventhal and Cameron, 1987), the decision to continue a pattern of behavior reflects an ongoing assessment of the behavioral, psychological, and physiological experiences that accompany the behavior change process. According to the model, people's assessment of these experiences is ultimately indexed by their satisfaction with the experiences resulting from the new pattern of behavior and people will maintain a change in behavior only if they are satisfied with what they have accomplished. The feeling of satisfaction indicates that the initial decision to change the behavior was correct and furthermore provides justification for the continued effort people must put forth to monitor their behavior and minimize vulnerability to relapse (for a more complete description of the model, see Rothman, 2000; Rothman et al., 2004).

Although there is evidence consistent with the premise that satisfaction is associated with behavioral maintenance in the health domain (e.g., Klem, Wing, McGuire, Seagle, and Hill, 1997; Urban, White, Anderson, Curry, and Kristal, 1992) as well as in the area of consumer behavior (e.g., Oliver, 1993), investigators have only begun to test systematically for dissociations between predictors of behavioral initiation and behavioral maintenance (see King, Rothman, and Jeffery, 2002). In order to test predictions regarding the differential determinants of initial and long-term behavior change, investigators have to capture the unique effect that a particular psychological state (e.g., self-efficacy) has on each phase of the behavior change process. To date, claims regarding the determinants of behavioral maintenance have relied on tests of whether a psychological state (e.g., self-efficacy at baseline) can predict a distal behavioral outcome (e.g., smoking status 18 months later). However, this analytic approach is inconclusive regarding the factors that underlie behavioral maintenance as it cannot determine whether, for example, people's initial feelings of self-efficacy influence their ability to maintain a behavior over and above its effect on their initial behavioral efforts. Across a series of intervention studies that have been designed to test predictions from the model in the contexts of smoking cessation and of weight loss, my colleagues and I have begun to accumulate evidence consistent with the model. For example, cessation self-efficacy has been shown to predict people's initial ability to quit smoking but not whether the quit is sustained. People's satisfaction with the outcomes afforded by cessation predicted whether people were able to sustain their quit over an extended period of time (Baldwin, Rothman, Hertel, Linde, Jeffry, Finch, and Lando, in press).

As efforts to understand the distinctions between the processes that guide behavioral initiation and behavioral maintenance move forward, it is critical that investigators examine how these processes operate in older adults. To date, investigators have found in samples of younger adults that people tend to have more difficulty maintaining than initiating a new pattern of behavior. Whether this pattern will hold for older adults is uncertain. Given the premise that older adults are somewhat less interested in new opportunities and find it more difficult to imagine the benefits afforded by a new behavior, it may be that older adults find it particularly hard to initiate new behaviors and thus greater attention must be paid to initiatives that can motivate them to take action.

However, the self-regulatory strategies that are typically employed by older adults may make them better able to maintain a new pattern of behavior (although declines in cognitive functioning may, over time, mitigate the impact of these strategies). To the extent that there may be greater continuity in the environments in which older adults live, it may be easier for them to develop habits. However, little is known about the process by which repeated behaviors become habits. My colleagues and I have suggested that what differentiates habits from behaviors that are maintained over time is that habits are behaviors for which people no longer feel any need to question their value (Rothman et al., 2004). For example, seat belt use may readily become a habit because people feel little need to continually reassess its worth. On the other hand, it may be difficult for a set of dietary behaviors to become a habit as people will continually reassess whether they are satisfied with the outcomes of the behavior. To the extent that habits are regulated by stored representations of the behavior, innovations in how people form and change implicit or automatically activated attitudes (Wilson, Lindsey, and Schooler, 2002) may provide critical insights into the design of initiatives that can create and sustain healthy habits.

If satisfaction proves to be a critical determinant of whether a new pattern of behavior is maintained, investigators need to formulate a better understanding of the factors that cause people to feel more or less satisfied with their actions. This is likely to be a daunting task as one would expect assessments of satisfaction to reflect not only the set of concerns highlighted by the behavioral domain but also the set of priorities specified by the individual. For example, people who want to lose weight in order to improve their social life will focus their assessment of their actions on a different set of criteria than will those who want to lose weight in order to be more physically active.

In order to apply this model to the behavioral practices of older adults, investigators need to develop a rich understanding of what older adults are likely to attend to when assessing the value of their behavior. According to socioemotional selectivity theory (Carstensen et al., 1999), older adults would be expected to base their evaluation on a behavior's ability to address or meet their emotional needs. To the extent that older adults focus their attention to a greater degree on their present psychological needs, they may find it particularly difficult to forestall an assessment of a behavior's value. This would lead to the prediction that older adults would have a particularly difficult time sustaining behaviors for which the initial costs are high and the focal benefits are delayed (e.g., smoking cessation). From the perspective of an intervention, older adults would therefore be likely to benefit from activities that both highlight any immediate benefits and heighten the critical long-term benefits afforded by the new behavior.

Older adults' ability to evaluate the consequences of their actions may also be constrained by cognitive impairments that can cause uncertainty as to whether the behavior has been performed (Purdie and McCrindle, 2002). If people fail to recognize that they have forgotten to perform a behavior (e.g., take medication), when they subsequently find that the benefits of the behavior are diminished, they will mistakenly conclude that the behavior is not effective. People's commonsense model of the health issue can also affect the conclusions they draw about their behavior as their model provides a framework for interpreting both the psychological and the physiological changes attributed to the behavior (Leventhal et al., 2001). For example, investigators have observed that patients misinterpret the feelings elicited by physical exertion as signs of cardiac distress and that this (mis)interpretation is associated with a reduction in activity (e.g., Petrie, Cameron, Ellis, Buick, and Weinman, 2002). Initiatives that shape what people expect to experience when engaging in a particular pattern of behavior may have the ability to increase the likelihood that people are satisfied with the actions they have taken and thus enhance the probability of sustained behavior change.

Taking the Next Steps: Enhancing Collaboration Between Theory and Practice

Given the critical impact that people's behavioral choices have on their health and well-being, the need for intervention strategies that can elicit changes in behavior continues unabated. Successfully meeting this challenge depends on advances in both theory and practice. Thus, we need to increase simultaneously the impact of our interventions and the relevance and precision of our theoretical models. Although there is widespread acknowledgment that theory and practice must progress in tandem, linking these efforts has proven to be a formidable challenge (Rothman, 2004; Suls and Rothman, 2004). One essential strategy is to improve the ways in which basic and applied behavioral scientists communicate with each other. In particular, the two broad groups of investigators must recognize and value the outcomes that can arise from close collaboration between theory and practice. On the intervention side, it is critical not only that intervention strategies be predicated on theoretical principles but also that their impact be assessed in a manner that can, in turn, inform theory. Investigators need to be able to articulate not only why an intervention will be effective but also how it will affect people's behavior. At the same time, theorists must specify the predicted relations in their models to a sufficient degree that the models can inform decisions regarding intervention design. Because interventions focus primarily on altering the status of a particular construct (e.g., perceptions of personal risk), it would be helpful if theorists elaborated more on the processes by which people formulate their beliefs. In this regard, social cognitive theory (Bandura, 1997) serves as an exemplary model as it clearly articulates the determinants of self-efficacy. By actively promoting the reciprocal relation between theory and practice, the information gleaned from intervention activities should lead to improvements in the quality and precision of our theoretical models—advances that, in turn, should enhance the development of new, innovative intervention strategies.

In the present context, efforts to apply current conceptualizations of behavioral decision making to older adults highlight the limits of our knowledge in this area. In particular, the less that is known about the processes underlying a given phenomenon, the more difficult it is to draw firm predictions about how or whether the effect might generalize new populations or situations. For instance, the applicability of message framing as a tool to motivate behavior change among older adults is constrained by limitations in our understanding of the processes that underlie its impact. The ability to specify the processes that underlie a particular intervention strategy also provides investigators with a framework within which to compare different types of intervention protocols. For example, an evaluation of a tailoring intervention might reveal not only that it was effective but also that its effectiveness could be attributed to its ability to heighten people's confidence that they could change their behavior. Although tailoring might prove to be an effective way to raise people's sense of personal efficacy, it is also quite possible that other intervention methods such as those that involve procedural or structural modification might prove to be a more effective way to target people's feelings of efficacy and, in turn, motivate behavior change. In the absence of any clear information about the underlying processes, it can prove to be quite difficult to compare and evaluate different intervention protocols.

If we are to successfully develop methods that can be used to motivate behavioral changes in older adults, investigators must embrace the value of a research program that addresses two distinct goals. The program must include activities that specify and detect both the psychological processes that regulate people's behavioral decisions and those that involve the implementation and evaluation of intervention strategies. It is hoped that the next generation of research in this area will be designed to meet these challenges.

REFERENCES

Ajzen, I. (1991). The theory of planned behavior. *Organizational Behavior and Human Decision Processes, 50*, 179-211.

Ajzen, I., and Fishbein, M. (1980). *Understanding attitudes and predicting social behavior.* Englewood Cliffs, NJ: Prentice Hall.

Apanovitch, A.M., McCarthy, D., and Salovey, P. (2003). Using message framing to motivate HIV-testing among low-income, ethnic minority women. *Health Psychology, 22*, 60-67.

Aronson, E. (1999). The power of self-persuasion. *American Psychologist, 54*, 875-884.

Aspinwall, L.G., and Brunhart, S.M. (1996). Distinguishing optimism from denial: Optimistic beliefs predict attention to health threats. *Personality and Social Psychology Bulletin, 22*, 993-1003.

Baldwin, A.S., Rothman, A.J., Hertel, A.W., Linde, J.A., Jeffery, R.W., Finch, E.A., and Lando, H. (in press). Specifying the determinants of behavior change initiation and maintenance: An examination of self-efficacy, satisfaction, and smoking cessation. Submitted to *Health Psychology*.

Bandura, A. (1997). *Self-efficacy: The exercise of control.* New York: W.H. Freeman.

Banks, S.M., Salovey, P., Greener, S., Rothman, A.J., Moyer, A., Beauvais, J., and Eppel, E. (1995). The effects of message framing on mammography utilization. *Health Psychology, 14*, 178-184.

Baumeister, R.F., Heatherton, T.F., and Tice, D. (1994). *Losing control: Why and how people fail at self-regulation.* San Diego: Academic Press.

Block, L.G., and Keller, P.A. (1995). When to accentuate the negative: The effects of perceived efficacy and message framing on intentions to perform a health-related behavior. *Journal of Marketing Research, 32*, 192-203.

Brug, J., Glanz, K., van Assema, P., Kok, G., and van Breukelen, G.J.P. (1998). The impact of computer-tailored feedback and iterative feedback on fat, fruit, and vegetable intake. *Health Education and Behavior, 25*, 517-531.

Brug, J., Steenhuis, I., van Assema, P., and De Vries, H. (1996). The impact of a computer-tailored nutrition intervention. *Preventative Medicine, 25*, 236-242.

Carstensen, L.L., Isaacowitz, D.M., and Charles, S.T. (1999). Taking time seriously: A theory of socioemotional selectivity. *American Psychologist, 54*, 165-181.

Cesario, J., Grant, H., and Higgins, E.T. (2004). Regulatory fit and persuasion: Transfer from "feeling right." *Journal of Personality and Social Psychology, 86*, 388-404.

Charles, S.T., and Carstensen, L.L. (1999). The role of time in the setting of social goals across the life span. In T.M. Hess and F. Blanchard-Fields (Eds.), *Social cognition and aging* (pp. 319-345). New York: Academic Press.

Cox, D., and Cox, A.D. (2001). Communicating the consequences of early detection: The role of evidence and framing. *Journal of Marketing, 65*, 91-103.

Croyle, R.T., Sun, Y.C., and Louie, D.H. (1993). Psychological minimization of cholesterol test results: Moderators of appraisal in college students and community residents. *Health Psychology, 12*, 503-507.

Detweiler, J.B., Bedell, B.T., Salovey, P., Pronin, E., and Rothman, A.J. (1999). Message framing and sun screen use: Gain-framed messages motivate beach-goers. *Health Psychology, 18*, 189-196.

Dijkstra, A., De Vries, H., and Roijackers, J. (1998a). Computerized tailored feedback to change cognitive determinants of smoking: A Dutch field experiment. *Health Education Research, 13*, 197-206.

Dijkstra, A., De Vries, H., and Roijackers, J. (1998b). Long-term effectiveness of computer-generated tailored feedback in smoking cessation. *Health Education Research, 13*, 207-214.

Ditto, P.H., and Croyle, R.T. (1995). Understanding the impact of risk factor test results: Insights from a basic research program. In R.T. Croyle (Ed.), *Psychosocial effects of screening for disease prevention and detection.* Oxford, England: Oxford University Press.

Ditto, P.H., and Lopez, D.F. (1992). Motivated skepticism: Use of differential decision criteria for preferred and nonpreferred conclusions. *Journal of Personality and Social Psychology, 63*, 568-584.

Eagly, A.H., and Chaiken, S. (1993). *The psychology of attitudes.* Orlando, FL: Harcourt, Brace, Jovanovich.

Elliot, A.J., and Church, M.A. (1997). A hierarchical model of approach and avoidance achievement motivation. *Journal of Personality and Social Psychology, 72*, 218-232.

Elliot, A.J., and McGregor, H.A. (1999). Test anxiety and the hierarchical model of approach and avoidance achievement motivation. *Journal of Personality and Social Psychology, 76*, 628-644.

Fredrickson, B.L., and Carstensen, L.L. (1990). Choosing social partners: How old age and anticipated endings make people more selective. *Psychology and Aging, 5*, 335-347.

Gerrard, M., Gibbons, F.X., Benthin, A.C., and Hessling, R.M. (1996). A longitudinal study of the reciprocal nature of risk behaviors and cognitions in adolescents: What you do shapes what you think, and vice versa. *Health Psychology, 16*, 344-354.

Gollwitzer, P.M. (1999) Implementation intentions: Strong effects of simple plans. *American Psychologist, 54*(7), 493-503.

Gross, J.J. (1998). Antecedent- and response-focused emotion regulation: Divergent consequences for experience, expression, and physiology. *Journal of Personality and Social Psychology, 74*, 224-237.

Gump, B.B., and Kulik, J.A. (1995). The effect of a model's HIV status of self-perceptions: A self-protective similarity bias. *Personality and Social Psychology Bulletin, 21*, 827-833.

Hooker, K. (1999). Possible selves in adulthood: Incorporating telenomic relevance into studies of the self. In T.M. Hess and F. Blanchard-Fields (Eds.), *Social cognition and aging* (pp. 99-124). New York: Academic Press.

Jeffery, R.W., Drewnowski, A., Epstein, L.H., Stunkard, A.J., Wilson, G.T., Wing, R.R., and Hill, D.R. (2000). Long-term maintenance of weight loss: Current status. *Health Psychology, 19*, 5-16.

Kalichman, S.C., and Coley, B. (1995). Context framing to enhance HIV-antibody-testing messages targeted to African American women. *Health Psychology, 14*, 247-254.

King, C., Rothman, A.J., and Jeffery, R.W. (2002). The challenge study: Theory-based interventions for smoking and weight loss. *Health Education Research, 17*(5), 522-530.

Klem, M.L., Wing, R.R., McGuire, M.T., Seagle, H.M., and Hill, J.O. (1997). A descriptive study of individuals successful at long-term maintenance of substantial weight loss. *American Journal of Clinical Nutrition, 66*, 239-246.

Kreuter, M.K., Bull, F.C., Clark, E.M., and Oswald, D.L. (1999). Understanding how people process health information: A comparison of tailored and non-tailored weight-loss materials. *Health Psychology, 18*, 487-494.

Kreuter, M.K., Oswald, D.L., Bull, F.C., and Clark, E.M. (2000). Are tailored health education materials always more effective than non-tailored materials? *Health Education Research, 15*, 305-315.

Kreuter, M.K., and Strecher, V.J. (1996). Do tailored behavior change messages enhance the effectiveness of health risk appraisals? Results from a randomized trial. *Health Education Research, 11*, 97-105.

Kunda, Z. (1990). The case for motivated reasoning. *Psychological Bulletin, 108*, 480-498.

Lalor, K.M., and Hailey, B.J. (1990). The effects of message framing and feelings of susceptibility to breast cancer on reported frequency of breast self-examination. *International Quarterly of Community Health Education, 10*, 183-192.

Lee, A.Y., and Aacker, J.L. (2004). Bringing the frame into focus: The influence of regulatory fit on processing fluency and persuasion. *Journal of Personality and Social Psychology, 86*, 205-218.

Lerman, C., and Rimer, B.K. (1995). Psychosocial impact of cancer screening. In R.T. Croyle (Ed.), *Psychosocial effects of screening for disease prevention and detection* (pp. 65-81). Oxford, England: Oxford University Press.

Lerman, C., Ross, E., Boyce, A., Gorchov, P.M., McLauglin, R., Rimer, B., and Engstrom, P. (1992). The impact of mailing psychoeducational materials to women with abnormal mammograms. *American Journal of Public Health, 82*, 729-730.

Leventhal, H., and Cameron, L. (1987). Behavioral theories and the problem of compliance. *Patient Education and Counseling, 10*, 117-138.

Leventhal, H., Nerenz, D.R., and Steele, D.J. (1984). Illness representations and coping with health threats. In A. Baum, S.E. Taylor, and J.E. Singer (Eds.), *Handbook of psychology and health* (vol. 4, pp. 219-252). Mahwah, NJ: Lawrence Erlbaum.

Leventhal, H., Rabin, C., Leventhal, E.A., and Burns, E. (2001). Health risk behaviors and aging. In J.E. Birren and K.W. Schaie (Eds.), *Handbook of the psychology of aging* (5th ed., pp. 186-214). New York: Academic Press.

Liberman, A., and Chaiken, S. (1992). Defensive processing of personally relevant health messages. *Personality and Social Psychology Bulletin, 18*, 669-679.

Linville, P.W., Fischer, G.W., and Fischhoff, B. (1993). AIDS risk perceptions and decision biases. In J.B. Pryor and G.D. Reeder (Eds.), *The social psychology of HIV infection* (pp. 5-38). Mahwah, NJ: Lawrence Erlbaum.

Maheswaran, D., and Meyers-Levy, J. (1990). The influence of message framing and issue involvement. *Journal of Marketing Research, 27*, 361-367.

Marlatt, G.A., and Gordon, J.R. (1985). *Relapse prevention: Maintenance strategies in the treatment of addictive behaviors*. New York: Guilford Press.

McGuire, W.J., and McGuire, C.V. (1991). The content, structure, and operation of thought systems. In R.S. Wyer, Jr. and T.K. Srull (Eds.), *Advances in social cognition* (vol. 4, pp. 1-78). Mahwah, NJ: Lawrence Erlbaum.

Meyerowitz, B.E., and Chaiken, S. (1987). The effect of message framing on breast self-examination attitudes, intentions, and behavior. *Journal of Personality and Social Psychology, 52*, 500-510.

Meyerowitz, B.E., Wilson, D.K., and Chaiken, S. (1991). *Loss-framed messages increase breast self-examination for women who perceive risk*. Paper presented at the annual convention of the American Psychological Society, June 13-16, Washington, DC.

Ockene, J.K., Emmons, K.M., Mermelstein, R.J., Perkins, K.A., Bonollo, D.S., Voorhees, C.C., and Hollis, J.F. (2000). Relapse and maintenance issues for smoking cessation. *Health Psychology, 19*, 17-31.

Oliver, R.L. (1993). Cognitive, affective and attribute bases of the satisfaction response. *Journal of Consumer Research, 30*, 418-430.

Petrie, K.J., Cameron, L.D., Ellis, C.J., Buick, D., and Weinman, J. (2002). Changing illness perceptions after myocardial infarction: An early intervention randomized controlled trial. *Psychosomatic Medicine, 64*, 580-586.

Petty, R.E., Barden, J., and Wheeler, S.C. (2002). The elaboration likelihood model of persuasion: Health promotions that yield sustained behavioral change. In R.J. DiClemente, R.A. Crosby, and M.C. Kegler (Eds.), *Emerging theories in health promotion practice and research* (pp. 71-99). San Francisco: Jossey-Bass.

Petty, R.E., and Cacioppo, J.T. (1990). Involvement and persuasion: Tradition versus integration. *Psychological Bulletin, 107*, 367-374.

Petty, R.E., and Wegener, D.T. (1998). Attitude change: Multiple roles for persuasion variables. In D. Gilbert, S. Fiske, and G. Lindzey (Eds.), *The handbook of social psychology* (4th ed., vol. 1, pp. 323-390). New York: McGraw-Hill.

Prochaska, J.O., DiClemente, C.C., and Norcross, J.C. (1992). In search of how people change: Applications to addictive behaviors. *American Psychologist, 47*, 1102-1114.

Prochaska, J.O., and Velicer, W.F. (1997). The transtheoretical model of health behavior change. *American Journal of Health Promotion, 12*, 38-48.

Prohaska, T.R., Keller, M.L., Leventhal, E.A., and Leventhal, H. (1987). Impact of symptoms and aging attribution on emotions and coping. *Health Psychology, 6*, 495-514.

Purdie, N., and McCrindle, A. (2002). Self-regulation, self-efficacy, and health behavior change in older adults. *Educational Gerontology, 28*, 379-400.

Rosenstock, I.M., Strecher, V.J., and Becker, M.H. (1988). Social learning theory and the health belief model. *Health Education Quarterly, 15*, 175-183.

Rothman, A.J. (2000). Toward a theory-based analysis of behavioral maintenance. *Health Psychology, 19*, 64-69.

Rothman, A.J. (2004). "Is there nothing more practical than a good theory?" Why innovations and advances in health behavior change will arise if interventions are used to test and refine theory. *International Journal of Behavioral Nutrition and Physical Activity, 1*, 11.

Rothman, A.J., Baldwin, A.S., and Hertel, A.W. (2004). Self-regulation and behavior change: Disentangling behavioral initiation and behavioral maintenance. In K. Vohs and R. Baumeister (Eds.), *The handbook of self-regulation* (pp. 130-148). New York: Guilford Press.

Rothman, A.J., Kelly, K.M, Hertel, A., and Salovey P. (2002). Message frames and illness representations: Implications for interventions to promote and sustain healthy behavior. In L.D. Cameron and H. Leventhal (Eds.), *The self-regulation of health and illness behavior* (pp. 278-296). London, England: Routledge.

Rothman, A.J., and Kiviniemi, M. (1999). "Treating people with health information": An analysis and review of approaches to communicating health risk information. *Journal of the National Cancer Institute Monographs, 25*, 44-51.

Rothman, A.J., Martino, S.C., Bedell, B.T., Detweiler, J.B., and Salovey, P. (1999). The systematic influence of gain- and loss-framed messages on interest in and use of different types of health behavior. *Personality and Social Psychology Bulletin, 25*, 1355-1369.

Rothman, A.J., Pronin, E., and Salovey, P. (1996). *The influence of prior concern on the persuasiveness of loss-framed messages about skin cancer*. Presented at the annual meeting of the Society of Experimental Social Psychology, October, Sturbridge, MA.

Rothman, A.J., and Salovey, P. (1997). Shaping perceptions to motivate healthy behavior: The role of message framing. *Psychological Bulletin, 121*, 3-19.

Rothman, A.J., Salovey, P., Antone, C., Keough, K., and Martin, C.D. (1993). The influence of message framing on intentions to perform health behaviors. *Journal of Experimental Social Psychology, 29*, 408-433.

Salovey, P., Rothman, A.J., Detweiler, J.B., and Steward, W. (2000). Emotional states and physical health. *American Psychologist, 55*, 110-121.

Salovey, P., Rothman, A.J., and Rodin, J. (1998). Health behavior. In D. Gilbert, S. Fiske, and G. Lindzey (Eds.), *Handbook of social psychology* (4th ed., vol. 2, pp. 633-683). New York: McGraw-Hill.

Schmid, T.L., Jeffery, R.W., and Hellerstedt, W.L. (1989). Direct mail recruitment to home-based smoking and weight control programs: A comparison of strengths. *Preventive Medicine, 18*, 503-517.

Schneider, T.R., Salovey, P., Apanovitch, A.M., Pizarro, J., McCarthy, D., Zullo, J., and Rothman, A.J. (2001). The effects of message framing and ethnic targeting on mammography use among low-income women. *Health Psychology, 20*, 256-266.

Siminoff, L.A., and Fettig, J.H. (1989). Effects of outcome framing on treatment decisions in the real world: Impact of framing on adjuvant breast cancer decisions. *Medical Decision Making, 9*, 262-271.

Skinner, C.S., Campbell, M.K., Rimer, B.K., Curry, S., and Prochaska, J.O. (1999). How effective is tailored print communication? *Annals of Behavioral Medicine, 21*, 290-298.

Skinner, C.S., Strecher, V.J., and Hospers, H. (1994). Physicians' recommendations for mammography: Do tailored messages make a difference? *American Journal of Public Health, 84*, 43-49.

Suls, J., and Rothman, A.J. (2004). Evolution of the psychosocial model: Implications for the future of health psychology. *Health Psychology, 23*, 119-125.

Taylor, S.E., Kemeny, M.E., Reed, G.M., Bower, J.E., and Gruenewald, T.L. (2000). Psychological resources, positive illusions, and health. *American Psychologist, 55*, 99-109.

Taylor, S.E., and Lobel, M. (1989). Social comparison activity under threat: Downward evaluation and upward contact. *Psychological Review, 96*, 569-575.

Tversky, A., and Kahneman, D. (1981). The framing of decisions and the rationality of choice. *Science, 221*, 453-458.

Urban, N., White, E., Anderson, G.L., Curry, S., and Kristal, A.R. (1992). Correlates of maintenance of a low-fat diet among women in the Women's Health Trial. *Preventive Medicine, 21*, 279-291.

U.S. Department of Health and Human Services. (2001). *Healthy people 2010: National health promotion and disease prevention objectives.* Washington, DC: U.S. Government Printing Office.

Wegener, D.T., and Petty, R.E. (1994). Mood management across affective states: The hedonic contingency hypothesis. *Journal of Personality and Social Psychology, 66*, 1034-1048.

Wegener, D.T., Petty, R.E., and Smith, S. (1996). Positive mood can increase or decrease message scrutiny: The hedonic contingency view of mood and message processing. *Journal of Personality and Social Psychology, 69*, 5-15.

Weinstein, N.D. (1988). The precaution adoption process. *Health Psychology, 7*, 355-386.

Weinstein, N.D. (1998). Accuracy of smokers' risk perceptions. *Annals of Behavioral Medicine, 20*, 1-8.

Weinstein, N.D., Rothman, A.J., and Sutton, S.R. (1998). Stage theories of health behavior. *Health Psychology, 17*, 290-299.

Williams, G.C., Ryan, R.M., Rodin, G.C., Grolnick, W.S., and Deci, E.L. (1998). Autonomous regulation and long-term medication adherence in adult outpatients. *Health Psychology, 17*, 269-276.

Wilson, T.D., Lindsey, S., and Schooler, T.Y. (2002). A model of dual attitudes. *Psychological Review, 107*, 101-126.

Worth, K.A., Sullivan, H.W., Hertel, A.W., Rothman, A.J., and Jeffery, R.W. (2005). Avoidance goals can be beneficial: A look at smoking cessation. *Basic and Applied Social Psychology, 27*(2), 107-116.

A Review of Decision-Making Processes: Weighing the Risks and Benefits of Aging

Mara Mather
University of California, Santa Cruz

INTRODUCTION

The ability to make decisions is a fundamental skill at any age, and it is especially crucial in our current society, which emphasizes independence throughout the life span. Older adults face decisions that can have a huge impact on the remaining years of their lives. Often their life circumstances are changing. A decision to retire is likely to be followed by the need to make many other decisions about how to structure everyday life. In addition, many everyday decisions—in order to maintain one's finances, relationships, and household—continue to be important throughout life. The physical toll of aging forces older adults to face difficult health care decisions, such as which medical procedure to try, what to do for a sick spouse, what type of health insurance to pay for, which medications to take, or how much effort to put into maintaining a healthy life-style. Within many older adults' lifetime, the health care system has shifted from a model in which the family doctor's advice was never challenged to one in which patients expect to be equal partners with their doctor in decision making. And those who are willing and able to tackle such decisions are more likely to get successful health care.

Despite growing interest and obvious practical implications, there are still relatively few studies investigating aging and decision making (for reviews see Peters, Finucane, MacGregor, and Slovic, 2000; Sanfey and Hastie, 2000; Yates and Patalano, 1999). It seems likely that the primary reason for this neglect is that older adults do not typically show obvious problems in making decisions. Certainly most older adults feel pretty confident about their ability to make decisions, a confidence that contrasts with their concerns about other cognitive abilities such as memory (Hertzog, Lineweaver, and McGuire, 1999; Princeton Survey Research, 1998). Another potential reason for the relative neglect of this topic is that decision making involves so many different subprocesses. For example, being able to keep multiple pieces of information in mind may be important for a decision between options. Thinking more than one step beyond the decision itself should help people examine the consequences of various possibilities and make the best decisions. An ability to deal with the emotional aspects of a decision is necessary in many cases. Based on the research reviewed in this paper, some of the processes involved with decision making show decline with age, whereas others remain stable or improve. To date, however, there has been very little research connecting age-related changes in the cognitive and emotional capabilities thought to underlie decision making with changes in decision making itself.

In this paper, I discuss two aspects of aging that seem particularly relevant for decision making. The first is older adults' increased effectiveness of emotion regulation. Both self-reports and actual emotional experience indicate that older adults are better at avoiding negative affect and maintaining positive affect (Carstensen, Pasupathi, Mayr, and Nesselroade, 2000; Gross et al., 1997). A desire to regulate emotions may influence decisions. For instance, avoiding regret and maximizing satisfaction are motivations behind many decisions (Loewenstein, Weber, Hsee, and Welch, 2001; Mellers and McGraw, 2001). In addition, the degree to which younger adults focus on emotion regulation influences their decision processes (Luce, 1998; Luce, Bettman, and Payne, 1997). Thus age-related changes in emotion may predict or help explain some age-related differences seen in decision making.

The second aspect I focus on is the cognitive neuroscience of aging. Certain regions of the brain deteriorate more with age than others, and thus the way that people make decisions may change as processes that rely on certain brain structures become less effective. In particular, aging tends to affect the frontal areas more than other regions of the brain. Frontal regions are essential for many of the more complex cognitive and emotional processes and are implicated in decision making. Understanding the impact of aging on the frontal regions of the brain may therefore help scientists predict and understand age differences in decision making.

After I review these two aspects of aging and their implications for decision making, I review several themes that emerge from the literature on aging and decision making. The first is a surprising lack of age differences in dealing with risky decisions, contrary to general stereotypes about increased cautiousness with age. Next, I review what seem to be the most frequently replicated age differences in decision making: older adults are more likely to avoid making decisions and to seek less information when faced with a decision. I also discuss age differences in memories of past decisions and how such differences might affect learning or future decisions. The causes of each of these age differences (or lack thereof) have not yet been identified, but I suggest ways in which they may be related to emotional and prefrontal functioning.

EMOTION AND OLDER ADULTS' DECISIONS

Emotions play a central role in many decisions (Damasio, 1994; Loewenstein and Lerner, 2000; Mellers and McGraw, 2001). On an intentional level, decision makers can take into account potential emotional reactions to the outcomes of their decisions (e.g., Bell, 1982; Josephs, Larrick, Steele, and Nisbett, 1992; Ritov, 1996). For example, people often attempt to choose options that minimize the chance that they will experience regret later (Mellers, Schwartz, and Ritov, 1999). But perhaps even more important are the unintentional influences of emotions on decisions. Affective judgments of objects and events are easily accessible and frequently serve as a cue to guide judgments and decisions (Finucane, Alhakami, Slovic, and Johnson, 2000; Slovic, Finucane, Peters, and MacGregor, 2002). And emotions that have nothing to do with the decision at hand can influence it (e.g., Isen, 2001; Lerner, Small, and Loewenstein, 2004). When experiencing a negative emotion because of a decision conflict, people change the way they examine and weigh features of choice alternatives in ways that help them feel better (e.g., Luce et al., 1997; Luce, Payne, and Bettman, 2000).

These links between emotion and decisions are relevant for aging research because emotional experience changes with age and these changes may influence decisions. For example, in a study in which participants were paged at random times throughout a week to indicate what emotions they were experiencing, older adults were more likely to maintain positive emotions over time (Carstensen et al., 2000). Their negative affect also lasted for a shorter time than that of younger adults. Older adults generally experience less negative affect than younger adults (Carstensen et al., 2000; Charles, Reynolds, and Gatz, 2001; Gross et al., 1997; Lawton, Kleban, and Dean, 1993; Lawton, Kleban, Rajagopal, and Dean, 1992). According to Carstensen's socioemotional selectivity theory (e.g., Carstensen, Isaacowitz, and Charles, 1999), this reduction in negative affect occurs because people change their goals as they approach the end of life and perceive limitations on their time. Specifically, when time is perceived as limited, such as when facing a terminal illness or a move to a new location, people focus more on achieving emotional satisfaction and meaning than on acquiring new information. Because of this shift in goals, older adults focus more on regulating emotion than younger adults do, which improves older adults' everyday emotional experience.

Recent studies suggest that this increased focus on regulating current emotion as people age influences attention and memory (for a review see Mather, 2004). In an attention task, older adults respond faster to dots that appear behind positive or neutral faces than those that appear behind negative faces, indicating they avoid attending to negative stimuli (Mather and Carstensen, 2003). When watching a slide show of emotional pictures, older adults show less activation in the amygdala (a region of the brain associated with emotional attention) in response to the negative pictures than to the positive pictures, whereas younger adults show similar amygdala activation levels for both types of emotional pictures (Mather et al., 2004).

A positivity effect is also evident in older adults' memory. Compared with younger or middle-aged adults, older adults show disproportionately poorer memory for negative pictures than for positive or neutral pictures (Charles, Mather, and Carstensen, 2003), are more likely to distort their autobiographical memories in a positive direction (Kennedy, Mather, and Carstensen, 2004), and are more likely to show memory distortion that favors chosen options over rejected options (Mather and Johnson, 2000). Remembering the past in a more positive light should help people feel better, and indeed older adults' mood improves after autobiographical recall (Kennedy et al., 2004). Younger or middle-aged adults exhibit just as much of a positivity bias as older adults if they are asked to think about how they feel about their choices (Mather and Johnson, 2000) or to fill out a brief mood scale every so often while filling out the memory questionnaire (Kennedy et al., 2004). This suggests that when emotional goals are more salient for younger adults, their memory biases resemble those of older adults.

Changes in the importance of emotional goals may also influence the way that decisions are made. In fact, some of the research inspired by socioemotional selectivity theory suggests changes across the life span in decisions about interpersonal relationships. Older adults are more likely than younger adults to choose to spend time with emotionally meaningful social partners (Fredrickson and Carstensen, 1990; Fung, Carstensen, and Lutz, 1999; Fung, Lai, and Ng, 2001). These familiar social partners are presumably the ones most likely to fulfill emotional needs. In contrast, younger adults do not show this preference unless they are told to imagine that their time is limited due to an upcoming geographical move (Fung et al., 1999). Imagining a different time frame also affects the older adults' preferences: when asked to imagine that their lives have been extended by 20 years, they no longer have a preference for familiar social partners (Fung et al., 1999). Consistent with these lab findings, cross-sectional studies of social networks indicate that while the number of peripheral social partners decreases with age, the size of the "inner circle" of emotionally close friends or family members remains constant with age (Lang and Carstensen, 1994).

An increased focus on emotional goals should have an impact on non-social decisions as well. Yet an increased role for emotion in decision making does not mean that decision quality will deteriorate. Despite our societal bias that rational and systematic processes lead to the best decisions, the quality of some decisions can suffer when people think systematically about them (Wilson and Schooler, 1991). Positive affect, in particular, can enhance decision making, leading to more creativity and efficiency, although it also increases risk aversion (Isen, 2001). In addition, as outlined in the next section, case studies of people with certain types of brain damage suggest that emotion plays an essential role in making good decisions.

THE PREFRONTAL CORTEX AND OLDER ADULTS' DECISIONS

Neural Substrates of Decision Making

Phineas Gage, one of the most famous neurological patients in history, was a railway worker whose frontal lobes were partially destroyed in an accident in 1848 (Damasio, Grabowski, Frank, Galaburda, and Damasio, 1994). A responsible, intelligent, and likable man before the accident, Gage lost control of his life after the accident. Though apparently not cognitively impaired, he became offensive and unreliable. Since this famous case, many physicians have noted that frontal lesions can be associated with deficits in rational decision making, emotional control, and social behavior. For example, patients with prefrontal lesions often show deficits in financial decision making (Goel, Grafman, Tajik, Gana, and Danto, 1998; Schindler, Ramchandani, Matthews, and Podell, 1995), which can be so extreme as to result in bankruptcy (Eslinger and Damasio, 1985). Yet not all frontal patients show obvious deficits in making decisions. Whether they will have difficulties can be predicted by the location of their brain lesions (Bechara, Damasio, Tranel, and Anderson, 1998). Two distinct regions within the prefrontal cortex contribute in different ways to decision processes: the orbitofrontal cortex and the dorsolateral prefrontal cortex (Krawczyk, 2002).

Case studies with patients clearly implicate the orbitofrontal cortex in both decision making and the processing of emotion. A reconstruction of Phineas Gage's brain, based on the damaged skull that was preserved by his doctor, revealed that the lesion damaged his orbitofrontal cortex (and other regions within the ventromedial prefrontal cortex) while sparing his dorsolateral prefrontal cortex (Damasio et al., 1994). Like Phineas Gage, modern-day patients with damage to the inner portion of the orbitofrontal cortex often make impulsive decisions that do not take into account long-term consequences. In a laboratory setting, this has been observed in studies using a gambling card game (Bechara, Damasio, Damasio, and Anderson, 1994).

In this game, participants are presented with four decks of cards and must choose one card at a time. Two decks contain many cards granting large gains in play money but also some cards that lead to a large penalty. These decks are disadvantageous in the long run. The other decks offer smaller immediate gains but also smaller losses and end up being advantageous in the long run. Participants are not told about the characteristics of the decks, but instead must learn about them through the process of sampling cards from each deck. Patients with medial orbitofrontal damage choose more cards from the risky decks even after they experience the large penalties. Control participants, in contrast, soon choose more cards from the more conservative, advantageous decks and begin to produce anticipatory skin conductance responses before they select a card from the risky decks (Bechara, Tranel, Damasio, and Damasio, 1996). The patients do not show any anticipatory arousal when selecting from the risky decks. This insensitivity to future consequences among the patients with medial orbitofrontal damage is also evident when the nature of the decks is changed so that the advantageous deck offers high immediate punishment but even higher future reward (Bechara, Tranel, and Damasio, 2000b) and is particularly striking when juxtaposed with their well-maintained performance on most other cognitive tasks (e.g., Bechara et al., 1998; Bechara, Tranel, and Damasio, 2000a).

In situations in which the reward system changes, patients with orbitofrontal lesions are unable to choose the correct action behaviorally, despite being able to describe what they should do (Rolls, Hornak, Wade, and McGrath, 1994), consistent with observations of their impulsive behaviors in real-world choices. More generally, the orbitofrontal cortex appears to monitor abstract rewards such as money or winning a competition, an important component of effective decision making (Breiter, Aharon, Kahneman, Dale, and Shizgal, 2001; Elliott, Dolan, and Frith, 2000; Elliott, Friston, and Dolan, 2000; Elliott, Newman, Longe, and Deakin, 2003; O'Doherty, Kringelbach, Rolls, Hornak, and Andrews, 2001; Thut et al., 1997; Zalla et al., 2000).

The dorsolateral prefrontal cortex also contributes to decision making, but not in ways that are as striking as those of the orbitofrontal cortex. In contrast to orbitofrontal lesion patients, dorsolateral prefrontal lesion patients are not impaired on the gambling task (Bechara et al., 1998) and are able to respond to changing reward contingencies (Rolls et al., 1994). Thus, the dorsolateral prefrontal cortex does not play a critical role in monitoring the longer-term future emotional outcome of events, or in associating pleasure or pain with abstract events. However, the dorsolateral prefrontal cortex plays a key role in the ability to maintain and manipulate information in working memory (Cohen et al., 1997; D'Esposito et al., 1995). This ability contributes to many aspects of decision making, such as tracking and integrating various features in order to make an overall evaluation. Working memory abilities may also be important for speculating about possible future outcomes, since such speculation often involves considering and integrating many different pieces of information.

Aging and Prefrontal Decline

With age, the volume of the brain declines at a rate of about 2 percent per decade (Raz, 2000). This decline in volume appears to be mostly the result of cell shrinkage and reductions in neural connections (Uylings, West, Coleman, De Brabander, and Flood, 2000). The neuron loss that does occur is selective, affecting some regions of the brain but not others. The region hardest hit by aging is the prefrontal cortex (Coffey et al., 1992; Cowell et al., 1994; DeCarli et al., 1994; Raz, 2000; Raz et al., 1997; Tisserand and Jolles, 2003; West, 1996). Although researchers do not yet fully understand why aging affects the prefrontal cortex more than other regions, it seems related to the later development of this region (Raz, 2000). Frontal regions continue to change and develop long after childhood is over (Bartzokis et al., 2003). But the benefits of such plasticity appear to come with a cost. In particular, myelination in the frontal regions has properties that allow it to continue developing into middle age but that may also make it more vulnerable to aging (Bartzokis et al., 2003). In addition, vascular disorders associated with aging, such as hypertension, appear to have more negative consequences for frontal regions than for other brain areas (Raz, Rodrigue, and Acker, 2003). Researchers have attributed many of the cognitive changes seen in normal aging to changes in the prefrontal cortex (Daigneault and Braun, 1993; Moscovitch and Winocur, 1995; West, 1996). Given the marked deficits in decision making seen in patients who have prefrontal (specifically orbitofrontal) lesions, like Phineas Gage, we might also expect to see changes in decision processes with age.

However, behaviorally, older adults could hardly look more different from patients with lesions in orbitofrontal regions. Unlike such patients, older adults in general do not have problems regulating their emotions or social behavior. In fact, as previously noted, older adults are generally better at avoiding negative affect and emotional outbursts than younger adults (Carstensen et al., 2000; Gross et al., 1997; Lawton et al., 1992). This suggests that not all functions subserved by prefrontal regions decline with age.

Although most studies investigating how aging affects prefrontal brain regions have not distinguished its subregions, behavioral data suggest that there is a dissociation. There are dramatic age-related declines in processes associated with the dorsolateral prefrontal cortex, such as working memory, but only minimal age-related declines in processes associated with the orbitofrontal cortex (MacPherson, Phillips, and Della Sala, 2002; Phillips and Della Sala, 1998). MacPherson et al. (2002) gave younger, middle-aged, and older adults two sets of tests: one associated with dorsolateral prefrontal function and the other associated with medial orbitofrontal function, based on prior patient and neuroimaging data. Performance declined with age for the dorsolateral measures but not for most of the orbitofrontal measures, suggesting that the two regions differ in their susceptibility to age-related changes. If this is the case, older adults should be as effective as younger adults at the emotional and social judgment aspects of decision making. In contrast, they should be less effective in aspects of decision making that require maintaining and manipulating multiple pieces of information.

Risky Decisions

A common stereotype of older adults is that they are risk avoidant (Okun, 1976). Because emotions play a central role in risky situations (Loewenstein et al., 2001), it is possible that age-related changes in emotions change the way risky decisions are made by older adults. Yet given the available evidence, it is difficult to make a clear prediction about how age-related changes in emotion will affect the way people deal with risk. Because positive affective experience remains mostly constant across the life span (Carstensen et al., 2000; Charles et al., 2001) or even increases slightly (Mroczek, 2001), the impact of positive affect on risky decisions (Isen, Nygren, and Ashby, 1988; Nygren, Isen, Taylor, and Dulin, 1996) is likely to remain constant with age. The decrease across the life span in negative emotions (such as fear, anger, sadness, and disgust) (Carstensen et al., 2000; Charles et al., 2001; Mroczek, 2001) does not lead to any clear predictions about risky decisions because different types of negative affect (such as fear and anger) affect risky decisions differently. Fear makes people more risk averse whereas anger makes them less risk averse (Lerner, Gonzalez, Small, and Fischhoff, 2003; Lerner and Keltner, 2001). Because both of these emotions decrease with age (Carstensen et al., 2000), their effects may tend to cancel each other out.

Indeed, survey data of financial behavior provide only mixed support for the stereotype of cautious older adults. Economists have noted that when the average age of Americans rises, the risk premiums for assets also rise (Bakshi and Chen, 1994), suggesting that as the population ages, risky investments become less popular. A number of studies have examined individual investors' risk tolerance by looking at the proportion of their assets invested in risky investments. Some of these studies have found that the proportion actually increases until about age 65, when it begins to decrease (Jianakoplos and Bernasek, 1998; Riley and Chow, 1992; Schooley and Worden, 1999). One study of university employees found that hypothetical asset allocations became more conservative with age (Dulebohn, 2002), whereas another study using a different sample of university employees found that, with age, people described themselves as more tolerant of risk in their financial decisions (Grable, 2000). A survey of high-level managers at Dutch bank and insurance companies revealed that older managers' business decisions were more aggressive than younger managers' decisions (Brouthers, Brouthers, and Werner, 2000). Conflicting results such as these may be due to factors confounded with age, such as wealth and the time horizon of the investment goals. Certainly the studies that show an inverse u-shaped function, with risk tolerance increasing in midlife and then decreasing after retirement (Jianakoplos and Bernasek, 1998; Riley and Chow, 1992; Schooley and Worden, 1999), suggest that asset allocation decisions are more influenced by changes in life circumstances than by age-related changes in information-processing strategies. Given the available evidence, we cannot rule out the possibility that younger adults would make similar financial decisions as older adults if they had the same amount of wealth and similar investment time horizons.

Gambling is a popular activity among older adults. A survey of activity directors at residential and assisted-care facilities and other senior centers revealed that bingo is the activity most participated in on-site, and that casino gambling is the most highly attended type of day-trip social activity (McNeilly and Burke, 2001). Playing bingo or the slots every so often is unlikely to cause serious financial or social problems, but gambling has its risks, especially if it becomes an addiction. Nationwide surveys indicate that rates of pathological gambling in the general population are lower for older adults than younger adults (National Opinion Research Center, 1999). However, this age effect is no longer significant when race, socioeconomic status, and gender are accounted for (Welte, Barnes, Wieczorek, Tidwell, and Parker, 2001). This finding suggests that when other factors are taken into account, age in itself does not predict rates of pathological gambling. For example, gender is one confound when looking at age trends, since a lower proportion of the older population is male and proportionately more males are pathological gamblers. Furthermore, the prevalence of gambling among older adults may not accurately reflect risk aversion because the gambling may instead serve as a social activity for older adults.

Evidence from experiments comparing individual decision-making strategies among younger and older adults provides even less support for the stereotype of cautious older adults. Two studies found no significant age differences in whether people selected cards from high-reward/high-risk decks in a gambling task (Kovalchik, Camerer, Grether, Plott, and Allman, 2005; MacPherson et al., 2002). A third study using the same gambling task even found that a small subset (14/40) of older adults failed to exhibit risk aversion, selecting more cards from the risky decks than from the more conservative, advantageous decks (Denburg, Tranel, Bechara, and Damasio, 2001), suggesting that some older adults' decision strategies may be even *more* risky than younger adults' strategies. In a task resembling blackjack, in which the goal was to obtain a hand of cards with the highest overall value but not to go over 21, both older and younger adults became more reluctant to take additional cards as the risk level increased (Dror, Katona, and Mungur, 1998). There were no age differences in risk taking or in the response times based on the level of risk. However, an exception is found in Chaubey (1974), who presented participants with tasks that varied in difficulty (e.g., hitting a glass with a ball from different distances), with the potential reward increasing with the task difficulty. Older adults chose to complete easier tasks than younger adults. The findings are difficult to interpret, however, because older adults also rated themselves as less likely to succeed at the tasks. For the most part, however, in laboratory studies of gambling, older adults are *not* more cautious than younger adults—instead older and younger adults appear to use similar strategies.

As highlighted by the gambling task (Bechara et al., 1994), an important component of many decisions involving risk is the ability to balance one's short-term and long-term interests. In order to prosper, some value needs to be placed on one's long-term interests. Yet most people value something that can be gained or experienced immediately much more than that same thing received at some time in the future. Indeed, people will pay exorbitant interest rates on credit cards so that they can purchase things immediately, even when the actual cost ends up being much higher than if they had waited and saved to purchase the same items.

Consistent with this general tendency, Green, Myerson, Lichtman, Rosen, and Fry (1996) found that both older and younger adults show "delay discounting," in which the current value of delayed rewards is worth less than their face value (e.g., a $10,000 reward in 10 years might be worth around $6,000 now). Green and colleagues found that income predicted delay discounting, whereas age itself did not. Both older and younger upper-income adults showed less delay discounting than lower-income older adults. This suggests that the impulsivity involved in financial decision making does not change across the life span as long as one's overall financial situation does not change.

A number of studies have used descriptions of choice dilemmas faced by hypothetical characters to examine older adults' decision-making strategies (Botwinick, 1966, 1969; Calhoun and Hutchison, 1981; Vroom and Pahl, 1971; Wallach and Kogan, 1961). For example, an "elderly man with eyesight becoming progressively worse has near blindness to look forward to at a later date. He has to decide about an eye operation which will result in restored vision if successful, or blindness if not" (Botwinick, 1966). Participants were asked to indicate the probability of success they would require before selecting the desired but risky alternative. Compared with younger adults, older adults were more likely to indicate they would not choose the risky alternative (having an eye operation) no matter what the probabilities (for a review see Okun, 1976). This appears to be the result of decision avoidance, because in a subsequent study in which participants were not given the option of totally avoiding the decisions, there were no age differences in how cautious people said they would be (Botwinick, 1969). A similar questionnaire assessed how people deal with uncertainty about risk for medical procedures (Curley, Eraker, and Yates, 1984). This questionnaire, administered to patients in hospital waiting rooms, revealed that uncertainty about the chances of success for a treatment affected younger and older adults' decisions in the same way. Thus, both when gambling and when deciding on a course of action in a hypothetical scenario, there do not appear to be age differences in risk taking. Perceptions of risk also do not seem to change with age. For example, after reading a vignette about a woman facing a decision about estrogen replacement therapy, estimates of the risk of the therapy did not differ for younger and older participants (Zwahr, Park, and Shifren, 1999). There is also a lack of change in perceptions of risk between adolescence and adulthood, despite stereotypes that adolescents see themselves as invulnerable (Beyth-Marom, Laurel, Fischhoff, Palmgren, and Quadrel, 1993; Quadrel, Fischhoff, and Davis, 1993).

In summary, this pattern of little or no age differences in risky decisions runs counter to popular beliefs that older adults are less likely to make risky decisions. Furthermore, the choice dilemma studies reveal an interesting age difference—older adults appear to be more reluctant than younger adults to make decisions in the first place.

Deciding Whether to Decide

In everyday life, when faced with a decision between two options, people often actually have a third option available to them: they can choose to not make a decision (Anderson, 2003). The choice dilemmas described in the preceding section suggest that older adults are more likely to avoid making a decision than younger adults (Okun, 1976). This tendency toward decision avoidance (or delegation) has been revealed in other studies as well. When faced with medical decisions, older adults are more likely than younger adults to indicate that they would rather not make the decisions themselves, instead leaving them up to the doctor (Cassileth, Zupkis,

Sutton-Smith, and March, 1980; Curley et al., 1984; Ende, Kazis, Ash, and Moskowitz, 1989; Steginga and Occhipinti, 2002). Similarly, older adults were more likely than younger adults to say they preferred not to have the responsibility for choosing a Medicare health plan (Finucane et al., 2002). Because many medical decisions are framed as a choice to take action (have surgery, take medication, etc.) or not, avoiding a decision can have the same result as deciding not to undergo treatment.

Researchers in Canada who were puzzled by the underutilization of total joint arthroplasty (a treatment for arthritis) provided an interesting example of decision avoidance (Hudak et al., 2002). They wondered why only 10 percent of older adults who were willing to consider total joint arthroplasty and were categorized as perfect clinical candidates for the treatment chose to have it. Interviews revealed that, instead of actually deciding against the treatment, the older adults tended to defer the decision until some undetermined later date. Thus, what appeared on the surface to be a decision was actually just an unwillingness to finalize the decision, making older adults appear to be risk avoidant.

This tendency to avoid decisions is somewhat puzzling, given that older adults appear to assess risk in a similar fashion to younger adults. Why is the act of decision making less attractive for older adults? One explanation may be found in the link between decision avoidance and emotion regulation. Among younger adults, the option of not making a decision at all is particularly attractive when the decision is emotion laden. For example, Beattie, Baron, Hershey, and Spranca (1994) asked participants to imagine that they had two children who both have an unusual disease and will die immediately without a bone marrow transplant. Participants rated the scenario in which they had to choose which child to donate their bone marrow to as less desirable than scenarios in which their bone marrow matched that of only one of the children and so they did not have to choose between their children. In general, the desire to avoid making a decision increases as the conflict between various options increases. For example, people are more likely to purchase a compact disc player if they find one attractive option on sale than if they find two attractive options on sale (Tversky and Shafir, 1992).

Does avoiding a decision make people feel upset by the lack of resolution? Quite the contrary—at least in the short run. People feel better after deciding *not* to make a decision in conflict-laden situations. When faced with a high-conflict decision, people who choose either not to make a decision or to stick with the status quo report less negative affect than people who choose other options (Luce, 1998). In addition, people who experience the most negative affect while considering options are most likely to decide to stick with the status quo (Luce, 1998).

A study examining problem-solving styles across the life span suggests that the emotional nature of problem situations becomes more salient as people age (Blanchard-Fields, Camp, and Casper Jahnke, 1995). In this study, participants read vignettes about problem situations and wrote essays about how they should be resolved. The vignettes varied in their level of emotional salience. For example, the following was a vignette with low emotional salience: "A father has a 16-year-old daughter who keeps taking his car several times a week. The family only has one car. What should he do?" The following was a vignette with high emotional salience: "A woman is married to an alcoholic. She feels no emotional support from the marriage. They lost their house and car. She has three children aged 3, 7, and 10 years. What should she do?" For scenarios with low and medium emotional salience, older adults were less likely than younger adults to suggest problem-focused action, such as self-initiated behaviors that would alter the situation. For such scenarios, older adults were more likely than younger adults to suggest strategies that avoided doing anything directly about the problem. For example, they might propose ways to suppress one's emotions or attend to things other than the problem situation. When confronted with problems with high emotional salience, younger adults' problem-solving strategies became more like those of the older adults, whereas older adults' strategies did not change much across the various levels of emotional salience. This pattern suggests that emotion is more likely to be a salient aspect of situations for older adults—and therefore their decision strategies are more likely to reflect emotion-focused processes, including attempts to avoid making a decision.

Although avoiding decisions may help regulate emotions in the short run, there are, of course, downsides. Avoiding decisions can lead to negative consequences when action is called for. An interesting point when considering age differences is that the negative consequences of decision avoidance often do not become apparent immediately but instead emerge over time. In the short run, actions are more likely to be regretted than inactions (Gilovich and Medvec, 1995). In contrast, in the long run, it is inactions that generate the most regret. For example, "Why did I choose to have dinner at such an expensive restaurant?" might indicate regret about a recent action, whereas "Why didn't I decide to buy real estate before the market took off?" is a regret about inaction over the past several decades. In further research, the influence of one's likely future perspective on the attractiveness of a decision should be examined. It may be that older adults prefer not to make stressful decisions because the possibility of near-term regret weighs more heavily than the possibility of distant-future regret.

Alternatively, it could be that older adults just don't trust themselves to make good decisions and therefore avoid making decisions when they can. In one study, older adults rated themselves as less analytical and more intuitive in their decision style (Finucane et al., 2002). This self-perception seems to accurately reflect the decline in executive processes mediated by the dorsolateral prefrontal cortex and the increased influence of emotional processes. In particular, older adults might be less confident than younger adults about their skills in certain domains. For example, making medical decisions may be particularly difficult for older adults because their generation was trained to believe that only doctors had the expertise to make such decisions. Yet active participation in medical decisions appears to have beneficial consequences, such as improved treatment effectiveness and lower postoperative depression (Zwahr, 1999).

Seeking Information

In everyday life, it often takes some effort to learn about the characteristics of choice options. The degree to which people seek information about their decision options varies widely. For example, to get a new refrigerator, some people might go into the nearest store that sells them and buy the least expensive one that is the right size. Others might seek more information by reading reviews and visiting several stores. Older adults' reduced working memory capacity may make it more difficult for them to hold multiple pieces of information in mind in order to make comparisons. This reduced capacity may lead them to seek less information when making a decision.

Consistent with this possibility, a number of studies have found that older adults seek less information than do younger adults when making decisions or solving problems. For example, Streufert, Pogash, Piasecki, and Post (1990) recruited mid-level managers to participate in an all-day group decision-making simulation and found that teams composed of older managers made fewer requests for additional information than younger teams and also made fewer decisions overall. Zwahr et al. (1999) found that, after reading a vignette about a medical decision, younger adults were more likely to decide to seek a second opinion or gather more information than were older adults. Older adults were more likely to select the proposed treatment or take no action. This suggests that when people do not make an immediate decision, younger adults might be postponing it to seek out additional information whereas older adults may simply be avoiding making the decision. A similar pattern of older adults requesting less information than younger adults while making medical decisions is seen in other studies (Ende et al., 1989; Leventhal, Leventhal, Schaefer, and Easterling, 1993; Meyer, Russo, and Talbot, 1995) and also extends to everyday problem solving (Berg, Meegan, and Klaczynski, 1999). Two studies examining decision information search patterns using a decision grid found that older adults examined less information in hypothetical decisions about purchasing a car and renting an apartment (Johnson, 1990, 1993).

One exception to the general pattern of reduced information seeking with age is a study in which tape recordings were made of patients interacting with their physicians (Beisecker and Beisecker, 1990). Hierarchical regression analyses revealed that older adults were more likely to make information-seeking comments than younger adults. Scores from scales measuring locus of authority and desire for information were entered first in the regression analysis, however, and so it is not clear whether a similar pattern would be seen without first accounting for these variables.

Although decreased working memory capacity may be an explanation for older adults' reduced information seeking, it remains to be tested fully. For example, do younger adults under divided attention conditions seek less information while making decisions? Would older adults seek more information if they had some sort of external memory aid so that they did not have to hold it all in mind at once? Johnson (1997) investigated the impact of a memory aid on information seeking during decision making but, since the control condition in her experiment did not replicate previous findings of age differences in information seeking, the findings are difficult to interpret. Further investigation is needed to understand whether reduced working memory capacity might be the cause of seeking less information.

Are age-related changes in emotional processes likely to have an impact on information seeking as well? There are some intriguing indications that they might. Older adults examining information in a decision grid in order to make a hypothetical choice among various cars spent a greater proportion of their time viewing positive features and a smaller proportion of their time viewing negative features than did younger adults (Mather, Knight, and McCaffrey, 2005). This finding suggests that some of older adults' reduced information-seeking tendencies might occur only in contexts where most of the available information is negative.

Age differences in emotional goals might also influence the strategies that people use to compare the various options in choices. There are a number of different strategies for comparing all of the various pieces of information involved in a choice. One possibility is the weighted additive strategy, which involves considering each alternative sequentially, multiplying each feature value (e.g., health plan A's value for location, cost, etc.) by the importance weight for that feature and then summing all the weighted values to compute an overall value for each alternative. The alternative with the highest overall value should be chosen. In this alternative-based strategy, an alternative's poor value for one feature can be compensated for by its good value for another feature. Other, often simpler, strategies involve making comparisons of features across alternatives. For example, one might choose the option with the best value on the most important feature (Tversky, 1969). That is, one might take the health plan with the lowest cost, regardless of how much coverage it promises or where its nearest clinic is located. Another feature-based strategy is to eliminate options that do not meet a minimum cutoff value for the most important feature, followed by eliminating those that do not meet the minimum for the second most important feature, and so on until only one option remains (Tversky, 1972). In these feature-based strategies, an option's good value on one feature cannot make up for its poor value on another feature. Thus the decision maker does not have to make explicit trade-offs between features.

Johnson (1990) found that older adults tended to use a feature-based strategy more than younger adults did when examining information about choice options. In Johnson's study, participants were shown a decision grid with concealed information about six cars. Comparative information was available for each car for nine different aspects, such as fuel economy and safety record. Each piece of information could be accessed by selecting its box in the grid. Younger adults tended to examine all the information about one car before shifting to examine information about another car. In contrast, older adults tended to examine all the information corresponding to a particular dimension (e.g., fuel economy information about each car) before shifting to examine information about another dimension.

A possible explanation for these results that was not suggested by Johnson is that these age differences are due to changes in the extent to which people engage in emotion regulation strategies. Luce et al. (1997) hypothesize that people cope with emotionally threatening decisions by altering their processing to reduce the amount of negative emotion experienced. Making explicit trade-offs between features is one of the most emotionally unpleasant aspects of decision processing. These trade-offs (e.g., taking a job that is farther away because it pays better) call attention to potential losses. In contrast, comparing the features across several alternatives reduces the salience of the fact that one feature must be given up in order to maximize another feature. Indeed, Luce et al. (1997) found that as decision tasks became more inherently emotion laden, participants shifted away from an alternative-based strategy to a feature-based strategy. In addition, this shift in strategies was not simply a result of reduced effort under emotional conditions. On the contrary, when presented with more emotional decisions, participants actually spent *more* time examining the features.

Interestingly, Johnson's frequently cited (1990) findings of age differences in search strategies have been difficult to replicate. Two subsequent studies by Johnson herself using similar materials (Johnson, 1993, 1997) and a study by Hartley (1990) found no age differences in search strategies. A recent study suggests these failures to replicate may be explained by individual difference factors (Mather et al., 2005). Participants in this study completed several tests associated with executive processes/frontal lobe function (the tasks tapped processes such as the ability to switch strategies and the ability to hold multiple pieces of information in mind) and were asked to make the same choice among cars that Johnson (1990) used. The older adults who did best on the executive function tasks (and therefore those best equipped to implement goals, including emotion regulation goals) were more likely to use feature-based decision comparison strategies. These findings suggest that older adults with the least decline in higher-order cognitive abilities may be the ones most likely to engage in strategies that help regulate emotion, such as feature-based comparison to decrease decision conflict. (For further discussion of the link between cognitive control and emotional regulation, see Mather and Carstensen, 2005.)

Repeated Decisions

It is hard to learn from past decisions unless one can gauge how effective they were. People tend to be overconfident when judging the quality of their own decisions (Lichtenstein and Fischhoff, 1977), but little is known about whether there are age differences in confidence about decisions. Several studies provide some initial evidence but it is somewhat contradictory. In a study in which participants were asked to come up with solutions for legal and financial problems, most of the older adults overestimated how many problems they had solved correctly (Devolder, 1993). In contrast, most younger adults underestimated how many problems they had solved correctly, a surprising finding given people's general tendency to be overconfident about their decisions. In another study, participants were asked to determine how much money a hypothetical person should contribute to his or her retirement savings plan, based on information about that person's financial situation (Hershey and Wilson, 1997). Younger adults appeared to be overconfident about their solutions unless they had completed a financial planning workshop, in which case they were underconfident. As a group, older adults did not appear to be overconfident or underconfident, either with or without the knowledge gained from the workshop. However, the results from this study are hard to interpret because participants each made only one rating on a scale of 1-7 to indicate how poor or good they thought the overall quality of their six solutions was. It would be interesting to repeat the study and then have participants estimate the dollar value of the discrepancy between their solution and the optimal solution.

Two studies that did not directly examine decision making also provide contradictory findings about people's confidence in their decision making. In both studies, participants were asked to rate their confidence in answers to general knowledge or trivia questions such as "Which city is farther north: (a) London or (b) New York?" In one study, older adults were just as overconfident in their responses as younger adults (Pliske and Mutter, 1996). However, in a second study, older adults made more extreme responses of "don't know" or "I'm sure" rather than intermediate confidence ratings (Kovalchik et al., 2005). In this study, older adults were also less overconfident than younger adults when they did give an intermediate confidence rating.

Two studies investigating age differences in memory for choices suggest that older adults may be more likely to repeatedly choose the same options because their memories are biased in favor of their past choices (Mather and Carstensen, 2004; Mather and Johnson, 2000). In these studies, participants made a series of two-option hypothetical choices, for example, between two job candidates or between two treatments for an illness. Each option was described with both positive and negative features. Later, participants were asked to make memory attributions about features from the previously considered choice options (e.g., does "easily discouraged" describe the first job candidate, the second job candidate, or is it a new feature?). In both studies, older adults were more likely than younger adults to have choice-supportive biases in their memory attributions. That is, they were more likely to attribute (and misattribute) positive features to chosen options than to rejected options—and more likely to attribute (and misattribute) negative features to rejected options than to chosen options.

This age difference in how much memory favors chosen options is not simply due to poorer memory among older adults; when older adults are tested after a shorter delay than younger adults to equate their overall accuracy, their memories are still more choice supportive than those of younger adults. In addition, when given a free recall test, older adults were more likely than younger adults to selectively remember the good things about chosen options and the bad things about rejected options (Mather and Carstensen, 2004). In everyday life, choices quite often involve options that have previously been chosen or rejected, such as entrees on a restaurant menu or items in a grocery store. Thus, because they are more likely to remember their choices favorably relative to forgone options, it is possible that older adults will be more likely than younger adults to repeatedly choose the same options. Remembering past choices in a favorable light should help people feel good. Thus, it may be older adults' greater focus on regulating emotion that leads to their choice supportive biases. Consistent with this possibility, if younger adults are asked to think about their feelings and reactions after making a choice, their later memories are as choice supportive as those of older adults who are not explicitly focused on emotion (Mather and Johnson, 2000).

Susceptibility to Scams

Although so far in this paper I have discussed decision making on an individual level, quite often there is social pressure to make certain decisions. It is particularly important to be able to identify and resist such pressure when it comes from someone attempting a scam. Older adults are frequently the target of scams, especially over the phone. One estimate is that over half of the targets for telemarketing scams were 50 or older (American Association of Retired Persons Foundation, 2003). Declines in memory and other cognitive abilities may increase older adults' susceptibility to such scams. For example, Jacoby (1999) describes a scam in which the perpetrator phones an older adult and elicits as much personal information as possible. Then in a callback the scammer asks questions based on the first phone call and, if the older adult fails to remember the previous conversation, the perpetrator makes a false claim about an earlier event. For example, he or she might claim to have received a check that was an overpayment and request a check for a lower amount. Because older adults appear to be more likely to be misled by false information in eyewitness testimony paradigms (Cohen and Faulkner, 1989; Mitchell, Johnson, and Mather, 2003), it seems possible that they are also more susceptible than younger adults to scams that make false suggestions about their past actions, although this possibility has not been tested.

The American Association of Retired Persons (AARP) recently conducted several studies to try to understand the personality and demographic characteristics associated with susceptibility to phone scams and to test various interventions to decrease susceptibility (AARP Foundation, 2003). Several hundred victims of one of two types of phone scams (a Canadian lottery scam in which victims were told they had won the Canadian lottery but needed to pay taxes to collect their winnings, or a movie investment scam involving the "next box office hit") were identified from lists seized by the Federal Bureau of Investigation and the California Department of Corporations. A nationally representative sample of adults aged 45 or older served as a control group.

The study revealed very different demographic characteristics for the lottery and the investment victims. Lottery victims averaged 74.5 years of age, were predominantly female, and typically had an income under $30,000. In contrast, investment victims tended to be under the age of 65 and male with incomes over $75,000. In addition, the investment victims' level of Internet use and level of education were greater than those of the general population. Thus, the first striking finding from this study is that there is no single demographic profile for older victims of phone scams; the profile varies widely depending on the type of scam. The report points out that "good con artists invest a lot of time figuring out which kinds of people are most vulnerable to which kinds of scams" (AARP Foundation, 2003, p. A-22). Personality questionnaires also revealed no defining characteristics of fraud victims in general. In fact, in some cases the two victim groups differed from the general population in opposite ways. For example, the lottery victims were more conforming and willing to go along with the crowd than the control group, whereas investment victims were less conforming.

In a separate series of studies conducted in collaboration with Anthony Pratkanis, an expert on persuasion, the AARP group used a "reverse boiler room" technique to try to reduce susceptibility to fraud. Trained volunteers called victims and potential victims from telemarketers' call lists and gave them information about telemarketing fraud. Control participants from the same sample population were called and simply asked about their favorite television program. A few days later, participants received a telephone solicitation and the response rate to this mock phone scam was measured. The results indicated that warning people about phone scams, getting them to generate advice for others about avoiding it, and demonstrating how easily they could fall prey to a scam were all effective techniques. On average, these techniques reduced susceptibility to mock telemarketing scams by about half.

The AARP research did not examine any cognitive variables and so does not provide any information about how cognitive decline might contribute to susceptibility to fraud. But the finding that some scams are actually more likely to work on middle-aged people with above-average education than on older adults in general indicates that cognitive decline cannot be a global explanation for why people become victims of fraud. Although the fact that the risk factors vary widely depending on the type of fraud makes addressing the problem more complex, it is good news for older adults that they are not necessarily the group most likely to fall for a scam.

CONCLUSION

When it comes to making decisions, older adults feel relatively confident about their abilities. When asked whether they expected to have problems making decisions as they got older, 37 percent of respondents between the ages of 35 and 49 said yes, whereas only 6 percent of the older adults said they have problems making decisions (Princeton Survey Research, 1998). Older adults' confidence in their decisions is mostly supported by the existing literature. With age, there are a number of things that change about the way people make decisions, but these changes often either lead to the same decisions (Johnson, 1990; Meyer et al., 1995; Stanley, Guido, Stanley, and Shortell, 1984; Walker, Fain, Fisk, and McGuire, 1997) or result in only subtle differences in the decisions made (Finucane et al., 2002). Under some experimental conditions, older adults make objectively better decisions than younger adults (Tentori, Osherson, Hasher, and May, 2001). Many studies have examined the decision-making competence of older adults to complete informed consent in medical contexts. While patients with dementia show impairments (for a review see Fitten, 1999), healthy older adults' decisions tend to be as reasonable as those made by younger adults (Fitten, Lusky, and Hamann, 1990; Marson, Ingram, Schmitt, and Harrell, 1994; Stanley et al., 1984). The most notable age difference is that older adults have poorer comprehension of medical treatments (Christensen, Haroun, Schneiderman, and Jeste, 1995; Sugarman, McCrory, and Hubal, 1998).

At the outset of this paper, I suggested that the pattern of changes in emotional processes and changes in the prefrontal brain region might explain why some aspects of decision making change with age while others do not. The evidence I reviewed suggests that when older adults do make decisions, they evaluate risk just as well as younger adults. The ability to weigh future consequences appropriately and not be driven solely by present gain requires an intact orbitofrontal cortex. Further research should help resolve whether the sparing of this particular region of the prefrontal cortex in aging can explain why the way that people deal with risky decisions does not change much with age. Instead, many of the changes in the way people make decisions appear to be subtle and may be related to changes in executive functioning and emotional processing.

Although older adults tend to evaluate risk in the same way as younger adults when they make decisions, they nevertheless appear to be risk avoidant because they avoid making decisions. Not taking risks that one should take, such as undergoing a potentially useful medical procedure that has some risks, can cause serious problems. Older adults' reluctance to make decisions may mean that they do not take appropriate risks. Among the decision processes discussed in this paper, this reluctance to make decisions is probably the age difference with the most significant consequences. Not making decisions can help people avoid conflict and negative emotions in the present, but it can also lead to missed opportunities as well as a greater risk of untreated disease. Of interest for future research is whether older adults' reluctance to make decisions stems from reduced confidence in their decision-making abilities, from reduced executive functioning that makes planning and executing decisions more difficult, or from a desire to avoid the negative emotions associated with making decisions.

Another age-related change that consistently appears across many studies is reduced information seeking when making a decision. It should be noted that there is no clear correlation between the amount of information sought and the quality of decisions. In some cases, seeking less information is simply an indication that one has more knowledge about the domain and so needs less input in order to decide. A question for future research is whether older adults seek less information because they have reduced working memory capacity or because they have different goals than younger adults do. Research has also revealed age differences in the way that people remember past decisions. These age-related patterns of memory bias may lead to consequences for choices that involve previously experienced options.

Although the field of aging and decision making has advanced to the point where it is possible to identify patterns of age differences that consistently appear across various studies, it is clear that more work is needed in order to explain these differences and to investigate their consequences. Particularly promising avenues for future research are the hypotheses that, compared with younger adults, older adults (1) rely more on emotional than on analytical processing to make decisions and (2) try to avoid negative affect when making decisions.

AUTHOR'S NOTE

Preparation of this report was supported in part by NSF Grant 0112284 and by NIA Grant 1R01AG025340-01A1. I thank George Loewenstein, Melissa Finucane, and Noah Mercer for their comments on earlier versions.

REFERENCES

American Association of Retired Persons Foundation. (2003). *Reducing participation in telemarketing fraud*. Washington, DC: Author.

Anderson, C.J. (2003). The psychology of doing nothing: Forms of decision avoidance result from reason and emotion. *Psychological Bulletin, 129*, 139-167.

Bakshi, G.S., and Chen, Z.W. (1994). Baby boom, population aging, and capital markets. *Journal of Business, 67*, 165-202.

Bartzokis, G., Cummings, J.L., Sultzer, D., Henderson, V.W., Nuechterlein, K.H., and Mintz, J. (2003). White matter integrity in healthy aging adults and patients with Alzheimer's disease: A magnetic resonance imaging study. *Archives of Neurology, 60*, 393-398.

Beattie, J., Baron, J., Hershey, J.C., and Spranca, M.D. (1994). Psychological determinants of decision attitude. *Journal of Behavioral Decision Making, 7*, 129-144.

Bechara, A., Damasio, A.R., Damasio, H., and Anderson, S.W. (1994). Insensitivity to future consequences following damage to human prefrontal cortex. *Cognition, 50*, 7-15.

Bechara, A., Damasio, H., Tranel, D., and Anderson, S.W. (1998). Dissociation of working memory from decision making within the human prefrontal cortex. *Journal of Neuroscience, 18*, 428-437.

Bechara, A., Tranel, D., and Damasio, H. (2000a). Characterization of the decision-making deficit of patients with ventromedial prefrontal cortex lesions. *Brain, 123*, 2189-2202.

Bechara, A., Tranel, D., and Damasio, A.R. (2000b). Poor judgment in spite of high intellect: Neurological evidence for emotional intelligence. In R. Bar-On and J.D.A. Parker (Eds.), *The handbook of emotional intelligence: Theory, development, assessment, and application at home, school, and in the workplace* (pp. 192-214). San Francisco: Jossey-Bass.

Bechara, A., Tranel, D., Damasio, H., and Damasio, A.R. (1996). Failure to respond autonomically to anticipated future outcomes following damage to prefrontal cortex. *Cerebral Cortex, 6*, 215-225.

Beisecker, A.E., and Beisecker, T.D. (1990). Patient information-seeking behaviors when communicating with doctors. *Medical Care, 28*, 19-28.

Bell, D.E. (1982). Regret in decision making under uncertainty. *Operations Research, 30*, 961-981.

Berg, C.A., Meegan, S.P., and Klaczynski, P. (1999). Age and experiential differences in strategy generation and information requests for solving everyday problems. *International Journal of Behavioral Development, 23*, 615-639.

Beyth-Marom, R., Laurel, A., Fischhoff, B., Palmgren, C., and Quadrel, M. (1993). Perceived consequences of risky behavior: Adolescents and adults. *Developmental Psychology, 29*, 549-563.

Blanchard-Fields, F., Camp, C., and Casper Jahnke, H. (1995). Age differences in problem-solving style: The role of emotional salience. *Psychology and Aging, 10*, 173-180.

Botwinick, J. (1966). Cautiousness in advanced old age. *Journal of Gerontology, 21*, 347-353.

Botwinick, J. (1969). Disinclination to venture responses vs. cautiousness in responding: Age differences. *Journal of Genetic Psychology, 115*, 55-62.

Breiter, H.C., Aharon, I., Kahneman, D., Dale, A., and Shizgal, P. (2001). Functional imaging of neural responses to expectancy and experience of monetary gains and losses. *Neuron, 30*, 619-639.

Brouthers, K.D., Brouthers, L.E., and Werner, S. (2000). Influences on strategic decision-making in the Dutch financial services industry. *Journal of Management, 26*, 863-883.

Calhoun, R.E., and Hutchison, S.L.J. (1981). Decision-making in old age: Cautiousness and rigidity. *International Journal of Aging and Human Development, 13*, 89-97.

Carstensen, L.L., Isaacowitz, D.M., and Charles, S.T. (1999). Taking time seriously: A theory of socioemotional selectivity. *American Psychologist, 54*, 165-181.

Carstensen, L.L., Pasupathi, M., Mayr, U., and Nesselroade, J.R. (2000). Emotional experience in everyday life across the adult life span. *Journal of Personality and Social Psychology, 79*, 644-655.

Cassileth, B.R., Zupkis, R.V., Sutton-Smith, K., and March, V. (1980). Information and participation preferences among cancer patients. *Annals of Internal Medicine, 92*, 832-836.

Charles, S.T., Mather, M., and Carstensen, L.L. (2003). Aging and emotional memory: The forgettable nature of negative images for older adults. *Journal of Experimental Psychology: General, 132*, 310-324.

Charles, S.T., Reynolds, C.A., and Gatz, M. (2001). Age-related differences and change in positive and negative affect over 23 years. *Journal of Personality and Social Psychology, 80*, 136-151.

Chaubey, N.P. (1974). Effect of age on expectancy of success and on risk-taking behavior. *Journal of Personality and Social Psychology, 29*, 774-778.

Christensen, K., Haroun, A., Schneiderman, L.J., and Jeste, D.V. (1995). Decision-making capacity for informed consent in the older population. *Bulletin of the American Academy of Psychiatry and the Law, 23*, 353-365.

Coffey, C.E., Wilkenson, W.E., Parashos, I.A., Soady, S.A., Sullivan, R.J., Patterson, L.J., Figiel, G.S., Webb, M.C., Spritzer, C.E., and Djang, W.T. (1992). Quantitative cerebral anatomy of the aging human brain: A cross-sectional study using magnetic resonance imaging. *Neurology, 42*, 527-536.

Cohen, G., and Faulkner, D. (1989). Age differences in source forgetting: Effects on reality monitoring and on eyewitness testimony. *Psychology and Aging, 4*, 10-17.

Cohen, J.D., Perlstein, W.M., Braver, T.S., Nystrom, L.E., Noll, D.C., Jonides, J., and Smith, E.E. (1997). Temporal dynamics of brain activation during a working memory task. *Nature, 386*(6625), 604-608.

Cowell, P.E., Turetsky, B.I., Gur, R.C., Grossman, R.I., Shtasel, D.L., and Gur, R.E. (1994). Sex differences in aging of the human frontal and temporal lobes. *Journal of Neuroscience, 14*, 4748-4755.

Curley, S.P., Eraker, S.A., and Yates, J.F. (1984). An investigation of patients' reactions to therapeutic uncertainty. *Medical Decision Making, 4*, 501-511.

Daigneault, S., and Braun, C.M.J. (1993). Working memory and the self-ordered pointing task: Further evidence of early prefrontal decline in normal aging. *Journal of Clinical and Experimental Neuropsychology, 15*, 881-895.

Damasio, A.R. (1994). *Descartes' error: Emotion, reason, and the human brain.* New York: Grosset/Putnam.

Damasio, H., Grabowski, T., Frank, R., Galaburda, A.M., and Damasio, A.R. (1994). The return of Phineas Gage: Clues about the brain from the skull of a famous patient. *Science, 264*, 1102-1105.

DeCarli, C., Murphy, D.G., Gillette, J.A., Haxby, J.V., Teichberg, D., Schapiro, M.B., and Horwitz, B. (1994). Lack of age-related differences in temporal lobe volume of very healthy adults. *American Journal of Neuroradiology, 15*(4), 689-696.

Denburg, N.L., Tranel, D., Bechara, A., and Damasio, A.R. (2001). Normal aging may compromise the ability to decide advantageously. *Brain and Cognition, 47*, 156-185.

D'Esposito, M., Detre, J.A., Alsop, D.C., Shin, R.K., Atlas, S., and Grossman, M. (1995). The neural basis of the central executive system of working memory. *Nature, 16*, 279-281.

Devolder, P.A. (1993). Adult age differences in monitoring of practical problem-solving performance. *Experimental Aging Research, 19*, 129-146.

Dror, I.E., Katona, M., and Mungur, K. (1998). Age differences in decision making: To take a risk or not? *Gerontology, 44*, 67-71.

Dulebohn, J.H. (2002). An investigation of the determinants of investment risk behavior in employer-sponsored retirement plans. *Journal of Management, 28*, 3-26.

Elliott, R., Dolan, R.J., and Frith, C.D. (2000). Dissociable functions in the medial and lateral orbitofrontal cortex: Evidence from human neuroimaging studies. *Cerebral Cortex, 10*, 308-317.

Elliott, R., Friston, K.J., and Dolan, R.J. (2000). Dissociable neural responses in human reward systems. *Journal of Neuroscience, 20*, 6159-6165.

Elliott, R., Newman, J.L., Longe, O.A., and Deakin, J.F.W. (2003). Differential response patterns in the striatum and orbitofrontal cortex to financial reward in humans: A parametric functional magnetic resonance imaging study. *Journal of Neuroscience, 23*, 303-307.

Ende, J., Kazis, L., Ash, A., and Moskowitz, M.A. (1989). Measuring patients' desire for autonomy: Decision-making and information-seeking preferences among medical patients. *Journal of General Internal Medicine, 4*, 23-30.

Eslinger, P., and Damasio, A.R. (1985). Severe disturbance of higher cognition after bilateral frontal lobe ablation: Patient EVR. *Neurology, 35*, 1731-1741.

Finucane, M.L., Alhakami, A., Slovic, P., and Johnson, S.M. (2000). The affect heuristic in judgments of risks and benefits. *Journal of Behavioral Decision Making, 13*, 1-17.

Finucane, M.L., Slovic, P., Hibbard, J.H., Peters, E., Mertz, C.K., and MacGregor, D.G. (2002). Aging and decision-making competence: An analysis of comprehension and consistency skills in older versus younger adults considering health-plan options. *Journal of Behavioral Decision Making, 15*, 141-164.

Fitten, L.J. (1999). Frontal lobe dysfunction and patient decision making about treatment and participation in research. In B.L. Miller and J.L. Cummings (Eds.), *The human frontal lobes* (pp. 277-287). New York: Guilford Press.

Fitten, L.J., Lusky, R., and Hamann, C. (1990). Assessing treatment decision-making capacity in elderly nursing home residents. *Journal of the American Geriatric Society, 38*, 1097-1104.

Fredrickson, B.L., and Carstensen, L.L. (1990). Choosing social partners: How old age and anticipated endings make people more selective. *Psychology and Aging, 5*, 335-347.

Fung, H.H., Carstensen, L.L., and Lutz, A.M. (1999). Influence of time on social preferences: Implications for life-span development. *Psychology and Aging, 14*, 595-604.

Fung, H.H., Lai, P., and Ng, R. (2001). Age differences in social preferences among Taiwanese and mainland Chinese: The role of perceived time. *Psychology and Aging, 16*, 351-356.

Gilovich, T., and Medvec, V.H. (1995). The experience of regret: What, when, and why. *Psychological Review, 102*, 379-395.

Goel, V., Grafman, J., Tajik, J., Gana, S., and Danto, D. (1998). A study of the performance of patients with frontal lobe lesions in a financial planning task. *Brain, 120*, 1805-1822.

Grable, J.E. (2000). Financial risk tolerance and additional factors that affect risk taking in everyday money matters. *Journal of Business and Psychology, 14*, 625-630.

Green, L., Myerson, J., Lichtman, D., Rosen, S., and Fry, A. (1996). Temporal discounting in choice between delayed rewards: The role of age and income. *Psychology and Aging, 11*, 79-84.

Gross, J.J., Carstensen, L.L., Pasupathi, M., Tsai, J., Skorpen, C.G., and Hsu, A.Y.C. (1997). Emotion and aging: Experience, expression, and control. *Psychology and Aging, 12*, 590-599.

Hartley, A.A. (1990). The cognitive ecology of problem solving. In L.W. Poon, D.C. Rubin, and B.A. Wilson (Eds.), *Everyday cognition in adulthood and late life* (pp. 300-329). Cambridge, England: Cambridge University Press.

Hershey, D.A., and Wilson, J.A. (1997). Age differences in performance awareness on a complex financial decision-making task. *Experimental Aging Research, 23*, 257-273.

Hertzog, C., Lineweaver, T.T., and McGuire, C.L. (1999). Beliefs about memory and aging. In F. Blanchard-Fields and T.M. Hess (Eds.), *Social cognition and aging* (pp. 43-68). New York: Academic Press.

Hudak, P.L., Clark, J.P., Hawker, G.A., Coyte, P.C., Mahomed, N.N., Kreder, H.J., and Wright, J.G. (2002). "You're perfect for the procedure! Why don't you want it?" Elderly arthritis patients' unwillingness to consider total joint arthroplasty surgery: A qualitative study. *Medical Decision Making, 22*(3), 272-278.

Isen, A.M. (2001). An influence of positive affect on decision making in complex situations: Theoretical issues with practical implications. *Journal of Consumer Psychology, 11*, 75-85.

Isen, A.M., Nygren, T.E., and Ashby, F.G. (1988). Influence of positive affect on the subject utility of gains and losses: It is just not worth the risk. *Journal of Personality and Social Psychology, 55*, 710-717.

Jacoby, L.L. (1999). Deceiving the elderly: Effects of accessibility bias in cued-recall performance. *Cognitive Neuropsychology, 16*, 417-436.

Jianakoplos, N.A., and Bernasek, A. (1998). Are women more risk averse? *Economic Inquiry, 36*, 620-630.

Johnson, M.M.S. (1990). Age differences in decision making: A process methodology for examining strategic information processing. *Journal of Gerontology: Psychological Sciences, 45*(2), P75-P78.

Johnson, M.M.S. (1993). Thinking about strategies during, before, and after making a decision. *Psychology and Aging, 8*, 231-241.

Johnson, M.M.S. (1997). Individual differences in the voluntary use of a memory aid during decision making. *Experimental Aging Research, 23*, 33-43.

Josephs, R.A., Larrick, R.P., Steele, C.M., and Nisbett, R.E. (1992). Protecting the self from the negative consequences of risky decisions. *Journal of Personality and Social Psychology, 62*, 26-37.

Kennedy, Q., Mather, M., and Carstensen, L.L. (2004). The role of motivation in the age-related positivity effect in autobiographical memory. *Psychological Science, 15*, 208-214.

Kovalchik, S., Camerer, C.F., Grether, D.M., Plott, C.R., and Allman, J.M. (2005). Aging and decision making: A broad comparative study of decision behavior in neurologically healthy elderly and young individuals. *Journal of Economic Behavior and Organization.*

Krawczyk, D.C. (2002). Contributions of the prefrontal cortex to the neural basis of human decision making. *Neuroscience and Biobehavioral Reviews, 26*, 631-664.

Lang, F.R., and Carstensen, L.L. (1994). Close emotional relationships in late life: How personality and social context do (and do not) make a difference. *Psychology and Aging, 9*, 315-324.

Lawton, M.P., Kleban, M.H., and Dean, J. (1993). Affect and age: Cross-sectional comparisons of structure and prevalence. *Psychology and Aging, 8*, 165-175.

Lawton, M.P., Kleban, M.H., Rajagopal, D., and Dean, J. (1992). Dimensions of affective experience in three age groups. *Psychology and Aging, 7*, 171-184.

Lerner, J.S., Gonzalez, R.M., Small, D.A., and Fischhoff, B. (2003). Effects of fear and anger on perceived risks of terrorism: A national field experiment. *Psychological Science, 14*, 144-150.

Lerner, J.S., and Keltner, D. (2001). Fear, anger, and risk. *Journal of Personality and Social Psychology, 81*, 146-159.

Lerner, J.S., Small, D.A., and Loewenstein, G. (2004). Heart strings and purse strings: Carryover effects of emotions on economic decisions. *Psychological Science, 15*, 337-341.

Leventhal, E.A., Leventhal, H., Schaefer, P., and Easterling, D. (1993). Conservation of energy, uncertainty reduction, and swift utilization of medical care among the elderly. *Journal of Gerontology: Psychological Sciences, 48*, 78-86.

Lichtenstein, S., and Fischhoff, B. (1977). Do those who know more also know more about how much they know? *Organizational Behavior and Human Decision Processes, 20*, 159-183.

Loewenstein, G.F., and Lerner, J. (2000). The role of emotion in decision making. In R. Davidson, H. Goldsmith, and R. Scherer (Eds.), *Handbook of affective science*. Oxford, England: Oxford University Press.

Loewenstein, G.F., Weber, E.U., Hsee, C.K., and Welch, N. (2001). Risk as feelings. *Psychological Bulletin, 127*, 267-286.

Luce, M.F. (1998). Choosing to avoid: Coping with negatively emotion-laden consumer decisions. *Journal of Consumer Research, 24*, 409-433.

Luce, M.F., Bettman, J.R., and Payne, J.W. (1997). Choice processing in emotionally difficult decisions. *Journal of Experimental Psychology: Learning, Memory, and Cognition, 23*, 384-405.

Luce, M.F., Payne, J.W., and Bettman, J.R. (2000). Coping with unfavorable attribute values in choice. *Organizational Behavior and Human Decision Processes, 81*, 274-299.

MacPherson, S.E., Phillips, L.H., and Della Sala, S. (2002). Age, executive function, and social decision making: A dorsolateral prefrontal theory of cognitive aging. *Psychology and Aging, 17*, 598-609.

Marson, D.C., Ingram, K.K., Schmitt, F.A., and Harrell, L.E. (1994). Determining the competency of Alzheimer patients to consent to treatment and research. *Alzheimer Disease and Associated Disorders, 8*, 5-18.

Mather, M. (2004). Aging and emotional memory. In D. Reisberg and P. Hertel (Eds.), *Memory and emotion* (pp. 272-307). London, England: Oxford University Press.

Mather, M., Canli, T., English, T., Whitfield, S.L., Wais, P., Ochsner, K.N., Gabrieli, J.D.E., and Carstensen, L.L (2004). Amygdala responses to emotionally valenced stimuli in older and younger adults. *Psychological Science, 15*, 259-263.

Mather, M., and Carstensen, L.L. (2003). Aging and attentional biases for emotional faces. *Psychological Science, 14*, 409-415.

Mather, M., and Carstensen, L.L. (2004). *Implications of the positivity effect for older people's memories about health care decisions.* Unpublished manuscript, Psychology Department, University of California, Santa Cruz.

Mather, M., and Carstensen, L.L. (2005). Aging and motivated cognition: The positivity effect in attention and memory. *Trends in Cognitive Science, 9*, 496-502.

Mather, M., and Johnson, M.K. (2000). Choice-supportive source monitoring: Do our decisions seem better to us as we age? *Psychology and Aging, 15*, 596-606.

Mather, M., Knight, M., and McCaffrey, M. (2005). The allure of the alignable: False memories of choice features. *Journal of Experimental Psychology: General, 134*(1), 38-51.

McNeilly, D.P., and Burke, W.J. (2001). Gambling as a social activity of older adults. *International Journal of Aging and Human Development, 52*, 19-28.

Mellers, B.A., and McGraw, A.P. (2001). Anticipated emotions as guides to choice. *Current Directions in Psychological Science, 10*, 210-214.

Mellers, B.A., Schwartz, A., and Ritov, I. (1999). Emotion-based choice. *Journal of Experimental Psychology: General, 128*, 332-345.

Meyer, B.J.F., Russo, C., and Talbot, A. (1995). Discourse comprehension and problem solving: Decisions about the treatment of breast cancer by women across the lifespan. *Psychology and Aging, 10*, 84-103.

Mitchell, K.J., Johnson, M.K., and Mather, M. (2003). Source monitoring and suggestibility to misinformation: Adult age-related differences. *Applied Cognitive Psychology, 17*, 107-119.

Moscovitch, M., and Winocur, G. (1995). Frontal lobes, memory, and aging. *Annals of the New York Academy of Sciences, 769*, 119-150.

Mroczek, D.K. (2001). Age and emotion in adulthood. *Current Directions in Psychological Science, 10*, 87-90.

National Opinion Research Center. (1999). *Gambling impact and behavior study.* Chicago: Author.

Nygren, T.E., Isen, A.M., Taylor, P.J., and Dulin, J. (1996). The influence of positive affect on the decision rule in risk situations: Focus on the outcome (and especially avoidance of loss) rather than probability. *Organizational Behavior and Human Decision Processes, 66*, 59-72.

O'Doherty, J., Kringelbach, M.L., Rolls, E.T., Hornak, J., and Andrews, C. (2001). Abstract reward and punishment representations in the human orbitofrontal cortex. *Nature Neuroscience, 4*, 95-102.

Okun, M.A. (1976). Adult age and cautiousness in decision: A review of the literature. *Human Development, 19*, 220-233.

Peters, E., Finucane, M., MacGregor, D., and Slovic, P. (2000). The bearable lightness of aging: Judgment and decision processes in older adults. In National Research Council, *The aging mind: Opportunities in cognitive research* (pp. 144-165). Committee on Future Directions for Cognitive Research on Aging, P. Stern and L.L. Carstensen (Eds.). Board on Behavioral, Cognitive, and Sensory Sciences. Washington, DC: National Academy Press.

Phillips, L.H., and Della Sala, S. (1998). Aging, intelligence, and anatomical segregation in the frontal lobes. *Learning and Individual Differences, 10*, 217-243.

Pliske, R.M., and Mutter, S.A. (1996). Age differences in the accuracy of confidence judgments. *Experimental Aging Research, 22*, 199-216.

Princeton Survey Research. (1998). *Images of aging: A report of research findings from a national survey*. Princeton, NJ: Author.

Quadrel, M., Fischhoff, B., and Davis, W. (1993). Adolescent (in)vulnerability. *American Psychologist, 48*, 102-116.

Raz, N. (2000). Aging of the brain and its impact on cognitive performance: Integration of structural and functional findings. In F.I.M. Craik and T.A. Salthouse (Eds.), *Handbook of aging and cognition* (2nd ed.). Mahwah, NJ: Lawrence Erlbaum.

Raz, N., Gunning, F.M., Head, D., Dupuis, J.H., McQuain, J., Briggs, S.D., Loken, W.J., Thornton, A.E., and Acker, J.D. (1997). Selective aging of the human cerebral cortex observed in vivo: Differential vulnerability of the prefrontal gray matter. *Cerebral Cortex, 7*, 268-282.

Raz, N., Rodrigue, K.M., and Acker, J.D. (2003). Hypertension and the brain: Vulnerability of the prefrontal regions and executive functions. *Behavioral Neuroscience, 117*, 1169-1180.

Riley, W.B.J., and Chow, K.V. (1992). Asset allocation and individual risk aversion. *Financial Analysts Journal, 48*, 32-38.

Ritov, I. (1996). Probability of regret: Anticipation of uncertainty resolution in choice. *Organizational Behavior and Human Decision Processes, 66*, 228-236.

Rolls, E.T., Hornak, J., Wade, D., and McGrath, J. (1994). Emotion-related learning in patients with social and emotional changes associated with frontal-lobe damage. *Journal of Neurology, Neurosurgery, and Psychiatry, 57*, 1518-1524.

Sanfey, A.G., and Hastie, R. (2000). Judgment and decision making across the adult life span: A tutorial review of psychological research. In D.C. Park and N. Schwarz (Eds.), *Cognitive aging: A primer* (pp. 253-273). Philadelphia: Psychology Press.

Schindler, B.A., Ramchandani, D., Matthews, M.K., and Podell, K. (1995). Competence and the frontal lobe: The impact of executive dysfunction on decisional capacity. *Psychosomatics, 36*, 400-404.

Schooley, D.K., and Worden, D.D. (1999). Investors' asset allocations versus life-cycle funds. *Financial Analysts Journal, 55*, 37-43.

Slovic, P., Finucane, M.L., Peters, E., and MacGregor, D. (2002). The affect heuristic. In T. Gilovich, D. Griffin, and D. Kahneman (Eds.), *Heuristics and biases: The psychology of intuitive judgment*. New York: Cambridge University Press.

Stanley, B., Guido, J., Stanley, M., and Shortell, D. (1984). The elderly patient and informed consent: Empirical findings. *Journal of the American Medical Association, 252*, 1302-1306.

Steginga, S.K., and Occhipinti, S. (2002). Decision making about treatment of hypothetical prostate cancer: Is deferring a decision an expert-opinion heuristic? *Journal of Psychosocial Oncology, 20*, 69-84.

Streufert, S., Pogash, R., Piasecki, M., and Post, G.M. (1990). Age and management team performance. *Psychology and Aging, 5*, 551-559.

Sugarman, J., McCrory, D.C., and Hubal, R.C. (1998). Getting meaningful informed consent from older adults: A structured literature review of empirical research. *Journal of the American Geriatrics Society, 46*, 517-524.

Tentori, K., Osherson, D., Hasher, L., and May, C. (2001). Wisdom and aging: Irrational preferences in college students but not older adults. *Cognition, 81*, 87-96.

Thut, G., Schultz, W., Roelcke, U., Nienhusmeier, M., Missimer, J., Maguire, R.P., and Leenders, K.L. (1997). Activation of the human brain by monetary reward. *Neuroreport, 8*(5), 1225-1228.

Tisserand, D.J., and Jolles, J. (2003). On the involvement of prefrontal networks in cognitive aging. *Cortex, 39*, 1107-1128.

Tversky, A. (1969). Intransitivity of preferences. *Psychological Review, 76*, 31-48.

Tversky, A. (1972). Elimination by aspects: A theory of choice. *Psychological Review, 79*, 281-299.

Tversky, A., and Shafir, E. (1992). The disjunction effect in choice under uncertainty. *Psychological Science, 3*(5), 305-309.

Uylings, H.B.M., West, M.J., Coleman, P.D., De Brabander, J.M., and Flood, D.G. (2000). Neuronal and cellular changes in the aging brain. In C.M. Clark and J.Q. Trojanowski (Eds.), *Neurodegenerative dementias* (pp. 61-76). New York: McGraw-Hill.

Vroom, V.H., and Pahl, B. (1971). Relationship between age and risk-taking among managers. *Journal of Applied Psychology, 55*, 399-405.

Walker, N., Fain, W.B., Fisk, A.D., and McGuire, C.L. (1997). Aging and decision making: Driving-related problem solving. *Human Factors, 39*, 438-444.

Wallach, M., and Kogan, N. (1961). Aspects of judgment and decision-making: Interrelationships and changes with age. *Behavioral Science, 6*, 23-36.

Welte, J., Barnes, G., Wieczorek, W., Tidwell, M.C., and Parker, J. (2001). Alcohol and gambling pathology among U.S. adults: Prevalence, demographic patterns and comorbidity. *Journal of Studies on Alcohol, 62*, 706-712.

West, R.L. (1996). An application of prefrontal cortex function theory to cognitive aging. *Psychological Bulletin, 120*, 272-292.

Wilson, T.D., and Schooler, J.W. (1991). Thinking too much: Introspection can reduce the quality of preferences and decisions. *Journal of Personality and Social Psychology, 60*, 181-192.

Yates, J.F., and Patalano, A.L. (1999). Decision making and aging. In D.C. Park, R.W. Morrell, and K. Shifren (Eds.), *Processing of medical information in aging patients: Cognitive and human factors perspectives* (pp. 31-54). Mahwah, NJ: Lawrence Erlbaum.

Zalla, T., Koechlin, E., Pietrini, P., Basso, G., Aquino, P., Sirigu, A., and Grafman, J. (2000). Differential amygdala responses to winning and losing: A functional magnetic resonance imaging study in humans. *European Journal of Neuroscience, 12*(5), 1764-1770.

Zwahr, M.D. (1999). Cognitive processes and medical decisions. In D.C. Park, R.W. Morrell, and K. Shifren (Eds.), *Processing of medical information in aging patients*. Mahwah, NJ: Lawrence Erlbaum.

Zwahr, M.D., Park, D.C., and Shifren, K. (1999). Judgments about estrogen replacement therapy: The role of age, cognitive abilities, and beliefs. *Psychology and Aging, 14*, 179-191.

A Social Psychological Perspective on the Stigmatization of Older Adults

Jennifer A. Richeson
Northwestern University
and
J. Nicole Shelton
Princeton University

INTRODUCTION

There is mounting evidence to suggest that older adults constitute a stigmatized group in the United States (and in most Western societies). Indeed, youth is of such value in U.S. culture that efforts to stay young fuel a multibillion dollar industry. The prevailing view is "If I can buy enough pills, cream, and hair, I can avoid becoming old" (Esposito, 1987). Certainly, individuals' efforts to avoid the near-certain, uncontrollable outcomes of old age (if one is lucky enough to survive) reveal the stigma and negative attitudes associated with advanced age. Similar to sexism or racism, "ageism" (Butler, 1969) refers to the negative attitudes, stereotypes, and behaviors directed toward older adults based solely on their perceived age. Evidence of ageism can be observed in any number of domains, including the workplace (e.g., Finkelstein, Burke, and Raju, 1995; McCann and Giles, 2002; Rosen and Jerdee, 1976) and health care facilities (e.g., Caporael and Culbertson, 1986; DePaola, Neimeyer, Lupfer, and Feidler, 1992). For instance, age discrimination in the workplace, such as mandatory retirement ages, led to the inclusion of age as a protected category with the Age Employment Discrimination Act of 1967. More subtle ageist behavior can be found in the expectancies that doctors hold regarding the capabilities of older individuals, attitudes that in turn shape treatment recommendations and decisions (e.g., Adelman, Greene, and Charon, 1991; Greene, Adelman, Charon, and Hoffman, 1986).

There have been numerous reviews of the literature from various fields documenting the differential, and sometimes expressively negative, treatment of older adults in many social domains (see Nelson, 2002). We do not repeat this information, but rather attempt to integrate that work with the emerging literature on the social psychology of stigma. Using a social-psychological approach, we explore the literature on age stigma with respect to both potential perpetrators (society, younger adults) and potential targets (older adults).[1] Specifically, in the first section we review the literature on perceivers of older adults—namely, younger adults—and their stereotypes, attitudes, and behaviors vis-à-vis older individuals. In the second section we focus on the targets—older adults—and their self-concepts, self-stereotyping, and coping in the face of ageism.

AGE STIGMA FROM THE PERCEIVER'S PERSPECTIVE

Chronological age, similar to sex and race, is a dimension on which individuals categorize others rather automatically (Brewer, 1988; Fiske, 1998). Cues to age are perceived from physical appearance, such as hair and facial morphology, as well as from verbal and nonverbal aspects of individuals' communications (Bieman-Copland and Ryan, 2001; Hummert, Garstka, and Shaner, 1997; Montepare and Zebrowitz-McArthur, 1988). Upon presentation of these cues, age is readily perceived, perhaps even unconsciously, often shaping interactions between younger and older individuals. For instance, younger individuals often use stereotypes associated with advanced age to make inferences regarding older adults' intentions, goals, wishes, and capacities and guide their behavior accordingly. First we examine the perceptions, attitudes, and stereotypes associated with older adults. Next, we consider the ways in which these stereotypes and attitudes shape behavior toward older adults. Last, we investigate potential directions for future research that may eventually change ageist stereotypes and attitudes.

Attitudes and Stereotypes

In general, individuals express predominantly negative attitudes and beliefs toward older adults, especially in comparison to their attitudes to-

[1]We would like to emphasize that our approach is not the only framework through which to investigate attitudes and stereotypes about aging and older adults. The structure of the review conforms to the norms of social psychological literature on social stigma. We acknowledge the limitations of such an approach, for instance, limiting the discussion of aging to stereotypes, attitudes, and discrimination; however, we believe that such a focus affords the integration of previous research on beliefs about aging and older adults with basic research and theoretical work on stigma in social psychology. Such an integration is likely to reveal both the consistencies as well as the contradictions between these literatures, as well as suggest new directions for investigation.

ward younger people. The difference between the attitudes of young and old is particularly pronounced when the general category of "older adults" is being considered rather than specific exemplars (Kite and Johnson, 1988; Palmore, 1990; see also Kite and Wagner, 2002, for a review). Numerous studies show, however, that older adults are not always perceived as a homogeneous group (Braithwaite, Gibson, and Holman, 1986; Brewer, Dull, and Lui, 1981; Brewer and Lui, 1984; Hummert, 1990; Hummert, Garstka, Shaner, and Strahm, 1994; Schmidt and Boland, 1986). The broad category of "older adults" consists of as few as three and as many as twelve subtypes (Hummert et al., 1994). Some work suggests that a large subset of older adults is perceived as "senior citizens" who are vulnerable, often lonely, physically and mentally impaired, and old-fashioned (Brewer et al., 1981). But at least two positive subtypes of older adults have also emerged in this work. The "perfect grandmother" subtype consists of women who are kind, serene, trustworthy, nurturing, and helpful. The "elder statesman" subtype consists of men who are competent, intelligent, aggressive, competitive, and intolerant. In addition to these, other well-replicated subtypes include the "golden ager," the shrew/curmudgeon, the John Wayne conservative, and the severely impaired (Hummert et al., 1994; Schmidt and Boland, 1986). The research on subtypes thus suggests that perceptions of older adults are both complex and differentiated, including both positive and negative exemplars.

The heterogeneity in attitudes and stereotypes toward different older adult subtypes has given rise to spirited debate as to whether ageism really exists. If perceptions about certain subtypes are positive, how can there be negative attitudes toward the group? Research conducted by Neugarten (1974) distinguishing between the "young-old" (i.e., individuals between 55 and 75 years old) and the "old-old" (i.e., individuals 75 years old and older) offers one explanation. Neugarten suggested that many of society's negative stereotypes about older people (e.g., being sick, poor, slow, miserable, disagreeable, and sexless) are based on observations of the old-old, and that these observations get overgeneralized to the young-old. Recent empirical investigations of this hypothesis suggest that various subtypes of older people reflect differences in chronological age (Hummert, 1990, 1994; Hummert, Garstka, Shaner, and Strahm, 1995). For instance, Hummert (1994) presented college students with photographs of older men and women whose facial features suggested three age ranges: young-old (55-64), middle-old (65-74), and old-old (75 years and over). Results revealed that physiognomic cues to advanced age (e.g., eye droop, wrinkled vs. smooth skin, grey hair) led to differing perceptions and stereotypes. Consistent with predictions, participants tended to pair photographs of young-old individuals with positive stereotypes, and to pair photographs of old-old individuals with negative stereotypes. This work suggests that the more positive subtypes of old age may be associated primarily with individuals in the early stages of older adulthood.

A different perspective on the heterogeneity of stereotypes of older adults stems from recent research finding that although certain subtypes of older adults are viewed more positively than others, positive stereotypes can also manifest in attitudes that are not positive (Fiske, Cuddy, Glick, and Xu, 2002). Fiske and colleagues (2002) argue that stereotypes of most social groups cluster on two dimensions—competence and warmth. Outgroups are perceived as high on one dimension but not the other, and in some cases they are perceived as low on both. Attitudes, emotions, and behaviors regarding out-groups are thought to follow these relative warmth and competence judgments (Fiske et al., 2002). Consider, for instance, the "perfect grandmother" subtype. Grandmothers are perceived positively as warm and likable, but they are also perceived as cognitively incompetent (Cuddy and Fiske, 2002). Low cognitive competence coupled with relatively high warmth results in pity, and, accordingly, grandmothers (and those perceived as grandmotherly) tend to be disrespected and denied opportunities in many domains. This type of research reveals the complexity of the relative positivity and negativity of various older adult subtypes, and the issue of ageism more generally.

Competence Stereotypes

Such variety in perceptions and subtypes of older adults suggests that there is not complete consensus regarding who belongs in the category or, by extension, what characteristics the members of the category possess. Nevertheless, research indicates that there are some consistent stereotypes of older individuals that shape perceptions. At the most general category level, older adults are stereotyped as deficient interpersonally, physically, and cognitively (e.g., Pasupathi, Carstensen, and Tsai, 1995). That is, older adults are expected to be slow or poor thinkers, movers, and talkers. Because age-related changes in cognitive function have been documented (Baltes, Lindenberger, and Staudinger, 1998; Salthouse, Hambrick, and McGuthry, 1998; Schaie, 1994), the "kernel of truth" in these stereotypes affords them particular strength. However, research taking more ecologically valid, adaptive approaches to the study of age-related cognitive differences suggests that stereotypes of cognitive functioning in older age are more severe than most actual deficits and, furthermore, that the stereotypes largely mask age-related cognitive performance gains (e.g., Adams, Labouvie-Vief, Hobart, and Dorosz, 1990; Blanchard-Fields and Chen, 1996; Colonia-Willner, 1998).

Forgetfulness. Among stereotypes about cognitive abilities, one of the most pernicious is forgetfulness (Bieman-Copland and Ryan, 1998; Ryan, Bieman-Copland, Kwong See, Ellis, and Anas, 2002). Erber and colleagues have conducted numerous studies regarding the forgetfulness stereotype (e.g., Erber, 1989; Erber, Caiola, and Pupo, 1994; Erber, Szuchman, and Prager, 2001; Erber, Szuchman, and Rothberg, 1990a, 1990b). The stereotype is widely held by both young and old (Parr and Siegert, 1993; Ryan, 1992), and is readily applied to explain "forgetful" behavior by older adults (Erber et al., 1994). Even identical behavior by older and younger individuals is attributed to mental deterioration for the older target but not the younger (Erber et al., 1990a, 1990b). In fact, rude and sometimes even criminal behavior on the part of older adults that can be attributed to forgetfulness tends to be excused as such (Erber et al., 2001). In general, the research suggests that older adults are thought to be forgetful due to biological changes associated with aging and therefore are not held accountable for forgetful behavior (e.g., missing an appointment, forgetting a birthday). Although this research reveals a potential benefit of being stereotyped as forgetful (i.e., lack of accountability for breaking social norms), the costs of the forgetfulness stereotype in other domains (e.g., the workplace) may outweigh the potential benefits.

Mental incompetence. Stereotypes about other mental capabilities of older adults have also been found to influence younger adults' interpretation of ambiguous events (Carver and de la Garza, 1984; Franklyn-Stokes, Harriman, Giles, and Coupland, 1988; Rubin and Brown, 1975; see also Giles, Coupland, Coupland, Williams, and Nussbaum, 1992, for a review). In these studies young adult participants read a brief description of a car accident involving a motorist of either one of two ages (22 or 84; Carver and de la Garza, 1984) or one of five ages (22, 54, 64, 74, or 84; Franklyn-Stokes et al., 1988). Participants were asked to rank order a set of provided questions that they would ask the motorist in order to discern the cause of the accident. In both studies, participants sought out stereotype-consistent information to shape their inquiries. Specifically, participants ranked statements about the motorist's physical, mental, and sensory state as more diagnostic the older the perceived age of the motorist, and they ranked alcohol consumption as more diagnostic the younger the perceived age of the motorist. In Franklyn-Stokes et al. (1988), the trends both for the motorist's capacity and for alcohol were linear, suggesting that ageist information seeking may take place "throughout the life span and [be] well grounded in middle age" (p. 420). This work suggests that stereotypes of older adults, similar to stereotypes of other groups, influence information processing, shaping what is both attended to and remembered about particular older adult targets (e.g., Hense, Penner, and Nelson, 1995).

Implicit or Unconscious Attitudes and Stereotypes

A growing body of research in social cognition suggests that individuals' attitudes and beliefs concerning various social groups (e.g., race, gender) can be activated without conscious awareness of the activation (e.g., Bargh and Chartrand, 1999; Fazio and Olson, 2003). Fazio, Jackson, Dunton, and Williams (1995) demonstrated, for instance, the automatic activation of racial attitudes. Specifically, white participants responded faster to negative target adjectives when they were preceded by primes that were photographs of blacks than when they were preceded by photographs of whites. Presumably, because participants held relatively negative attitudes toward blacks, it was easier for them to process, and therefore respond to, adjectives that were also negative (i.e., congruent with the valence of the racial prime).

Perdue and Gurtman (1990) found a similar reaction time bias when evaluating words that were primed with the words "young" or "old": individuals took longer to identify positive words when presented after the word "old" than when presented after the word "young." Differential automatic evaluations of racial, gender, and age groups have also been detected using a method developed by Greenwald and his colleagues (the Implicit Association Test, or IAT) (Dasgupta and Greenwald, 2001; Dasgupta, McGhee, Greenwald, and Banaji, 2000; Greenwald, McGhee, and Schwartz, 1998; Hummert, Garstka, O'Brien, Greenwald, and Mellott, 2002; Nosek, Banaji, and Greenwald, 2002). Specifically, both young and older participants have been found to associate "pleasant" words more readily with pictures of younger adults than with pictures of older adults (Hummert et al., 2002; Nosek et al., 2002.) The differential ease with which pleasantness is associated with young rather than old reflects an automatic age bias against older adults (see Levy and Banaji, 2002, for a review).

Like stereotypes, attitudes about older adults also differ depending on the subtype brought to mind (Hummert, 1990; Schmidt and Boland, 1986). For instance, a recent study found that the "perfect grandparent" subtype yielded less automatic age bias than either the general category "the elderly" or the negative "old curmudgeon" subtype (Jelenec and Steffens, 2002). Interestingly, the general category of "the elderly" yielded attitudes as negative as the curmudgeon subtype, suggesting that many younger individuals may automatically think of negative subtypes when generating attitudes about older adults. Consistent with this hypothesis, recent work finds that young perceivers view negative exemplars of the older adult category to be more typical (more like older adults in general) than positive exemplars (Chasteen, 2000; Chasteen and Lambert, 1997; but see also Hummert, 1990).

Gender Differences. Although only a few studies have considered the effect of target sex or gender in perceptions of older individuals, beliefs about older women and men appear to differ at least on some dimensions (Canetto, Kaminski, and Felicio, 1995; Kite, Deaux, and Miele, 1991; Kogan and Mills, 1992; but see also O'Connell and Rotter, 1979). Sontag (1979) suggested that there is a double standard of aging in that women are judged more harshly than men, and some support for this view has been found in the ages selected for the onset of older adult status for men and women (e.g., Dravenstedt, 1976; Zepelin, Sills, and Heath, 1986-1987) as well as in attractiveness ratings (Deutch, Zalenski, and Clarke, 1986). In a study of stereotyping, Hummert and colleagues (1997) also found gender differences. Perceivers associated positive stereotypes with photographs of "young-old" and "middle-old" women less than with similarly aged men, but they associated "old-old" men with positive stereotypes less often than for similarly aged women.

In contrast to this work, O'Connell and Rotter (1979) found little evidence that gender interacts with age in shaping evaluations of older adults. Specifically, they found that 25- and 55-year-old men were rated as more competent than women of those ages, but there were no differences in the competence judgments of 75-year-old men and women. Taken together, these studies suggest that future research is necessary to elucidate how age and gender may interact to shape perceptions. Similarly, there is a dearth of research examining the combined effects of age and other basic categories (e.g., race, sexual orientation) on stereotypes of and attitudes about older adults. It is likely that the combination of these factors, rather than age alone, shapes attitudes and behavior toward individuals (e.g., Conway-Turner, 1995).

Behavior Toward Older Adults

Stereotypes such as forgetfulness and mental deficiency generate negative expectancies for older adults that often translate into behavior with respect to housing availability, in the workplace, during medical encounters, and perhaps even with family and friends. As are racial minorities, older adults are susceptible to housing discrimination. One study found, for example, that rooms previously advertised as available for rent were more likely to be described as unavailable when an older person inquired about availability than when a younger person made the inquiry (Page, 1997). Even children have been found to discriminate against older adults (Isaacs and Bearison, 1986). Children (ages 4, 6, or 8) were asked to work on a jigsaw puzzle with either an old (age 75) or a young (age 35) confederate. Results revealed that the children sat farther away from, made less eye contact with, spoke fewer words to, initiated less conversation with, and asked for less help from the older confederate compared to the younger confederate.

There is also evidence that older adults face discriminatory treatment in medical encounters with both nurses and physicians. Perhaps because these professionals consistently see some of the most impaired older adults, negative attitudes toward older adults in general are common among health care workers (e.g., DePaola et al., 1992; Kahana and Kiyak, 1984; Penner, Ludenia, and Mead, 1984; Sherman, Roberto, and Robinson, 1996). The impact of these negative attitudes can be found in the treatment of nursing home residents (Baltes, 1988; Baltes, Burgess, and Stewart, 1980) and in physicians' diagnoses of older adults' medical problems (Adelman et al., 1991; Adelman, Greene, Charon, and Friedman, 1992; Greene et al., 1986; Greene, Adelman, Charon, and Friedman, 1989; Lasser, Siegel, Dukoff, and Sunderland, 1988). For instance, depression often goes unnoticed in older adults or gets misdiagnosed as dementia (Lamberty and Bieliauskas, 1993), and older adults with acute and chronic pain are sometimes mistreated (Gagliese and Melzack, 1997) or overlooked for preventive measures such as routine screenings because of physicians' beliefs about the course of normal aging (Derby, 1991). Negative beliefs among medical care workers are particularly worrisome in that expectations can become self-fulfilling prophecies (Learman, Avorn, Everitt, and Rosenthal, 1990).

These studies present just a few domains in which older adults may face discrimination (see Pasupathi and Lockenhoff, 2002, for a review). However, not all behavior that differs between young and older adults is discriminatory, making the issue of distinguishing between discriminatory and appropriately differentiated behavior rather complex. In order to develop interventions that reduce harm to, but maximize benefits for, older adults, disambiguating negative discriminatory and beneficial age-differentiated behavior is of paramount importance. In the section that follows, we present the case of disentangling patronizing from accommodating intergenerational communications in order to reveal the nuances associated with many forms of age-differentiated behavior.

Patronizing Versus Accommodating Speech

Research on intergenerational interactions suggests that negative stereotypes and attitudes toward older adults can manifest in patronizing behavior (Hummert, Shaner, Garstka, and Henry, 1998; Ruscher, 2001; Williams and Nussbaum, 2001). One form of patronizing behavior is known as secondary baby talk or elderspeak (Caporael, 1981; Culbertson and Caporael, 1983; Kemper, Finter-Urczyk, Ferrell, Harden, and Billington, 1998). Elderspeak is a simplified speech register that is characterized by slowed speech with exaggerated intonation, higher pitch, simplified grammar, limited vocabulary, and the use of short sentences (Caporael and Culbertson, 1986; Kemper, 1994). Elderspeak has been observed in a number of naturalistic settings, such as residential care facilities for older adults (Ashburn and Gordon, 1981; Caporael and Culbertson, 1986; see Ryan, Hummert, and Boich, 1995, for a review), as well as in laboratory interactions between young and older adults (e.g., Kemper, Vandeputte, Rice, Cheung, and Gubarchuk, 1995; Thimm, Rademacher, and Kruse, 1998).

Patronizing behaviors can reveal ageism insofar as they communicate to older adults that they are no longer the equals of middle-aged adults and therefore their opinions, capabilities, and choices are unworthy of serious consideration (Caporael and Culbertson, 1986; Kemper, 1994; Ryan, Hamilton, and Kwong See, 1994). Indeed, research has linked elderspeak and similar speech accommodations with the speakers' beliefs about the functional ability of older adults (Caporael, Lukaszewski, and Culbertson, 1983) and with their holding negative stereotypical perceptions of older adult listeners (Hummert et al., 1998; Thimm et al., 1998). Furthermore, the use of baby talk with high-functioning older adults has been found to have negative consequences, such as lower self-esteem (O'Connor and Rigby, 1996), feelings of humiliation and dependency (Caporael et al., 1983; Ryan et al., 1994), and increased feelings of communicative incompetence (Kemper et al., 1995). For instance, older adults who participated in a communication task with young adults who used elderspeak reported that they experienced more communication problems during the interaction and were more likely to perceive themselves as cognitively impaired (Kemper et al., 1995; Kemper, Othick, Gerhing, Gubarchuk, and Billington, 1998; Kemper, Othick, Warren, Gubarchuk, and Gerhing, 1996). This work suggests that the misapplication of stereotypes about old age to high-functioning older adults can have deleterious consequences for those individuals' actual level of functioning and mental health.

Similar to the issues underlying the "kernel of truth" of competence stereotypes, elderspeak is ambiguous in that there seem to be both costs and benefits (Caporael et al., 1983; Cohen and Faulkner, 1986; Kemper et al., 1995, 1996). Kemper and colleagues (1995) found that when younger adults spontaneously used elderspeak during a task that involved providing older adults with verbal instructions for finding a destination on a map, their older adult participants benefited in the form of improved task performance. And using a form of elderspeak with older adults suffering from Alzheimer's disease has been found to improve communication between caregivers and patients (Ripich, 1994). Given the negative psychosocial but positive performance consequences of elderspeak, Ryan and colleagues (1995) argued that there exists a "communicative predicament of aging" (p. 1). Specifically, elderspeak directed to high-functioning older adults is perceived as patronizing and seems to decrease their perceived communicative self-efficacy, but failure to use some form of elderspeak may undermine the actual communicative efficacy of lower-functioning older adults.

In a series of elegant experiments, Kemper and her colleagues (1995, 1996, 1998a, 1998b, 1999) sought to examine the components of elderspeak that underlie the positive benefits of communication but are not accompanied by negative psychosocial consequences. This work finds that providing semantic elaborations and simplifying speech by reducing the use of subordinate embedded clauses, but not by shortening speech segments, results in better performance by older adults (Kemper and Harden, 1999). Using short sentences, speaking in a slow rate, and using a high pitch do not benefit older adults, and instead result in negative self-perceptions as well as negative perceptions of the speaker by the older adult (Kemper and Harden, 1999). This work suggests that there is a form of elderspeak that is not perceived as condescending or patronizing and that is an appropriate and beneficial accommodation for healthy older adults. Similarly, older adults with Alzheimer's disease may also reveal improved performance on communication tasks with some but not all aspects of elderspeak. Small, Kemper, and Lyons (1997) found, for instance, that repeating and paraphrasing sentences improved patients' sentence comprehension, but saying the sentences more slowly did not.

Clearly this research has important practical implications for caregivers, family members, and researchers. Treatment and diagnosis disparities (e.g., misdiagnosed pain, depression) could stem from ineffective physician-patient communication (Grant, 1996; Greene et al., 1986; Lagana and Shanks, 2002; Radecki, Kane, Solomon, and Mendenhall, 1988; Revenson, 1989; but see also Hooper, Comstock, Goodwin, and Goodwin, 1982). This work also highlights the need for research to disambiguate stereotypes from actual group differences, in order to develop interventions that address actual needs without reinforcing group stereotypes and that therefore are not rejected as patronizing. Other age-differentiated behaviors must also be examined with similar scrutiny in order to disambiguate discrimination from beneficial differentiation.

Interventions

Given the aforementioned research suggesting that older adults constitute a devalued group in U.S. society and culture, it is fitting to devote some attention to potential interventions. In the research literature on racial prejudice and intergroup conflict, increased contact between members of different groups has been heralded as the "gold standard" route to prejudice reduction (Allport, 1954; Pettigrew and Tropp, 2000). However, research examining the impact of intergenerational contact on attitudes toward older adults has yielded mixed results (Lutsky, 1980). Some work finds that frequent contact with an older adult person leads to more positive attitudes toward older adults more generally (Cummings, Williams, and Ellis, 2003; Gatz, Popkin, Pino, and VandenBos, 1984; Hale, 1998). For instance, children in daily contact with older adults at their preschool were found to hold positive attitudes toward older adults, whereas children without such contact held vague or indifferent attitudes (Caspi, 1984). In contrast, other studies have found either no relationship or a negative relationship between contact frequency and the positivity of attitudes toward older adults (Ivester and King, 1977). Consistent with revisions to Allport's original contact hypothesis, however, most research suggests that quality of contact, rather than frequency, predicts subsequent attitudes (Knox, Gekoski, and Johnson, 1986). This suggests that greater, positive intergenerational contact is a promising route to the reduction of negative stereotypes, attitudes, and discrimination. Consequently, additional research on the dynamics of intergenerational interactions that foster positive contact experiences is essential (e.g., Coupland, Coupland, Giles, Henwood, and Wiemann, 1988; Giles, Fox, Harwood, and Williams, 1994).

A different approach to reducing negative attitudes and stereotypes concerning older adults can be drawn from recent work examining the effects of exposure to atypical or counterstereotypical older adults (e.g., Duval, Ruscher, Welsh, and Catanese, 2000). For example, Dasgupta and Greenwald (2001) found that young adult participants revealed less automatic age bias if they had recently been exposed to admired older adult exemplars (e.g., Mother Theresa) and disliked young exemplars (e.g., Tonya Harding), compared to recent exposure to disliked older adult exemplars and admired young exemplars. Research in other domains finds similar results (e.g., Blair, Ma, and Lenton, 2001; Lowery, Hardin, and Sinclair, 2001; Rudman, Ashmore, and Gary, 2001). Specifically, imagining a capable woman reduced automatic gender stereotyping (Blair et al., 2001), and exposure to a black individual in a high-status, counterstereotypical role reduced whites' automatic racial bias (Lowery et al., 2001; Richeson and Ambady, 2003). Taken together, this research suggests that exposure to atypical exemplars of stigmatized groups may reduce bias and stereotyping toward those groups.

Emerging Themes and Directions for Future Research

The research examined above suggests overwhelmingly that, although it is true that aging has certain negative consequences, people (namely, younger adults) who exhibit negative stereotypes, attitudes, and behavior toward older adults overestimate, overgeneralize, and overaccommodate the extent of actual impairments and difficulties. Even "positive" stereotypes of older adults can manifest in patronizing behaviors and contribute to the inadequate treatment of older people (Cuddy and Fiske, 2002). In nearly every situation in which contact between older and younger adults is possible, if not required (e.g., workplace, health care, housing), research suggests that older adults face discrimination. Combating such widespread discrimination will require the concerted efforts of researchers in multiple disciplines and content areas, in collaboration with practitioners.

One dominant theme that emerges from the research reviewed is the complexity and "porous" nature of age categories: they are far more differentiated, permeable, and transient than many other social categories, like race. Fruitful avenues for future exploration are likely to arise from the fact that the young will eventually become old. For instance, does the fact that one will eventually join the stigmatized group influence the stereotyping process? Perhaps stereotyping of older adults is perceived as relatively more permissible because individuals expect to join the group. Or, rather, anxiety and apprehension associated with aging could exacerbate stereotyping and prejudice toward older people; indeed, some preliminary research suggests that this is the case (Chasteen, 2000). Future research should disambiguate and compare stereotypes about aging and stereotypes about older adults, if indeed these are dissociable constructs.

These future directions assume a motivational basis underlying stereotyping and prejudice, focusing on the potentially self-protective function of age bias (Snyder and Miene, 1994). By contrast, considerable research in social psychology suggests that stereotyping also serves the purpose of cognitive efficiency (Macrae, Milne, and Bodenhausen, 1994). In what ways are age stereotypes and perceptions cognitively efficient, especially given that they become more complex as individuals age (Hummert et al., 1994)? Does information processing proceed more smoothly and efficiently after knowing age information, as does other social category information? What cues to age are more likely to activate age stereotypes? Facial photographs? Speech patterns? How do occupational labels affect perceptions of older adult targets? The category of "older adults" is particularly complex and basic research should systematically examine the differences between older adult targets of varying ages (e.g., young-old, middle-old, and old-old).

Another important question is "How old is old?" As life expectancies increase, will the lower boundary of the older adult category also increase? Or will the category become increasingly differentiated, much like racial categories in Brazil? Furthermore, given the research on the association between chronological age and negative stereotypes, will perceptions of older adults become more negative as older adults get even older? Social psychology has failed to regularly include age categories in examinations of the basic processes of categorization, stereotype activation, and stereotype application. Such investigations are essential in order to understand how age alone and in connection with other group memberships affects perception, cognition, and information processing. These investigations will also suggest interventions that can reduce stereotyping and prejudice against older adults.

A second theme emerging from the research is the importance of disambiguating behavior that stems from negative stereotypes from that which represents proper adaptations and accommodations to correlates of advanced age. This effort has been and will continue to be served by research that takes an adaptive approach to age differences in cognition, decoupling the myths and realities included in stereotypes of older adults and aging (e.g., Blanchard-Fields and Chen, 1996). The present review suggests, however, that much of this work on adaptive cognition has not yet penetrated many of the more robust negative stereotypes of older adults. Consequently, social psychological research on attitudes and attitude change may prove particularly important in communicating new findings about the actual capabilities of older adults to physicians, older-adult residential facility workers, employers, coworkers, and the general public. As with the problem of elderspeak, social psychologists, aging researchers, and practitioners can work together to devise messages, images, and interventions that provide accurate information about aging and older adults without promoting and reinforcing negative stereotypes.

Although the research on the attitudes of younger adults provides fruitful avenues for future investigations, research must also examine those of older adults as well. Consequently, the next section of our review examines the effects of age stigma on the self-perceptions, attitudes, and behaviors of older adults.

AGE STIGMA FROM THE PERSPECTIVE OF OLDER ADULTS

In this section, we focus on older adults' perspectives on aging. First, we examine the self-concept and identity of older adults. Next, we review the literature on self-stereotyping by older adults and its implications for mental and physical health. We then review the consequences of exposure to age stereotypes for older adults, considering cognitive, behavioral, and mental health outcomes. Last, we examine the coping strategies older adults use to contend with ageism.

Identity and Self-Concept

The self-concept refers to a set of concepts that individuals have about their physical, psychological, and social attributes. The self-concept involves individuals' evaluations of who they are, including their evaluations of abilities, competencies, successes, and failures. How do older adults respond when asked the question "Who am I?" Similarly, how do older adults perceive their future selves? Moreover, how do older adults experience and evaluate their lives? Are they satisfied or are they depressed?

One intriguing issue in this research area is that, although many older adults acknowledge that their chronological age is older than that of others, and older than in previous life stages, they do not consider themselves "old" (Linn and Hunter, 1979; Neugarten and Hagestad, 1976). Instead, they perceive themselves as "young." Moreover, although older adults are more likely than college students to describe themselves in terms of ageist stereotypes, they are just as likely as college students to describe themselves in terms of youthful traits, like bold or impatient (Mueller, Wonderlich, and Dugan, 1986). The gap between actual and perceived age is also reflected in the fact that individuals select increasingly higher chronological ages as the onset of "old age" as they themselves get older (Seccombe and Ishii Kuntz, 1991). In other words, 65 no longer seems old when one is 60, compared to when one was 35.

Additional evidence of the disconnect between actual age and perceived age can be garnered from research employing implicit measures of group identification. Hummert and colleagues (2002) found, for example, that older adults associate self-related words (e.g., me, mine) with the category "young" more rapidly than they associate these words with the category "old." Although such out-group identification could be viewed as maladaptive, the research suggests otherwise. Identifying with youth rather than old age is correlated with higher scores on tests of physical and emotional health (Hummert et al., 2002; Tuckman and Lavell, 1957). Thus, despite perceivers' efforts to categorize older adults as old based on chronological age, many older adults eschew the label, and this resistance to such labeling seems to have positive consequences.

Although older adults do not always perceive themselves as old, chronological age predicts interesting differences between the self-views of younger and older adults. For instance, because older adults have had a lifetime to accumulate self-knowledge, they have a more secure and complex view of the self, compared to younger adults (Perlmutter, 1988). Moreover, there is considerable stability in self-perceptions and identity from mid-life to late life. Whitbourne and Sneed (2002) suggest that older adults are able to maintain a consistent identity by assimilating age-related changes into their existing self-concepts, and only shifting their self-views through a process called "accommodation" when assimilation is no longer possible. The balance between assimilation and accommodation results in an older adult who does not deny age-related changes and maintains a stable sense of self.

Debunking the misperception that old age is a stagnant developmental period, research on possible selves suggests that old age is a time when people are still developing and expanding upon their identities. Older adults think not only about their past selves but also about possible future selves. Possible selves involve self-knowledge pertaining to one's potential and future (Markus and Nurius, 1986). Possible selves represent both what people would like to become ("hoped-for" selves) and what they are afraid of becoming ("feared selves"; Cross and Markus, 1991). Possible selves are important because they guide people's behaviors in terms of what activities and goals they approach or avoid. For example, if an older adult visualizes a possible self who is not financially dependent on his or her family, then the person may decide not to retire at the conventional retirement age. Possible selves are also important because they provide an interpretive context for the current self. For example, an older adult with a "financially independent" possible self will attach a different interpretation to moving in with his or her children than will an older adult without such a possible self.

Although research suggests that older adults tend to have fewer possible selves than young adults (Cross and Markus, 1991; Markus and Herzog, 1991), the possible selves they tend to hold reflect a variety of domains. Specifically, issues related to health, family, leisure, lifestyle, and independence influence common possible selves held by older adults (Frazier, Hooker, Johnson, and Kaus, 2000; Frazier, Johnson, Gonzalez, and Kafka, 2002; Waid and Frazier, 2003). Research indicates, furthermore, that health-related possible selves are the most prevalent visualized by older adults (Holahan, 1988; Hooker, 1992; Hooker and Kaus, 1992, 1994). Similarly, research suggests that older adults often focus desired possible selves on achievement in current roles, such as "being useful and able to help others," and focus feared possible selves, by contrast, on interpersonal relationships and on physical health, such as "living in a nursing home" (Cross and Markus, 1991). The maintenance of healthy possible selves is a significant predictor of successful aging through the promotion of health-enhancing and health-protecting behaviors among older adults (Holahan, 1988; Hooker, 1992; Hooker and Kaus, 1992, 1994; Markus and Herzog, 1991).

Although older adults are less confident about achieving desired possible selves compared to younger adults (Cross and Markus, 1991), they tend to be more active in taking steps to bring about their most important desired selves and to prevent their most important feared selves from occurring (Cross and Markus, 1991). Because many of the possible selves held by older adults involve outcomes and circumstances that are not always under a person's control (e.g., becoming a widow), realistic pessimism may be warranted and quite adaptive.

Implications of Self-Stereotyping

Older adults are typically aware that although people hold positive and negative stereotypes about their age group, the negative stereotypes shape the predominant view (Kite and Johnson, 1988). Unlike some stigmatized groups, however, older adults often endorse these negative stereotypes and views of aging (Heckhausen, Dixon, and Baltes, 1989; Hummert et al., 1994; Kite et al., 1991). For instance, Hummert and colleagues (1994) found that the negative perceptions of older adults (e.g., despondent, socially isolated, physically and psychologically impaired) among older, middle-aged, and young adults do not differ substantially. Additionally, Luszcz (1983, 1985-1986) found that older adults viewed other older adults as less likable, more depressed, and more dependent than middle-aged adults.

Although older adults share many of the same stereotypes of aging and of older adults as others, their overall perception of the category "old" is more complex than that held by others. Older adults use a greater variety of traits to describe older people, and have more subcategories of older people than do younger adults (Brewer and Lui, 1984; Heckhausen et al., 1989). The findings are mixed, however, regarding whether this differentiation includes more positive or negative subcategories. Hummert and colleagues (1994) found that older adults' subcategories were just as likely to include negative as well as positive stereotypes. By contrast, other researchers find that these subcategories tend to include more positive descriptions (Harris, 1975; Kite et al., 1991). Brewer and Lui (1984) found that older adults identify with one of the positive subtypes, thus differentiating themselves from negative subtypes.

Despite the finding that older adults, on average, hold unfavorable attitudes about the category "old" that are similar to those held by others, there are individual differences in the extent to which older adults hold these negative views, and these differences in self-perceptions have been found to predict important health outcomes. For instance, older adults with more positive self-perceptions and views of aging have better physical health and better survival rates than those with more negative self-perceptions and views, even after controlling for appropriate variables such as gender and socioeconomic status (Levy, Slade, and Kasl, 2002; Levy, Slade, Kunkel, and Kasl, 2002). Similarly, negative views about aging predict low self-esteem and high levels of depression among older adults (Bengtson, Reedy, and Gordon, 1985; Coleman, Aubin, Ivani-Chalian, Robinson, and Briggs, 1993). Taken together, this research suggests that negative views of aging and negative self-stereotyping may be harmful to individuals' health.

Consequences of Exposure to Ageist Stereotypes

Recent research suggests that exposure to ageist stereotypes can affect the mental and physical health and capabilities of older adults. Levy, Hausdorff, Hencke, and Wei (2000) found that exposing older adults to negative age stereotypes at a subliminal level led to a heightened cardiovascular response (measured by systolic blood pressure, diastolic blood pressure, and heart rate) to the stress of mathematical and verbal challenges, compared to that of older adults exposed to positive stereotypes about aging. In addition, exposure to age stereotypes has been shown to influence older adults' will to live (Levy, Ashman, and Dror, 1999-2000), walking speed (Hausdorff, Levy, and Wei, 1999), and handwriting (Levy, 2000). Specifically, the handwriting of older adults who had been subliminally primed with negative stereotypes of old age was judged to be older, shakier, and relatively more deteriorated than the handwriting of older adults who had been subliminally primed with positive age stereotypes (Levy, 2000).

The effects of exposure to age stereotypes have also been implicated in the performance of older adults on tests of memory (Hess, Auman, Colcombe, and Rahhal, 2003; Levy and Langer, 1994; Stein, Blanchard-Fields, and Herzog, 2002). For instance, Hess and colleagues (2003) found that concerns about negative age stereotypes can undermine older adults' memory performance through stereotype threat effects (Steele, Spencer, and Aronson, 2002). That is, older adults who were explicitly exposed to the stereotype that older adults have memory impairments (threat condition) performed more poorly on a subsequent recall task, compared to older adults who were exposed either to more optimistic information about aging and memory or to no information. Consistent with stereotype threat theory (Steele et al., 2002), both the importance of memory performance to participants and the activation of the negative memory stereotype predicted the subsequent performance of participants in the threat condition.

Similarly, there is some initial research suggesting that more subtle or implicit exposure to negative age stereotypes may also undermine performance on some memory tests, compared to implicit exposure to either positive stereotypes (Levy, 1996) or stereotype-irrelevant words (Stein et al., 2002). Although these latter studies on implicit self-stereotyping are promising, Stein and colleagues (2002) caution against their overinterpretation or application given the small sample sizes, apparent fragility of the findings, and modest effect sizes. Consistent with this work, however, a cross-cultural study revealed that older adults from cultures in which aging is viewed more positively (i.e., China and the American deaf community) performed better on a memory test than did older American hearing individuals (Levy and Langer, 1994; but see also Yoon, Hasher, Feinberg, Rahhal, and Winocur, 2000). There were no differences, however, in the memory performance among youth from the three cultures. Taken together, these findings suggest that being exposed to negative age stereotypes, or living in a culture that endorses the negative stereotypes, may undermine older adults' ability to perform optimally on memory tests.

Taken as a whole, this research suggests that exposure to age stereotypes can influence older adults' performance in a variety of domains. The findings are quite provocative when contrasted to the traditional views of aging that attribute the cognitive, psychological, and behavioral declines associated with advanced age exclusively to biological factors. Instead, this work suggests that negative stereotypes may explain some of the age-related variance in cognitive and physical task performance that has been attributed to biological differences (e.g., Baltes et al., 1998). It is important to note, however, that this line of research does not deny that there are biological changes associated with aging. Instead, it underscores the need to consider both biological and social/contextual factors in order to form a complete understanding of the age-related cognitive and behavioral changes that shape the life experiences and opportunities of older adults (e.g., Blanchard-Fields and Chen, 1996).

Coping with a Negative Age Identity

Despite the prevalence of negative self-relevant stereotypes, most older adults have a positive sense of subjective well-being (Haug, Belkgrave, and Gratton, 1984; Mroczek and Kolarz, 1998). Diener and Shuh (1998), for example, found that the later adult years are associated with increased feelings of life satisfaction. Similarly, Thunher (1983) found no changes in happiness during the 8 years following retirement, when the stigma of "too old" becomes salient. Moreover, Levy and Langer (1994) found that the self-esteem of American and Chinese older adults did not differ from that of young adults in those cultures. These findings are consistent with research on other stigmatized groups, such as blacks and women (Crocker and Major, 1989).

How do older adults maintain positive well-being in the face of stressors associated with aging? Research indicates that stigmatized individuals do not passively accept society's negative stereotypes, prejudice, and discrimination (Zebrowitz, 2003; see also Crocker, Major, and Steele, 1998; Miller and Major, 2000, for reviews). Instead they use a variety of strategies to respond to and cope with prejudice and stigma-related stress. Here, we use Miller and Meyers' (1998) theoretical framework of compensatory strategies as a way to understand older adults' strategies for coping with stigma-related stress. Miller and Meyers suggest that the strategies individuals use to cope with a devalued social identity can be categorized into two groups: (1) primary compensatory strategies and (2) secondary compensatory strategies. Through primary compensatory strategies, individuals reduce the threat posed by prejudice by engaging in behaviors that enable them to achieve desired outcomes in spite of their stigma. Secondary compensatory strategies, by contrast, allow individuals to change their perceptions of outcomes that have been tainted by stigma. In essence, primary compensatory strategies are used to prevent negative outcomes related to stigma, while secondary compensatory strategies change one's feelings about negative outcomes once they have occurred. In the sections that follow, we examine older adults' maintenance of positive self-views through the application of these compensatory strategies.[2]

Primary Compensatory Strategies

In order to ward off the application of negative stereotypes, individuals may rely on primary compensatory strategies. One common primary strategy is self-presentation (Leary and Kowalski, 1990). Although its focus is not stigma, socioemotional selectivity theory (Carstensen, 1991) makes predictions that are compatible with primary compensatory strategies. We consider below the relevance of these two theories to coping with age stigma.

Self-presentation. According to self-presentation theory, people want to maintain positive self-views and are motivated to convey certain impressions of themselves to others. One way older adults cope with the stereotypes about their group is by monitoring and controlling how others perceive them. In a recent review, Martin, Leary, and Rejeski (2000) suggest that the self-presentational concerns of older adults can be categorized into three themes: (1) physical appearance, (2) competence and reliance, and (3) behavioral norms. Managing physical appearance and perceptions of competence and reliance are most consistent with primary compensatory strategies. Specifically, older individuals may attempt to manage or alter their physical appearance because it is relatively easy to categorize people as young or old upon first sight, which, in turn, may prompt the activation, and perhaps application, of negative age stereotypes. Older adults may also employ impression management strategies in order to avoid the potential costs associated with appearing incompetent and dependent. For example,

[2]The compensatory strategies theorized by Miller and Meyers (1998) are conceptually similar to the control strategies proposed by Heckhausen (1997; Heckhausen and Schultz, 1993). Nevertheless, we make use of the Miller and Meyers framework because of its focus on stigma.

some older adults who suffer from urinary incontinence restrict their daily activities in order to remain near a bathroom (Mitteness, 1987). Similarly, older adults with hearing impairments may pretend to have heard conversations by nodding, smiling, and acting pleasantly during social interactions (Hallberg and Carlsson, 1991).

Although some of the self-presentational strategies older adults use may be successful, they may also come with negative consequences. Martin and colleagues (2000) suggest that some of the tactics may inadvertently cause individuals to engage in more risk-taking behaviors. For example, older adults who want to portray a physically fit or self-reliant image may attempt tasks that are beyond their capabilities, such as walking quickly or lifting heavy objects. Martin and colleagues (2000) suggest that some of these tactics may also lead to higher health risks. For example, an older adult who does not want to be mocked at the gym for not having a youthful body may opt not to exercise at all, becoming sedentary and not benefiting from the advantages of exercise. Thus, the person has avoided a circumstance in which she or he could be the target of prejudice, but has also increased his or her risk for health problems. Engaging in impression management can be a double-edged sword for older adults, as well as for other stigmatized groups (Crocker et al., 1998), because of the complexities associated with coping with a devalued social identity.

Socioemotional Selectivity Theory. Socioemotional selectivity theory (SST) construes older adults as active agents who construct their social worlds to fulfill their social and emotional needs. SST also posits that the perception of time as limited, not age, plays a central role in the selection and pursuit of social goals (Carstensen, 1991, 1995; Carstensen, Isaacowitz, and Charles, 1999). When time is perceived to be expansive, people give more consideration to the acquisition of knowledge, whereas when time is perceived to be limited, people give more consideration to seeking emotional comfort. Older adults perceive their time as limited, and consequently make choices that maximize positive emotions. Fredrickson and Carstensen (1990), for example, found that older adults show a bias for interacting with familiar, close social partners, whereas younger individuals show a preference for interacting with novel social partners. Similarly, in a sample of 69- to 104-year-olds, Lang and Carstensen (1994) found that although the older adults had fewer peripheral social partners compared to the younger adults, there was no difference between the two groups in the number of close social partners.

Drawing on the theories of self-presentation and socioemotional selectivity sketched above, one could hypothesize that avoiding social interactions with strangers is a primary compensatory strategy. Interactions with strangers, and particularly young adult strangers, are more likely to pose a threat to one's self-definition and require effort to ward off or disconfirm negative stereotypes. When older adults are involved in social interactions with close others, however, aging stereotypes are often less relevant and the interactions are more likely to affirm the self. Efforts to reduce one's chances of being a target of prejudice, in other words, are consistent with older adults' placing greater emphasis on emotional comfort, a tenet of socio-emotional selectivity theory.

Secondary Compensatory Strategies

When individuals do become the target of prejudice, they may rely on secondary compensatory strategies to help them change the way they feel about the social situation. Secondary compensatory strategies can be categorized into three groups: (1) psychological disengagement, (2) disidentification, and (3) social comparison. We briefly describe each in the context of the experiences of older adults.

Psychological Disengagement. Psychological disengagement occurs when stigmatized individuals disengage their self-esteem from outcomes in the domains in which they are expected to perform poorly (see Steele et al., 2002). Research indicates that some older adults also psychologically disengage from traits and domains that are negatively associated with their group (Brandtstaedter and Greve, 1994; Heckhausen and Brim, 1997; Luszcz and Fitzgerald, 1986). Older adults, compared to middle-aged adults, for example, place less importance on goals related to work and finances, two domains in which older adults are perceived to have diminished capacity. Because one's self-esteem is no longer tied to the domains in which the group is stereotyped to perform poorly, psychological disengagement helps individuals maintain a positive social identity. In addition to disengaging from devalued domains, older adults may opt to strengthen their connection to domains in which they have acquired knowledge and competence. Ryff (1989) suggests that such compensation plays a major role in the positive psychological adjustment of older adults.

Disidentification. Instead of disengaging from a stereotyped domain, some individuals choose to disidentify with their stigmatized group (Steele, 1997). Extreme forms of disidentification include "passing" as a member of a nonstigmatized group, while less extreme forms include de-emphasizing the group's importance to one's overall self-concept. Disidentification among older adults is evident in certain behaviors, such as lying about one's age, dying one's hair, and using antiaging wrinkle creams. The finding that many older adults do not consider themselves "old" could also be taken as evidence of disidentification. Recall, for instance, that older adults tended to identify with younger adults more than with older adults on an implicit identity measure (Hummert et al., 2002). Moreover, this out-group identification was most pronounced for older adults with high self-esteem. Whether these data are indicative of disidentification from the group, or rather a failure of individuals to identify with the group initially, the outcome seems to be positive psychological well-being.

Social Comparison. Stigmatized individuals have also been found to use social comparisons in order to protect their identity and self-worth (Crocker et al., 1998). Individuals can affirm their self-worth by making downward comparisons with others (i.e., comparison with individuals who are worse off than they) or by limiting their social comparisons to intragroup, rather than intergroup, contexts. Research regarding older adults' use of social comparisons, however, is quite complex, and may not follow the patterns found for other stigmatized groups, highlighting the need for social stigma researchers in social psychology to examine this group.

According to research on social comparisons, downward comparisons involve comparing the self with another person who is inferior to oneself in a given domain (Wood, 1989). Although some older adults engage in downward comparisons, many individuals are more likely to engage in *social downgrading*, which refers to comparing the self to a negatively biased view of one's group (Heckhausen and Brim, 1997). In other words, individuals downgrade the abilities of other group members, thus allowing them to maintain positive self-views by comparison. Older adults, for instance, often have biased, negative expectations about what other people their age are able to do, allowing them to feel relatively superior about their own abilities (Heckhausen and Krueger, 1993). Similar to the self-enhancement function of the more common "better-than-average" effect, older adults seem to affirm their self-worth by believing they are better than "most people their age" (Celejewski and Dion, 1998; Heckhausen and Brim, 1997; Pinquart, 2002).

Research suggests that stigmatized individuals often compare their outcomes to *similar* others in order to maintain a positive identity (Crocker et al., 1998). In contrast, older adults make more social comparisons with *dissimilar* others as a way of affirming their uniqueness (Suls and Mullen, 1982). In addition, older adults use temporal comparisons as opposed to interpersonal comparisons in order to maintain positive self-views (Suls and Mullen, 1982). Temporal comparisons are evaluations based on what one could do before, compared to what one can do in the present. Older adults use such comparisons to remind themselves that, although certain behaviors are challenging now, they were able to perform these behaviors successfully in the past. Temporal comparisons allow for positive self-views that are grounded in one's prior accomplishments.

As with primary compensatory strategies, however, secondary strategies can come with costs. For instance, psychological disengagement from domains in which older adults are stereotyped to perform poorly is likely to yield underperformance in those very domains, thus reinforcing the stereotypes. Furthermore, many of the negative stereotypes of older adults fall in domains that are essential for independence and healthful living. Disengaging self-esteem from their performance in these domains may relegate older adults to premature dependence. Disengagement from the identity may undermine the collective power of older adults insofar as individuals must be identified with a group in order to engage in action on its own behalf. Additionally, group identification seems to provide a buffer against the negative mental health consequences of discrimination (Garstka, Schmitt, Branscombe, and Hummert, 2004). Lastly, the use of temporal social comparisons and social downgrading may limit individuals' growth and personal development. Ideally, researchers, advocates, and practitioners can work in collaboration with older adults to find a balance between accurate self-views and effective self-protection from the negative impact of age stigma.

Emerging Themes and Directions for Future Research

Several themes emerge from research on older adults and stigma. First, unlike many other stigmatized groups, older adults often do not think of themselves as members of the group, and, perhaps by extension, endorse negative stereotypes about aging. This is probably due to the fact that this is one of the few stigmatized groups in which individuals gradually enter over time, and the boundaries of the group are both porous and ambiguous. That is, at one point individuals are out-group members who hold negative stereotypes about the group. As time progresses, however, individuals find themselves as candidates for in-group membership, and must wrestle with whether or not they identify with the group, and whether the prevailing negative stereotypes apply to them. Perhaps as a solution to this dilemma, older adults have complex views both of themselves and of their age group, and these views incorporate both negative and positive stereotypes.

Future research is needed on the processes by which these more complex views are incorporated in individuals' self-concepts. For example, at what period of life does this process begin? How stressful or disruptive is the process? What contextual factors shape the outcome of this process? Moreover, how do individuals negotiate the "transition" from nonstigmatized middle-aged adult to stigmatized older adult? Are individuals who are members of a stigmatized group based on some other dimension of identity (e.g., race, sexual orientation) better or less able to cope with this transition (e.g., McDougall, 1993)?

A second theme that emerges from the research is that features of the social context can shape, in part, older adults' social identity, physical health, and cognitive task performance. This idea is consistent with research on adult social cognition that examines cognitive changes and performance within the framework of adaptive functioning (e.g., Blanchard-Fields and Chen, 1996), as well as research revealing contextual effects on older adults' memory performance, such as the presence of a child as opposed to a young-adult listener (Adams, Smith, Pasupathi, and Vitolo, 2002). Similarly, the research by Hess and colleagues (2003) and Levy and colleagues (see Levy, 2003, for a review) suggests that older adults' cognition, behavior, and mental health may be influenced by exposure to negative stereotypes in the social context. Building on this work, future research should investigate how cues in the social contexts of older adults outside the laboratory may be changed in ways that will improve their well-being.

The final theme that emerges from this research is that of coping strategies. Older adults are faced with a unique set of physical changes that influence their use of coping strategies to contend with stigma-related stress. Research examining older adults' coping behavior in the face of negative age stereotypes should also adopt an adaptive framework. Consistent with the social psychological research on social stigma, it is likely that this research will reveal both costs and benefits of several coping mechanisms that must be negotiated. Future research should examine these negotiations. In addition, personality and motivational factors are likely to contribute to the particular coping strategy that individuals select in a given context. Given that older adults were once younger adults, and have acquired their stigma later in life, they are likely to use their coping strategies later. Other stigmatized groups, such as ethnic minorities and gay individuals, seem to adopt coping strategies relatively early on in order to negotiate prejudice. Consequently, research on the specific strategies used by older adults, as well as comparative work with the strategies used by other stigmatized groups, is warranted.

In sum, the message of the work reviewed in the second section of this paper is a call for additional research on older adults and the effects of ageism. The findings of such research will be essential to the development of societal-level intervention programs and strategies to reduce and eventually eradicate ageism, lessening the burden on older adults of developing strategies to cope with and combat ageism on their own.

GENERAL CONCLUSIONS

The purpose of our review was to examine previous research on the stigmatization of older adults and to consider the consequences of ageism for the opportunities and life outcomes of older individuals. The first section reviewed the research literature on the stereotypes, attitudes, and behavior of younger adults with respect to older adults. The second section reviewed literature on older adults' self-concepts, self-stereotypes, and coping in the face of ageism. Overwhelmingly, research from both perspectives reveals that ageist beliefs can negatively influence the life outcomes of older adults, directly as well as through expectancy effects and self-stereotyping. In addition, the reviewed literature reveals important complexities and nuances of age stigma. For instance, not all age-differentiated behavior is the result of negative stereotypes and some such behavior may even be beneficial for older adults. Furthermore, research suggests that many older adults are remarkably resilient in the face of negative stereotypes, employing a variety of coping strategies designed to protect their self-esteem and well-being.

As life expectancy increases, it is neither just nor desirable for society to undermine the effectiveness of such a large component of the population. For instance, when stereotypes lead individuals to restrict themselves to domains in which their groups are not stereotyped negatively, those individuals lose their freedom to participate fully in society and society loses potentially unique contributions to those domains. Consequently, we propose that future research conduct a thorough, systematic examination of the nuances, varieties, and multiple dynamics of ageism. This examination must be grounded in basic science, drawing on the accumulated research of related fields (e.g., gerontology, communication) as well as paying particular attention to the idiosyncrasies associated with advanced age. The present review captures only some of what the social psychology of stigma has to offer to research on aging. We believe that only such a contextualized, interdisciplinary approach will unearth feasible and effective solutions to reduce or even eliminate ageism and its deleterious consequences for older and younger adults alike.

REFERENCES

Adams, C., Labouvie-Vief, G., Hobart, C.J., and Dorosz, M. (1990). Adult age group differences in story recall style. *Journal of Gerontology, 45*(1), P17-P27.

Adams, C., Smith, M.C., Pasupathi, M., and Vitolo, L. (2002). Social context effects on story recall in older and younger women: Does the listener make a difference? *Journal of Gerontology: Psychological Sciences, 57*(1), P28-P40.

Adelman, R.D., Greene, M.G., and Charon, R. (1991). Issues in the physician-elderly patient interaction. *Aging and Society, 2*, 127-148.

Adelman, R.D., Greene, M.G., Charon, R., and Friedman, E. (1992). The content of physician and elderly patient interaction in the medical primary care encounter. *Communication Research, 19*, 370-380.

Allport, G.W. (1954). *The nature of prejudice*. Reading, MA: Addison-Wesley.

Ashburn, G., and Gordon, A. (1981). Features of a simplified register in speech to elderly conversationalists. *International Journal of Psycholinguistics, 8*, 7-31.

Baltes, M.M. (1988). The etiology and maintenance of dependency in the elderly: Three phases of operant research. *Behavior Therapy, 19*, 301-319.

Baltes, M.M., Burgess, R., and Stewart, R. (1980). Independence and dependence in self-care behaviors in nursing home residents: An operant-observational study. *International Journal of Behavioral Development, 3*, 489-500.

Baltes, P.B., Lindenberger, U., and Staudinger, U.M. (1998). Life-span theory in developmental psychology. In R.M. Lerner (Ed.), *Handbook of child psychology: Theoretical models of human development* (vol. 1, pp. 1029-1143). New York: Wiley.

Bargh, J.A., and Chartrand, T.L. (1999). The unbearable automaticity of being. *American Psychologist, 54*, 462-479.

Bengtson, V.L., Reedy, M.N., and Gordon, C. (1985). Aging and self-conceptions: Personality processes and social contexts. In J. Birren and K. Schaie (Eds.), *Handbook of the psychology of aging* (pp. 544-593). New York: Van Nostrand Reinhold.

Bieman-Copland, S., and Ryan, E.B. (1998). Age-biased interpretation of memory successes and failures in adulthood. *Journal of Gerontology: Psychological Sciences, 53*(2), P105-P111.

Bieman-Copland, S., and Ryan, E.B. (2001). Social perceptions of failures in memory monitoring. *Psychology and Aging, 16*, 357-361.

Blair, I.V., Ma, J.E., and Lenton, A.P. (2001). Imagining stereotypes away: The moderation of implicit stereotypes through mental imagery. *Journal of Personality and Social Psychology, 81*, 828-841.

Blanchard-Fields, F., and Chen, Y. (1996). Adaptive cognition and aging. *American Behavioral Scientist, 39*, 231-248.

Braithwaite, V., Gibson, D., and Holman, J. (1986). Age stereotyping: Are we oversimplifying the phenomenon? *International Journal of Aging and Human Development, 22*, 315-325.

Brandtstaedter, J., and Greve, W. (1994). The aging self: Stabilizing and protective processes. *Developmental Review, 14*, 52-80.

Brewer, M.B. (1988). A dual-process model of impression formation. In T.K. Srull and R.S. Wyer (Eds.), *Advances in social cognition* (vol. 1, pp. 1-36). Mahwah, NJ: Lawrence Erlbaum.

Brewer, M.B., Dull, V., and Lui, L.L. (1981). Perceptions of the elderly: Stereotypes as prototypes. *Journal of Personality and Social Psychology, 41*, 656-670.

Brewer, M.B., and Lui, L.N. (1984). Categorization of the elderly by elderly: Effects of perceiver's category membership. *Personality and Social Psychology Bulletin, 10*, 585-595.

Butler, R.N. (1969). Age-ism: Another form of bigotry. *Gerontologist, 9*, 243-246.

Canetto, S.S., Kaminski, P.L., and Felicio, D.M. (1995). Typical and optimal aging in women and men: Is there a double standard? *International Journal of Aging and Human Development, 40*, 187-207.

Caporael, L.R. (1981). The paralanguage of caregiving: Baby talk to the institutionalized aged. *Journal of Personality and Social Psychology, 40*, 876-884.

Caporael, L.R., and Culbertson, G.H. (1986). Verbal response modes of baby talk and other speech at institutions for the aged. *Language and Communication, 6*, 99-112.

Caporael, L.R., Lukaszewski, M., and Culbertson, G. (1983). Secondary baby talk: Judgments by institutionalized elderly and their caregivers. *Journal of Personality and Social Psychology, 44*, 746-754.

Carstensen, L.L. (1991). Selectivity theory: Social activity in life-span context. *Annual Review of Gerontology and Geriatrics, 11*, 195-217.

Carstensen, L.L. (1995). Evidence for a life-span theory of socioemotional selectivity. *Current Directions in Psychological Science, 4*, 151-156.

Carstensen, L.L., Isaacowitz, D.M., and Charles, S.T. (1999). Taking time seriously: A theory of socioemotional selectivity. *American Psychologist, 54*, 165-181.

Carver, C.S., and de la Garza, N.H. (1984). Schema-guided information search in stereotyping and the elderly. *Journal of Applied Social Psychology, 14*, 69-81.

Caspi, A. (1984). Contact hypothesis and inter-age attitudes: A field study of cross-age contact. *Social Psychology Quarterly, 47*, 74-80.

Celejewski, I., and Dion, K.K. (1998). Self-perception and perception of age groups as a function of the perceiver's category membership. *International Journal of Aging and Human Development, 47*, 205-216.

Chasteen, A.L. (2000). The role of age and age-related attitudes in perceptions of elderly individuals. *Basic and Applied Social Psychology [Special Issue: The Social Psychology of Aging], 22*, 147-156.

Chasteen, A.L., and Lambert, A.J. (1997). Perceptions of disadvantage versus conventionality: Political values and attitudes toward the elderly versus blacks. *Personality and Social Psychology Bulletin, 23*, 469-481.

Cohen, G., and Faulkner, D. (1986) Memory for proper names: Age differences in retrieval. *British Journal of Developmental Psychology, 4*, 187-197.

Coleman, P.G., Aubin, A., Ivani-Chalian, C., Robinson, M., and Briggs, R. (1993). Predictors of depressive symptoms and low self-esteem in a follow-up study of elderly people over ten years. *International Journal of Geriatric Psychiatry, 8*, 343-349.

Colonia-Willner, R. (1998). Practical intelligence at work: Relationship between aging and cognitive efficiency among managers in a bank environment. *Psychology of Aging, 13*, 45-57.

Conway-Turner, K. (1995). Inclusion of black studies in gerontology courses: Uncovering and transcending stereotypes. *Journal of Black Studies, 25*, 577-588.

Coupland, N., Coupland, J., Giles, H., Henwood, K., and Wiemann, J. (1988). Elderly self-disclosure: Interactional and intergroup issues. *Language and Communication, 8*, 109-133.

Crocker, J., and Major, B. (1989). Social stigma and self-esteem: The self-protective properties of social stigma. *Psychological Review, 96*, 608-630.

Crocker, J., Major, B., and Steele, C.M. (1998). Social stigma. In D. Gilbert, S.T. Fiske, and G. Lindzey (Eds.), *Handbook of social psychology* (4th ed.). Boston: McGraw-Hill.

Cross, S., and Markus, H.R. (1991). Possible selves across the life span. *Human Development, 34*, 230-255.

Cuddy, A.J.C., and Fiske, S.T. (2002). Doddering but dear: Process, content, and function in stereotyping of older persons. In T.D. Nelson (Ed.), *Stereotyping and prejudice against older persons* (pp. 3-26). Cambridge, MA: MIT Press.

Culbertson, G.H., and Caporael, L.R. (1983). Baby talk speech to the elderly: Complexity and content of messages. *Personality and Social Psychology Bulletin, 9*, 305-312.

Cummings, S.M., Williams, M.M., and Ellis, R.A. (2003). Impact of an intergenerational program on 4th graders' attitudes toward elders and school behaviors. *Journal of Human Behavior in the Social Environment, 6*, 91-107.

Dasgupta, N., and Greenwald, A.G. (2001). On the malleability of automatic attitudes: Combating automatic prejudice with images of admired and disliked individuals. *Journal of Personality and Social Psychology, 81*, 800-814.

Dasgupta, N., McGhee, D.E., Greenwald, A.G., and Banaji, M.R. (2000). Automatic preference for white Americans: Eliminating the familiarity explanation. *Journal of Experimental Social Psychology, 36*, 316-328.

DePaola, S.J., Neimeyer, R.A., Lupfer, M.B., and Feidler, J. (1992). Death concern and attitudes towards the elderly in nursing home personnel. *Death Studies, 16*, 537-555.

Derby, S.E. (1991). Ageism in cancer care of the elderly. *Oncology Nursing Forum, 18*, 921-926.

Deutch, F.M., Zalenski, C.M., and Clarke, M.E. (1986). Is there a double standard of aging? *Journal of Applied Social Psychology, 16*, 771-785.

Diener, E., and Shuh, E. (1998). Age and subjective well-being: An international analysis. *Annual Review of Gerontology and Geriatrics, 17*, 304-324.

Dravenstedt, J. (1976). Perceptions of onsets of young adulthood, middle age, and old age. *Journal of Gerontology, 31*, 53-57.

Duval, L.L., Ruscher, J.B., Welsh, K., and Catanese, S.P. (2000). Bolstering and undercutting use of the elderly stereotype through communication of exemplars: The role of speaker age and exemplar stereotypicality. *Basic and Applied Social Psychology [Special Issue: The Social Psychology of Aging], 22*, 137-146.

Erber, J.T. (1989). Young and older adults' appraisal of memory failures in young and older adult target persons. *Journal of Gerontology, 44*, 170-175.

Erber, J.T., Caiola, M.A., and Pupo, F.A. (1994). Age and forgetfulness: Managing perceivers' impressions of targets' capability. *Psychology and Aging, 9*, 554-561.

Erber, J.T., Szuchman, L.T., and Prager, I.G. (2001). Ain't misbehavin': The effects of age and intentionality on judgments about misconduct. *Psychology and Aging, 16*, 85-95.

Erber, J.T., Szuchman, L.T., and Rothberg, S.T. (1990a). Age, gender, and individual differences in memory failure appraisal. *Psychology and Aging, 5*, 600-603.

Erber, J.T., Szuchman, L.T., and Rothberg, S.T. (1990b). Everyday memory failure: Age differences in appraisal and attribution. *Psychology and Aging, 5*, 236-241.

Esposito, J.L. (1987). *The obsolete self: Philosophical dimensions of aging*. Los Angeles: University of California Press.

Fazio, R.H., Jackson, J.R., Dunton, B.C., and Williams, C.J. (1995). Variability in automatic activation as an unobtrusive measure of racial attitudes: A bona fide pipeline? *Journal of Personality and Social Psychology, 69*, 1013-1027.

Fazio, R.H., and Olson, M.A. (2003). Implicit measures in social cognition research: Their meaning and uses. *Annual Review of Psychology, 54*, 297-327.

Finkelstein, L.M., Burke, M.J., and Raju, N.S. (1995). Age discrimination in simulated employment contexts: An integrative analysis. *Journal of Applied Psychology, 60*, 652-663.

Fiske, S.T. (1998). Stereotyping, prejudice, and discrimination. In D.T. Gilbert, S.T. Fiske, and G. Lindzey (Eds.), *The handbook of social psychology* (4th ed., vol. 2, pp. 357-411). New York: McGraw-Hill.

Fiske, S.T., Cuddy, A.J.C., Glick, P., and Xu, J. (2002). A model of stereotype content as often mixed: Separate dimensions of competence and warmth respectively follow from status and competition. *Journal of Personality and Social Psychology, 82*, 878-902.

Franklyn-Stokes, A., Harriman, J., Giles, H., and Coupland, N. (1988). Information seeking across the lifespan. *Journal of Social Psychology, 128*, 419-421.

Frazier, L.D., Hooker, K., Johnson, P.M., and Kaus, C.R. (2000). Continuity and change in possible selves in later life: A 5-year longitudinal study. *Basic and Applied Social Psychology, 22*, 237-243.

Frazier, L.D., Johnson, P., Gonzalez, G., and Kafka, C. (2002). Psychosocial influences on possible selves: A comparison of three cohorts of older adults. *International Journal of Behavioral Development, 26*, 308-317.

Fredrickson, B.L., and Carstensen, L.L. (1990). Choosing social partners: How old age and anticipated endings make us more selective. *Psychology and Aging, 5*, 335-347.

Gagliese, L., and Melzack, R. (1997). Chronic pain in elderly people. *Pain, 70*, 3-14.

Garstka, T.A., Schmitt, M.T., Branscombe, N.R., and Hummert, M.L. (2004). How young and older adults differ in their responses to perceived age discrimination. *Psychology and Aging, 19*, 326-335.

Gatz, M., Popkin, S., Pino, C., and VandenBos, G. (1984). Psychological interventions with older adults. In J.E. Birren and K.W. Schaie (Eds.), *Handbook of the psychology of aging* (2nd ed., pp. 755-787). New York: Reinhold.

Giles, H., Coupland, N., Coupland, J., Williams, A., and Nussbaum, J. (1992). Intergenerational talk and communication with older people. *International Journal of Aging and Human Development, 34*, 271-297.

Giles, H., Fox, S., Harwood, J., and Williams, A. (1994). Talking age and aging talk: Communicating through the life span. In M. Hummert, J. Wiemann, and J. Nussbaum (Eds.), *Interpersonal communication in older adulthood: Interdisciplinary theory and research* (pp. 130-161). New York: Sage.

Grant, L.D. (1996). Effects of ageism on individual and health care providers' responses to healthy aging. *Health and Social Work, 21*, 9-15.

Greene, M.G., Adelman, R., Charon, R., and Friedman, E. (1989). Concordance between physicians and their older and younger patients in the primary medical encounter. *Gerontologist, 29*, 808-813.

Greene, M.G., Adelman, R., Charon, R., and Hoffman, S. (1986). Ageism in the medical encounter: An exploratory study of the doctor-elderly relationship. *Language and Communication, 6*, 113-124.

Greenwald, A.G., McGhee, D.E., and Schwartz, J.L.K. (1998). Measuring individual differences in implicit cognition: The Implicit Association Test. *Journal of Personality and Social Psychology, 74*, 1464-1480.

Hale, N.M. (1998). Effects of age and interpersonal contact on stereotyping of the elderly. *Current Psychology, 17*, 28-47.

Hallberg, L., and Carlsson, S. (1991). A qualitative study of strategies for managing a hearing impairment. *British Journal of Audiology, 25*, 201-211.

Harris, L. (1975). *The myth and reality of aging in America*. Washington, DC: National Council on the Aging.

Haug, M., Belkgrave, L., and Gratton, B. (1984). Mental health and the elderly: Factors in stability and change. *Journal of Health and Social Behavior, 25*, 100-115.

Hausdorff, J.M., Levy, B.R., and Wei, J.Y. (1999). The power of ageism on physical function of older persons: Reversibility of age-related gait changes. *Journal of the American Geriatrics Society, 47*, 1346-1349.

Heckhausen, J. (1997). Developmental regulation across adulthood: Primary and secondary control of age-related challenges. *Developmental Psychology, 33*, 176-187.

Heckhausen, J., and Brim, O.G. (1997). Perceived problems for self and others: Self-protection by social downgrading throughout adulthood. *Psychology and Aging, 12*, 610-619.

Heckhausen, J., Dixon, R., and Baltes, P.B. (1989). Gains and losses in development throughout adulthood as perceived by different adult age groups. *Developmental Psychology, 25*, 109-121.

Heckhausen, J., and Krueger, J. (1993). Developmental expectations for the self and most other people: Age grading in three functions of social comparison. *Developmental Psychology, 29*, 539-548.

Heckhausen, J., and Schulz, R. (1993). Optimization by selection and compensation: Balancing primary and secondary control in life span development. *International Journal of Behavioral Development [Special Issue: Planning and Control Processes Across the Life Span], 16*, 287-303.

Hense, R.L., Penner, L.A., and Nelson, D.L. (1995). Implicit memory for age stereotypes. *Social Cognition, 13*, 399-415.

Hess, T., Auman, C., Colcombe, S., and Rahhal, T. (2003). The impact of stereotype threat on age differences in memory performance. *Journal of Gerontology: Psychological Sciences, 58*(1), P3-P11.

Holahan, C.K. (1988). Relation of life goals at age 70 to activity participation and health and psychological well-being among Terman's gifted men and women. *Psychology and Aging, 3*, 286-291.

Hooker, K. (1992). Possible selves and perceived health in older adults and college students. *Journal of Gerontology, 47*, 85-95.

Hooker, K., and Kaus, C.R. (1992). Possible selves and health behaviors in later life. *Journal of Aging and Health, 4*, 390-411.

Hooker, K., and Kaus, C.R. (1994). Health-related possible selves in young and middle adulthood. *Psychology and Aging, 9*, 126-133.

Hooper, E.M., Comstock, L.M., Goodwin, J.M., and Goodwin, J.S. (1982). Patient characteristics that influence physician behavior. *Medical Care, 20*, 630-638.

Hummert, M.L. (1990). Multiple stereotypes of elderly and young adults: A comparison of structure and evaluations. *Psychology and Aging, 5*, 82-193.

Hummert, M.L. (1994). Physiognomic cues and the activation of stereotypes of the elderly in interaction. *International Journal of Aging and Human Development, 39*, 5-20.

Hummert, M.L., Garstka, T.A., O'Brien, L.T., Greenwald, A.G., and Mellott, D.S. (2002). Using the Implicit Association Test to measure age differences in implicit social cognitions. *Psychology and Aging, 17*, 482-495.

Hummert, M.L., Garstka, T.A., and Shaner, J.L. (1997). Stereotyping of older adults: The role of target facial cues and perceiver characteristics. *Psychology and Aging, 12*, 107-114.

Hummert, M.L., Garstka, T.A., Shaner, J.L., and Strahm, S. (1994). Stereotypes of the elderly held by young, middle-aged, and elderly adults. *Journal of Gerontology: Psychological Sciences, 49*(5), P240-P249.

Hummert, M.L., Garstka, T.A., Shaner, J.L., and Strahm, S. (1995). Judgments about stereotypes of the elderly: Attitudes, age associations and typicality ratings of young, middle-aged, and elderly adults. *Research on Aging, 17*, 168-189.

Hummert, M.L., Shaner, J.L., Garstka, T.A., and Henry, C. (1998). Communication with older adults: The influence of age stereotypes, context and communicator age. *Human Communication Research, 25*, 124-151.

Isaacs, L., and Bearison, D. (1986). The development of children's prejudice against the aged. *International Journal of Aging and Human Development, 23*, 175-194.

Ivester, C., and King, K. (1977). Attitudes of adolescents toward the aged. *The Gerontologist, 17*, 85-89.

Jelenec, P., and Steffens, M.C. (2002). Implicit attitudes toward elderly women and men. *Current Research in Social Psychology, 7*, 275-293.

Kahana, E., and Kiyak, H. (1984). Attitudes and behavior of staff in facilities of the aged. *Research on Aging, 6*, 395-416.

Kemper, S. (1994). "Elderspeak": Speech accommodations to older adults. *Aging and Cognition, 1*, 17-28.

Kemper, S., Finter-Urczyk, A., Ferrell, P., Harden, T., and Billington, C. (1998). Using elderspeak with older adults. *Discourse Processes, 25*, 55-73.

Kemper, S., and Harden, T. (1999). Experimentally disentangling what's beneficial about elderspeak from what's not. *Psychology and Aging, 14*, 656-670.

Kemper, S., Othick, M., Gerhing, H., Gubarchuk, J., and Billington, C. (1998). The effects of practicing speech accommodations to older adults. *Applied Psycholinguistics, 19*, 175-192.

Kemper, S., Othick, M., Warren, J., Gubarchuk, J., and Gerhing, H. (1996). Facilitating older adults' performance on a referential communication task through speech accommodations. *Aging, Neuropsychology, and Cognition, 3*, 37-55.

Kemper, S., Vandeputte, D., Rice, K., Cheung, H., and Gubarchuk, J. (1995). Spontaneous adoption of elderspeak during referential communication tasks. *Journal of Language and Social Psychology, 14*, 40-59.

Kite, M.E., Deaux, K., and Miele, M. (1991). Stereotypes of young and old: Does age outweigh gender? *Psychology and Aging, 6*, 19-27.

Kite, M.E., and Johnson, B.T. (1988). Attitudes toward older and younger adults: A meta-analysis. *Psychology and Aging, 3*, 233-244.

Kite, M.E., and Wagner, L.S. (2002). Attitudes toward older adults. In T.D. Nelson (Ed.), *Ageism: Stereotyping and prejudice against older persons* (pp. 129-161). Cambridge, MA: MIT Press.

Knox, V.J., Gekoski, W.L., and Johnson, E.A. (1986). Contact with and perceptions of the elderly. *The Gerontologist, 26*, 309-313.

Kogan, N., and Mills, M. (1992). Gender influences on age cognitions and preferences: Sociocultural or sociobiological? *Psychology and Aging, 7*, 98-106.

Lagana, L., and Shanks, S. (2002). Mutual biases underlying the problematic relationship between older adults and mental health providers: Any solution in sight? *International Journal of Aging and Human Development, 55*, 271-295.

Lamberty, G.J., and Bieliauskas, L.A. (1993). Distinguishing between depression and dementia in the elderly: A review of neuropsychological findings. *Archives of Clinical Neurology, 8*, 149-170.

Lang, F.R., and Carstensen, L.L. (1994). Close emotional relationships in late life: Further support for proactive aging in the social domain. *Psychology and Aging, 9*, 315-324.

Lasser, R., Siegel, E., Dukoff, R., and Sunderland, T. (1988). Diagnosis and treatment of geriatric depression. *CNS Drugs, 9*, 17-30.

Learman, L.A., Avorn, J., Everitt, D.E., and Rosenthal, R. (1990). Pygmalion in the nursing home: The effects of caregiver expectations on patient outcomes. *Journal of the American Geriatric Society, 38*, 797-803.

Leary, M.R., and Kowalski, R.M. (1990). Impression management: A literature review and two-component model. *Psychological Bulletin, 107*, 34-47.

Levy, B.R. (1996). Improving memory in old age through implicit self-stereotyping. *Journal of Personality and Social Psychology, 71*, 1092-1107.

Levy, B.R. (2000). Handwriting as a reflection of aging self-stereotypes. *Journal of Geriatric Psychiatry, 33*, 81-94.

Levy, B.R. (2003). Mind matters: Cognitive and physical effects of aging self-stereotypes. *Journal of Gerontology: Psychological Sciences, 58*(4), P203-P211.

Levy, B.R., Ashman, O., and Dror, I. (1999-2000). To be or not to be: The effects of aging self-stereotypes on the will-to-live. *Omega: Journal of Death and Dying, 40*, 409-420.

Levy, B.R., and Banaji, M.R. (2002). Implicit ageism. In T. Nelson (Ed.), *Ageism: Stereotypes and prejudice against older persons* (pp. 49-75). Cambridge, MA: MIT Press.

Levy, B.R., Hausdorff, J.M., Hencke, R., and Wei, J.Y. (2000). Reducing cardiovascular stress with positive self-stereotypes of aging. *Journal of Gerontology: Psychological Sciences, 55*(4), P205-P213.

Levy, B.R., and Langer, E. (1994). Aging free from negative stereotypes: Successful memory in China and among the American deaf. *Journal of Personality and Social Psychology, 66*, 989-997.

Levy, B.R., Slade, M.D., and Kasl, S.V. (2002). Longitudinal benefit of positive self-perceptions of aging on functional health. *Journal of Gerontology: Psychological Sciences, 57*(5), P409-P417.

Levy, B.R., Slade, M.D., Kunkel, S.R., and Kasl, S.V. (2002). Longevity increased by positive self-perceptions of aging. *Journal of Personality and Social Psychology, 83*, 261-270.

Linn, M., and Hunter, K. (1979). Perception of age in the elderly. *Journal of Gerontology, 34*, 46-53.

Lowery, B.S., Hardin, C., and Sinclair, S. (2001). Social influence effects on automatic racial prejudice. *Journal of Personality and Social Psychology, 81*, 842-855.

Luszcz, M.A. (1983). An attitudinal assessment of perceived intergenerational affinities linking adolescence and old age. *International Journal of Behavioral Development, 6*, 221-231.

Luszcz, M.A. (1985-1986). Characterizing adolescents, middle-aged, and elderly adults: Putting the elderly into perspective. *International Journal of Aging and Human Development, 22*, 105-121.

Luszcz, M.A., and Fitzgerald, K.M. (1986). Understanding cohort differences in cross-generational, self, and peer perceptions. *Journal of Gerontology, 41*, 234-240.

Lutsky, N. (1980). Attitudes toward old age and elderly persons. In C. Eisdorfer (Ed.), *Annual review of gerontology and geriatrics* (vol. 1, pp. 287-336). New York: Springer.

Macrae, C.N., Milne, A.B., and Bodenhausen, G.V. (1994). Stereotypes as energy-saving devices: A peek inside the cognitive toolbox. *Journal of Personality and Social Psychology, 66*, 37-47.

Markus, H.R., and Herzog, A.R. (1991). The role of the self-concept in aging. *Annual Review of Gerontology and Geriatrics, 11*, 110-143.

Markus, H.R., and Nurius, P. (1986). Possible selves. *American Psychologist, 41*, 954-969.

Martin, K.A., Leary, M.R., and Rejeski, W.J. (2000). Self-presentational concerns in older adults: Implications for health and well-being. *Basic and Applied Social Psychology, 22*, 169-179.

McCann, R., and Giles, H. (2002). Ageism in the workplace: A communication perspective. In T.D. Nelson (Ed.), *Ageism: Stereotyping and prejudice against older persons* (pp. 163-199). Cambridge, MA: MIT Press.

McDougall, G.J. (1993). Therapeutic issues with gay and lesbian elders. *Clinical Gerontologist [Special Issue: The Forgotten Aged, Ethnic, Psychiatric, and Societal Minorities], 14*, 45-57.

Miller, C.T., and Major, B. (2000). Coping with stigma and prejudice. In T. Heatherton, R. Kleck, M. Hebl, and J. Hull (Eds.), *The social psychology of stigma* (pp. 243-272). New York: Guilford Press.

Miller, C.T., and Meyers, A.M. (1998). Compensating for prejudice: How heavyweight people (and others) control outcomes despite prejudice. In J. Swim and C. Stangor (Eds.), *Prejudice: The target's perspective*. New York: Academic Press.

Mitteness, L.S. (1987). The management of urinary incontinence by community-living elderly. *The Gerontologist, 27*, 185-193.

Montepare, J.M., and Zebrowitz-McArthur, L. (1988). Impressions of people created by age-related qualities of their gaits. *Journal of Personality and Social Psychology, 55*, 547-556.

Mroczek, D.K., and Kolarz, C.M. (1998). The effect of age on positive and negative affect: A developmental perspective on happiness. *Journal of Personality and Social Psychology, 75*, 1333-1349.

Mueller, J.H., Wonderlich, S., and Dugan, K. (1986). Self-referent processing of age-specific material. *Psychology and Aging, 1*, 293-299.

Nelson, T.D. (2002). *Ageism: Stereotyping and prejudice against older persons*. Cambridge, MA: MIT Press.

Neugarten, B. (1974, September). Age groups in American society and the rise of the young-old. *Annals of the American Academy of Political and Social Science*, 187-198.

Neugarten, B.L., and Hagestad, G.O. (1976). Age and the life course. In R.H. Binstock and E. Shanas (Eds.), *Handbook of aging and the social sciences*. New York: Van Nostrand Reinhold.

Nosek, B.A., Banaji, M.R., and Greenwald, A.G. (2002). Harvesting implicit group attitudes and beliefs from a demonstration website. *Group Dynamics [Special Issue: Groups and Internet], 6*, 101-115.

O'Connell, A.N., and Rotter, N.G. (1979). The influence of stimulus age and sex on person perception. *Journal of Gerontology, 34*, 220-228.

O'Connor, B.P., and Rigby, H. (1996). Perceptions of baby talk, frequency of receiving baby talk, and self-esteem among community and nursing home residents. *Psychology and Aging, 11*, 147-154.

Page, S. (1997). Accommodating the elderly: Words and actions in the community. *Journal of Housing for the Elderly, 12*, 55-61.

Palmore, E.D. (1990). *Ageism, negative and positive*. New York: Springer.

Parr, W.V., and Siegert, R. (1993). Adults' conceptions of everyday memory failures in others: Factors that mediate the effects of target age. *Psychology and Aging, 8*, 599-605.

Pasupathi, M., Carstensen, L.L., and Tsai, J.L. (1995). Ageism in interpersonal settings. In B. Lott and D. Maluso (Eds.), *The social psychology of interpersonal discrimination* (pp. 160-182). New York: Guilford Press.

Pasupathi, M., and Lockenhoff, C.E. (2002). Ageist behavior. In T.D. Nelson (Ed.), *Ageism: Stereotyping and prejudice against older persons* (pp. 201-246). Cambridge, MA: MIT Press.

Penner, L.A., Ludenia, K., and Mead, G. (1984). Staff attitudes: Image or reality. *Journal of Gerontological Nursing, 10*, 110-117.

Perdue, C.W., and Gurtman, M.B. (1990). Evidence for the automaticity of ageism. *Journal of Experimental Social Psychology, 26*, 199-216.

Perlmutter, M. (1988). Cognitive potential throughout life. In J. Birren and V. Bengtson (Eds.), *Emergent theories of aging* (pp. 247-268). New York: Springer.

Pettigrew, T.F., and Tropp, L.R. (2000). Does intergroup contact reduce prejudice: Recent meta-analytic findings. In S. Oskamp (Ed.), *Reducing prejudice and discrimination. The Claremont Symposium on Applied Social Psychology* (pp. 93-114). Mahwah, NJ: Lawrence Erlbaum.

Pinquart, M. (2002). Good news about the effects of bad old-age stereotypes. *Experimental Aging Research, 28*, 317-336.

Radecki, S.E., Kane, R.L., Solomon, D.H., and Mendenhall, R.C. (1988). Do physicians spend less time with older patients? *Journal of the American Geriatrics Society, 36*, 713-718.

Revenson, T.A. (1989). Compassionate stereotyping of elderly patients by physicians: Revising the social contact hypothesis. *Psychology and Aging, 4*, 230-234.

Richeson, J.A., and Ambady, N. (2003). Effects of situational power on automatic racial prejudice. *Journal of Experimental Social Psychology, 39*, 177-183.

Ripich, D.N. (1994). Functional communication with AD patients: A caregiver training program. *Alzheimer's Disease and Related Disorders, 8*, 95-109.

Rosen, B., and Jerdee, T.H. (1976). The nature of job-related age stereotypes. *Journal of Applied Psychology, 61*, 180-183.

Rubin, K.H., and Brown, I.D. (1975). A life-span look at person perception and its relationship to communicative interaction. *Journal of Gerontology, 30*, 461-468.

Rudman, L.A., Ashmore, R.D., and Gary, M.L. (2001). "Unlearning" automatic biases: The malleability of implicit prejudice and stereotypes. *Journal of Personality and Social Psychology, 81*, 856-868.

Ruscher, J.B. (2001). *Prejudiced communication: A social psychological perspective.* New York: Guilford Press.

Ryan, E.B. (1992). Beliefs about memory changes across the lifespan. *Journal of Gerontology: Psychological Sciences, 47*, P96-P101.

Ryan, E.B., Bieman-Copland, S., Kwong See, S., Ellis, C.H., and Anas, A.P. (2002). Age excuses: Conversational management of memory failures in older adults. *Journal of Gerontology: Psychological Sciences, 57*, P256-P267.

Ryan, E.B., Hamilton, J.M., and Kwong See, S. (1994). Patronizing the old: How do younger and older adults respond to baby talk in the nursing home? *International Journal of Aging and Human Development, 39*, 21-32.

Ryan, E.B., Hummert, M.L., and Boich, L.H. (1995). Communication predicaments of aging: Patronizing behavior toward older adults. *Journal of Language and Social Psychology, 14*, 144-166.

Ryan, E.B., Meredith, S.D., MacLean, M.J., and Orange, J.B. (1995). Changing the way we talk with elders: Promoting health using the communication enhancement model. *International Journal of Aging Human Development, 41*, 87-105.

Ryff, C.D. (1989). In the eye of the beholder: Views of psychological well-being among middle-aged and older adults. *Psychology and Aging, 4*, 195-210.

Salthouse, T.A., Hambrick, D.Z., and McGuthry, K.E. (1998). Shared age-related influences on cognitive and noncognitive variables. *Psychology and Aging, 13*, 486-500.

Schaie, K.W. (1994). The course of adult intellectual development. *American Psychologist, 49*, 304-313.

Schmidt, D.F., and Boland, S.M. (1986). Structure of perceptions of older adults: Evidence for multiple stereotypes. *Psychology and Aging, 1*, 255-260.

Seccombe, K., and Ishii Kuntz, M. (1991). Perceptions of problems associated with aging: Comparisons among four older age cohorts. *Gerontologist, 31*, 527-533.

Sherman, M.M., Roberto, K.A., and Robinson, J. (1996). Knowledge and attitudes of hospital personnel towards older adults. *Gerontology and Geriatrics Education, 16*, 25-35.

Small, J.A., Kemper, S., and Lyons, K. (1997). Sentence comprehension in Alzheimer's disease: Effects of grammatical complexity, speech rate, and repetition. *Psychology and Aging, 12*, 1-11.

Snyder, M., and Miene, P.K. (1994). Stereotyping of the elderly: A functional approach. *British Journal of Social Psychology [Special Issue: Stereotypes: Structure, Function and Process], 33*, 63-82.

Sontag, S. (1979). The double standard of aging. In J. Williams (Ed.), *Psychology of women* (pp. 462-478). New York: Academic Press.

Steele, C.M. (1997). A threat in the air: How stereotypes shape intellectual identity and performance. *American Psychologist, 52*, 613-629.

Steele, C.M., Spencer, S., and Aronson, J. (2002). Contending with group image: The psychology of stereotype and social identity threat. In M.P. Zanna (Ed.), *Advances in experimental social psychology* (vol. 34, pp. 379-440). San Diego: Academic Press.

Stein, R., Blanchard-Fields, F., and Herzog, C. (2002). The effects of age-stereotype priming on the memory performance of older adults. *Experimental Aging Research, 28*, 169-181.

Suls, J., and Mullen, B. (1982). From the cradle to the grave: Comparison and self-evaluation across the life span. In J. Suls (Ed.), *Psychological perspectives on the self* (vol. 1, pp. 97-128). Mahwah, NJ: Lawrence Erlbaum.

Thimm, C., Rademacher, U., and Kruse, L. (1998). Age stereotypes and patronizing messages: Features of age-adapted speech in technical instructions to the elderly. *Journal of Applied Communication Research [Special Issue: Applied Research in Language and Intergenerational Communication], 26*, 66-82.

Thunher, M. (1983). Turning points and developmental change: Subjective and "objective" assessments. *American Journal of Orthopsychiatry, 53*, 52-60.

Tuckman, J., and Lavell, M. (1957). Self-classification as old or not old. *Geriatrics, 12*, 666-671.

Waid, L.D., and Frazier, L.D. (2003). Cultural differences in possible selves during later life. *Journal of Aging Studies, 17*, 251-268.

Whitbourne, S.K., and Sneed, J.R. (2002). The paradox of well-being, identity processes, and stereotype threat: Ageism and its potential relationships to the self in later life. In T. Nelson (Ed.), *Ageism: Stereotypes and prejudice against older persons* (pp. 247-273). Cambridge, MA: MIT Press.

Williams, A., and Nussbaum, J.F. (2001). *Intergenerational communication across the lifespan.* Mahwah, NJ: Lawrence Erlbaum.

Wood, J.V. (1989). Theory and research concerning social comparison of personal attributes. *Psychological Bulletin, 106*, 231-248.

Yoon, C., Hasher, L., Feinberg, F., Rahhal, T.A., and Winocur, G. (2000). Cross-cultural differences in memory: The role of culture-based stereotypes about aging. *Psychology and Aging, 15*, 694-704.

Zebrowitz, L.A. (2003). Aging stereotypes—Internalization or inoculation? A commentary. *Journal of Gerontology: Psychological Sciences, 58*, 214-215.

Zepelin, H., Sills, R.A., and Heath, M.W. (1986-1987). Is age becoming irrelevant? An exploratory study of perceived age norms. *International Journal of Aging and Human Development, 24*, 241-256.

Measuring Psychological Mechanisms

Committee on Aging Frontiers in Social Psychology, Personality, and Adult Developmental Psychology

INTRODUCTION

Most social research on aging attempts to characterize behavioral patterns in a population. The bulk of this research relies on information provided by samples of individuals through surveys or interviews. Thus, the accuracy and quality of self-reported information are critical for the interpretation of social science findings in multiple disciplines. Psychological research has revealed problems with a heavy reliance on self-reported information and identified some solutions. In addition, psychologists have invested considerable efforts in developing methods that circumvent self-reports and reveal social and cognitive processes that may be out of conscious awareness. In doing so, psychological science has developed a number of measurement tools and analytic approaches that allow for relatively nuanced assessments of cognition, emotion, and behavior that are of use not only to psychologists, but also to sociologists, demographers, economists, and health professionals.

In a nutshell, people are quite good at providing accurate information about concrete matters, like occupation or marital status. Self-reports are also well suited to assess explicit beliefs, like political opinions or values. However, psychological research has shown that survey responses can vary as a function of the context in which the questions are embedded and can even be influenced by extraneous—and seemingly innocuous—factors like the weather (Schwarz, this volume). Moreover, reliance on self-reported information presumes considered self-knowledge. In many cases, questions seek information that people do not have, even when they believe that they do: why they exercise or don't, whether they are racist or ageist, or whether they are more easily persuaded by certain kinds of messages than others. Thus, whereas self-reported information is well suited to answer certain questions, it is seriously limited in answering others.

This paper briefly reviews some methodological and analytical approaches that hold significant promise for the field of aging research, including the measurement of implicit constructs and experience sampling. The measurement of change over time, which is essential to a deep understanding of aging, is also an area in which rapid progress is being made. This overview is followed by three short papers: two address measurement concerns and ways to minimize bias in self-reports; the third looks at the emerging use of neuroscience in social cognition research on aging. Breakthroughs in thought and theory often occur after improvements in measurement techniques and methodology are made; some of the latest developments discussed briefly here illustrate the potential for psychological research on aging.

MEASURING IMPLICIT CONSTRUCTS

Explicit constructs and processes are those that are subject to conscious awareness and direct self-report; *implicit* constructs and processes are not. There has been a recent explosion of interest in social psychology in the area of implicit social cognition, with the term being used in several different ways (see Petty, Wheeler, and Tormala, 2003). Some researchers are interested in implicit constructs such as attitudes, goals, and motives. For example, do people have evaluative predispositions of which they are unaware (e.g., an implicit attitude such as an unrecognized dislike of old people)? Other researchers are interested in implicit biases, in which people are perfectly aware of their attitudes or motives but do not know where they come from, or in implicit effects, in which people are aware of their attitudes or motives but do not know what effect those attitudes or motives have on their thoughts and actions.

To examine implicit constructs and processes, social psychologists have developed a battery of implicit measures that do not call for conscious self-reports of the construct or process. The earliest such measures were in essence disguised self-reports (e.g., thematic apperception tests) or behavioral observations (e.g., how close one sat next to a stranger) from which researchers inferred an underlying attitude or motive. Recently, implicit measures based on reaction times have demonstrated considerable utility in predicting behaviors that could not be predicted by direct self-reports (e.g., Dovidio, Kawakami, and Gaertner, 2002). Furthermore, even when direct self-reports were useful in predicting behavior, implicit measures have been shown to account for additional variance (e.g., Vargas, von Hippel, and Petty, 2004).

Two measures have captured the bulk of recent research attention. One measure is based on priming procedures, which were developed initially by cognitive psychologists. With this measure, participants are presented with different stimuli (e.g., elderly or young faces—the primes) and then asked to indicate the evaluative meaning (i.e., good/bad) of various words (e.g., dirt or flower) as quickly as possible by pressing an appropriate response key on a computer. Reaction times for the classification of the words are assessed. To the extent that elderly faces facilitate responses to negative words or inhibit responses to positive words in comparison to young faces, one can infer that a negative attitude toward the elderly is automatically activated when the face appears (e.g., Fazio, Sanbonmatsu, Powell, and Kardes, 1996).

The second measure is the implicit association test (Greenwald, McGhee, and Schwartz, 1998). It assesses the strength of association between a target concept (e.g., the elderly) and an attribute dimension (e.g., good/bad) by examining the speed with which participants can use two response keys to categorize words (or pictures) when each key is assigned a dual meaning (e.g., elderly/good versus young/bad). If people are classifying young (e.g., spring break) and old (e.g., retirement) terms or positive (e.g., flower) and negative (e.g., dirt) words, the question is whether it is easier to do so when elderly is paired with good or with bad on the response keys. The relative pattern of reaction times to the categorization task is informative with respect to whether the category of elderly is more closely associated with good or bad. Both the priming measure and the implicit association test have been used successfully in research on prejudice toward a wide variety of social groups (see recent reviews by Blair, 2002; Fazio and Olson, 2003).

Interestingly, although implicit and explicit measures typically produce the same pattern of evaluations for common objects (e.g., ice cream), implicit measures for evaluations of prejudice have not correlated very well with more traditional explicit measures. There are at least two popular explanations for this. One relies on the idea that the implicit measures are accurate and the explicit measures are misleading. For example, a person might not want to report prejudice toward a minority group for fear of social rejection. A second possibility, however, is that both attitudes are valid (Wilson, Lindsey, and Schooler, 2000). Indeed, some research has demonstrated that each type of measure can predict different behaviors. Explicit measures tend to predict deliberative behaviors better than implicit measures, while implicit measures tend to predict spontaneous behaviors better than explicit ones (e.g., Dovidio, Kawakami, Johnson, Johnson, and

Howard, 1997). The same explanation applies for measures of implicit and explicit motives (e.g., McClelland, Koestner, and Weinberger, 1989).

In addition to using implicit measures, social psychologists have also used various experimental procedures to invoke implicit processes. Perhaps the most notable in this regard is the work on priming. In this work, researchers attempt to subtly activate various concepts (e.g., stereotypes of the elderly) and examine their effects on behavior. For example, participants have been asked to unscramble sentences with elderly content (e.g., retired Florida Ted to) and have been exposed to a subliminal presentation of elderly-related words (e.g., wrinkled, retire; see Bargh and Chartrand, 2000, for a review). Subtly activating stereotypes—whether about oneself or others—can influence behavior (see Steele, Spencer, and Aronson, 2002; Wheeler and Petty, 2001). In one study, for example (Dijksterhuis, Aarts, Bargh, and van Knippenberg, 2000), researchers assessed the extent to which people automatically associated the elderly with forgetfulness. People who made a strong association between the elderly and forgetfulness showed memory impairment themselves when they were primed with the elderly category.

Many challenges remain in this area. For example, measurement of implicit constructs in multigroup studies of culture, ethnicity, and race is an especially difficult methodological problem. Methods must be developed for conducting multigroup comparisons, contrasting results about implicit constructs both within and between group studies, improving the reliability and validity of existing measures, and promoting the development of new constructs for understanding culture, ethnicity, and race in older adults.

EXPERIENCE SAMPLING

Much of what is known about aging comes from surveys that assess constructs of interest by administering a single item (or a handful of items) in the form of questionnaires administered years apart. Data are usually characterized by age differences in measures of central tendencies (e.g., means, medians, etc.). Although the approach has generated important information about both stability and change over time (see reviews by Costa and McCrae, 1997; Ryff, Kwan, and Singer, 2001), recent research suggests that assessing daily experiences further strengthens predictions about social behavior and allows for closer examination of links between constructs and experiences (Almeida and Kessler, 1998; Kahneman, Krueger, Schkade, Schwarz, and Stone, 2004).

However, there are at least two major types of intraindividual variability: within-person changes over relatively long periods of time that may or may not be reversible, such as those seen in development; and within-person changes that are more fluid, such as mood states (see Nesselroade,

2001). Experience sampling also allows for an examination of variability across a week, a day, or an even shorter interval. Experience-sampling approaches are found primarily in the research literatures on personality, emotion, and human abilities (see, e.g., Carstensen, Pasupathi, Mayr, and Nesselroade, 2000; Fleeson, 2001; Hultsch, MacDonald, and Dixon, 2002; Schwartz, Neale, Marco, Shiffman, and Stone, 1999). Variability within an individual across relatively short intervals, such as a day or a week, has proven to be a powerful predictor of such outcomes as divorce and mortality, among others.

The study of intraindividual variability has contributed importantly to our understanding of personality and emotions and the ways in which they change over time. For example, variability in reports about self-concept across a week-long sampling period predicts the intensity with which people experience both positive and negative emotions (Charles and Pasupathi, 2003). From a developmental perspective, we have also learned that phenomena apparent at the intraindividual level may not necessarily be reflected in mean changes in performance across a group or even within the same individual across time. In the study by Charles and Pasupathi (2003), for example, there was less variability in older adults than in younger adults. Similarly, Mroczek and Spiro (2003) report individual differences in the rate of age-related change of the personality traits of extraversion and neuroticism.

Studies of the relationship between personality and intraindividual variability in emotional experience found that emotional variability over time is related to withdrawal from life (Eaton and Funder, 2001; Larsen, 2000), and the same research also shows that each of three different aspects of emotional experience (valence, intraindividual variability, and rate of change) correlate with different, specific personality variables (extraversion, repression, and fearfulness and hostility toward others, respectively), and that these relationships are not consistent across gender. Eid and Diener (1999), demonstrated that intraindividual variability in affect is distinct enough to be considered a unique trait, separate from measures of neuroticism and other personality factors and that variations in intraindividual organization of behavior variation across situations is reflected in distinctive profiles of situation-behavior relationships (Shoda, Mischel, and Wright, 1994).

Intraindividual variability appears to be a rich resource for behavioral prediction. For example, the lability of self-esteem predicts vulnerability to depression (Butler, Hokanson, and Flynn, 1994). As Nesselroade (2001) points out, intraindividual methodologies allow for the integration of idiographic (concerning discrete or unique facts or events) and nomothetic (concerning the discovery of scientific laws) emphases in the study of behavior. An experience-sampling study that included the full adult age range found that older adults experienced more complex combinations of emotions than younger adults and were more likely to experience positive and negative emotions simultaneously (Carstensen et al., 2000). Complexity of experience was related to superior regulation of emotion. Thus, information garnered from repeated sampling provides a richer account of the strategies people use that result in better or poorer self-regulation. Certain types of intraindividual variability may also be predictors of cognitive dysfunction and even death. For example, Hultsch, MacDonald, Hunter, Levy-Bencheton, and Strauss (2000) found that greater individual variability on tests of several cognitive domains characterized those older adults with mild dementia. Eizenman, Nesselroade, Featherman, and Rowe (1997) found that within-person variation over weekly measurements of perceived locus of control predicted mortality status 5 years later.

Progress in analytical approaches to intraindividual variability has been rapid in recent years (see Nesselroade and Ram, 2004), pointing to new ways to model individual growth (i.e., multilevel model or random effects model) (Eid and Diener, 1999; Mroczek and Spiro, 2003) by parsing average trends and isolating individual variability, and also pointing to novel ways to understand dynamic change (McArdle and Hamagami, 2004; Boker and Bisconti, 2005; Boker, Neale, and Rausch, 2004).

SOCIAL NEUROSCIENCE

The addition of brain imaging techniques to the methodological arsenal has greatly increased the power of measurement approaches in psychology. Jointly using brain and behavioral data, scientists have advanced the understanding of the specific processes involved in behavioral responses. There has been a growing interdisciplinary effort by social psychologists and cognitive neuroscientists to use methods such as functional brain imaging (e.g., positron emission tomography [PET], functional magnetic resonance imaging [fMRI], and magnetoencephalogram [MEG]) to study social cognition (Adolphs, 2003; Heatherton, Macrae, and Kelley, 2004; Ochsner and Lieberman, 2001). The cognitive neuroscience of aging has benefited enormously from these methods and the social neuroscience of aging is expected to do the same.

Rapid progress is already being made in identifying the neural basis of social cognition in younger populations. There have been three special issues of neuroscience journals dedicated to social neuroscience, and the *Journal of Cognitive Neuroscience* has added the topic to its core publication mission. The field is likely to grow rapidly as the methods of cognitive neuroscience provide social psychologists with new tools to understand human nature. Researchers have identified a number of brain regions that support social capacities, such as recognition of faces and their emotional expressions, theory of mind, social emotions (e.g., empathy), judgments of attractiveness, cooperation, and so forth. It is crucial both for social psychologists to recognize that brain mechanisms are involved in producing social behaviors, and for neuroscientists to appreciate that brains function in social contexts that fundamentally constrain behavior. For example, studies in social cognitive neuroscience demonstrate that the category of "people" is given privileged status by the brain as it processes objects in its environment: that is, there is a distinct functional neuroanatomy for semantic judgments made about people that is distinct from similar judgments made about other objects (Mitchell, Heatherton, and Macrae, 2002).

Social brain science is providing new insights into long-standing questions regarding social behavior. One such question concerns the mechanisms that support the self-reference memory enhancement effect, in which information encoded with reference to the self is better remembered than information encoded with reference to other people. This question remained unresolved because the competing theories made identical behavioral predictions (i.e., better memory performance for material related to self). A resolution came about when Kelley and colleagues (2002), using fMRI, found that an area of the medial prefrontal cortex was uniquely associated with self-referential processing. This team of researchers subsequently found that activity in this region predicted whether or not people remembered traits they had processed with reference to self (Macrae, Kelley, and Heatherton, 2004).

Another exciting area of research reveals that different brain regions are involved in the anticipation and the experience of reward. Reward anticipation is likely involved in drug addiction, gambling, and other tasks in which people work to achieve a desired state (Knutson and Peterson, 2005). Experiments of this type characterize the emerging field of neuroeconomics. Knutson, Westdorp, Kaiser, and Hommer (2000) have devised a very creative procedure, referred to as the monetary incentive delay task, in which participants "play a game" during which they are led to anticipate winning or losing money. Using fMRI technology, the researchers have examined activation in the nucleus accumbens as volunteers play the "game." Their initial findings suggest that while the medial caudate is activated proportionally in anticipation of both rewards and punishments and their magnitudes, the ventral striatal nucleus accumbens is activated proportionately only with the amount of an anticipated reward, not with a punishment (Knutson, Adams, Fong, and Hommer, 2001). While most psychological and pharmaceutical treatments for psychopathology focus on dampening negative emotions, this work lays the foundation for ways to modify behavior by recruiting positive emotional systems.

Very few studies have applied social neuroscience to questions about aging, but intriguing results have emerged from those that have. For example, one study finds that in older adults brain regions involved in storing emotion memories respond little to negative images but are activated in response to positive images (Mather et al., 2004). Cognitive aging researchers have also demonstrated neural compensation: on tasks that place a significant demand on controlled and deliberative processes, older adults show bilateral frontal activation while younger people show laterality (Park, Polk, Mikels, Taylor, and Marshuetz, 2001; Reuter-Lorenz, 2002).

The investigation of the role of neural plasticity in social tasks may be particularly interesting. The literature is replete with examples showing that older adults arrange their environment to be supportive, to recruit other cognitive resources, and to use others in such tasks as collaborative problem solving (Dixon, 2000). It appears also that compensation occurs at a neural level, but this requires more investigation.

REFERENCES

Adolphs, R. (2003). Cognitive neuroscience of human social behavior. *Nature Reviews Neuroscience, 4*, 165-178.

Almeida, D.M., and Kessler, R.C. (1998). Everyday stressors and gender differences in daily distress. *Journal of Personality and Social Psychology, 75*(3), 670-680.

Bargh, J.A., and Chartrand, T.L. (2000). The mind in the middle: A practical guide to priming and automaticity research. In H.T. Reiss and C.M. Judd (Eds.), *Handbook of research methods in social and personality psychology*. New York: Cambridge University Press.

Blair, I. (2002). The malleability of automatic stereotypes and prejudice. *Personality and Social Psychology Review, 6*, 242-261.

Boker, S.M., and Bisconti, T.L. (2005). Dynamical systems modeling in aging research. In C.S. Bergeman and S.M. Boker (Eds.), *Quantitative methodology in aging research*. Mahwah, NJ: Lawrence Erlbaum.

Boker, S.M., Neale, M.C., and Rausch, J. (2004). Latent differential equation modeling with multivariate multi-occasion indicators. In K. van Montfort, H. Oud, and A. Satorra (Eds.), *Recent developments on structural equation models: Theory and applications* (pp. 151-174). Amsterdam: Kluwer.

Butler, A.C., Hokanson, J.E., and Flynn, H.A. (1994). A comparison of self-esteem lability and low trait self-esteem as vulnerability factors for depression. *Journal of Personality and Social Psychology, 66*(1), 166-177.

Carstensen, L.L., Pasupathi, M., Mayr, U., and Nesselroade, J.R. (2000). Emotional experience in everyday life across the adult life span. *Journal of Personality and Social Psychology, 79*(4), 644-655.

Charles, S.T., and Pasupathi, M. (2003). Age-related patterns of variability in self-descriptions: Implications for everyday affective experience. *Psychology and Aging, 18*, 524-536.

Costa, P.T., and McCrae, R.R. (1997). Longitudinal stability of adult personality. In R. Hogan, J.A. Johnson, and S.R. Briggs (Eds.), *Handbook of personality psychology* (pp. 269-290). San Diego, CA: Academic Press.

Dijksterhuis, A., Aarts, H., Bargh, J.A., and van Knippenberg, A. (2000). On the relation between associative strength and automatic behavior. *Journal of Experimental Social Psychology, 36*(5), 531-544.

Dixon, R.A. (2000). Concepts and mechanisms of gains in cognitive aging. In D.C. Park and N. Schwarz (Eds.), *Cognitive aging: A primer* (pp. 23-41). Philadelphia: Psychology Press.

Dovidio, J.F., Kawakami, K., and Gaertner, S.L. (2002). Implicit and explicit prejudice and interracial interactions. *Journal of Personality and Social Psychology, 82*, 62-68.

Dovidio, J.F., Kawakami, K., Johnson, C., Johnson, B., and Howard, A. (1997). On the nature of prejudice: Automatic and controlled processes. *Journal of Experimental Social Psychology, 3*(5), 510-540.

Eaton, L.G., and Funder, D.C. (2001). Emotional experience in daily life: Valence, variability, and rate of change. *Emotion,* (4), 413-421.

Eid, M., and Diener, E. (1999). Intraindividual variability in affect: Reliability, validity, and personality correlates. *Journal of Personality and Social Psychology, 76*(4), 662-676.

Eizenman, D.R., Nesselroade, J.R., Featherman, D.L., and Rowe, J.W. (1997). Intraindividual variability in perceived control in an older sample: The MacArthur successful aging studies. *Psychology and Aging, 12*(3), 489-502.

Fazio, R.H., and Olson, M. (2003). Implicit measures in social cognition research: Their meaning and use. *Annual Review of Psychology, 54*, 297-327.

Fazio, R.H., Sanbonmatsu, D.M., Powell, M.C., and Kardes, F.R. (1996). On the automatic activation of attitudes. *Journal of Personality and Social Psychology, 50*, 229-238.

Fleeson, W. (2001). Towards a structure- and process-integrated view of personality: Traits as density distributions of states. *Journal of Personality and Social Psychology, 80*, 1011-1027.

Greenwald, A.G., McGhee, D.E., and Schwartz, J.L.K. (1998). Measuring individual differences in implicit cognition: The implicit association test. *Journal of Personality and Social Psychology, 74*, 1464-1480.

Heatherton, T.F., Macrae, C.N., and Kelley, W.M. (2004). What the social brain sciences can tell us about the self. *Current Directions in Psychological Science, 13*(5), 190-193.

Hultsch, D.F., MacDonald, S.W., and Dixon, R.A. (2002). Variability in reaction time performance of younger and older adults. *Journals of Gerontology Series B: Psychological Sciences and Social Sciences, 57*(2), P101-P115.

Hultsch, D.F., MacDonald, S.W., Hunter, M.A., Levy-Bencheton, J., and Strauss, E. (2000). Intraindividual variability in cognitive performance in older adults: Comparison of adults with mild dementia, adults with arthritis, and healthy adults. *Neuropsychology, 14*, 588-598.

Kahneman, D., Krueger, A., Schkade, S., Schwarz, N., and Stone, A. (2004). A survey method for characterizing daily life experience: The day reconstruction method. *Science, 306*, 1776-1780.

Kelley, W.M., Macrae, C.N., Wyland, C.L., Caglar, S., Inati, S., and Heatherton, T.F. (2002). Finding the self? An event-related fMRI study. *Journal of Cognitive Neuroscience, 14*, 785-794.

Knutson, B., Adams, C.M., Fong, G.W., and Hommer, D. (2001). Anticipation of increasing monetary reward selectively recruits nucleus accumbens. *Journal of Neuroscience, 21*(16), RC159.

Knutson, B., and Peterson, R. (2005). Neurally reconstructing expected utility. *Games and Economic Behavior, 52*, 305-315.

Knutson, B., Westdorp, A., Kaiser, E., and Hommer, D. (2000). FMRI visualization of brain activity during a monetary incentive delay task. *Neuroimage, 12*, 20-27.

Larsen, R.J. (2000). Toward a science of mood regulation. *Psychological Inquiry, 11*(3), 129-141.

Macrae, C.N., Kelley, W.M., and Heatherton, T.F. (2004). A self less ordinary: The medial prefrontal cortex and you. *The new cognitive neurosciences* (3rd ed.). Cambridge, MA: MIT Press.

Mather, M., Canli, T., English, T., Whitfield, S., Wais, P., Ochsner, K., Gabrieli, J.D., and Carstensen, L.L. (2004). Amygdala responses to emotionally valenced stimuli in older and younger adults. *Psychological Science, 15*(4), 259-263.

McArdle, J.J., and Hamagami, F. (2004). Methods for dynamic change hypotheses. In K. van Montfort, J. Oud, and A. Satorra (Eds.), *Recent developments on structural equation models: Theory and applications* (pp. 295-335). Dordrecht, Netherlands: Kluwer Academic Publishers.

McClelland, D.C., Koestner, R., and Weinberger, J. (1989). How do self-attributed and implicit motives differ? *Psychological Review, 96*, 690-702.

Mitchell, J.P., Heatherton, T.F., and Macrae, C.N. (2002). Distinct neural systems subserve person and object knowledge. *Proceedings of the National Academy of Sciences, 99*, 15238-15243.

Mroczek, D.K., and Spiro, A. (2003). Modeling intraindividual change in personality traits: Findings from the normative aging study. *Journals of Gerontology Series B: Psychological Sciences and Social Sciences, 58B*(3), P153-P165.

Nesselroade, J.R. (2001). Intraindividual variability in development within and between individuals. *European Psychologist, 6*(3), 187-193.

Nesselroade, J.R., and Ram, N. (2004). Studying intraindividual variability: What we have learned that will help us understand lives in context. *Research in Human Development, 1*, 9-29.

Ochsner, K., and Lieberman, M. (2001). The emergence of social cognitive neuroscience. *American Psychologist, 56*, 717-734.

Park, D.C., Polk, T.A., Mikels, J.A., Taylor, S.F., and Marshuetz, C. (2001). Cerebral aging: Integration of brain and behavioral models of cognitive function. *Dialogues in Clinical Neuroscience, 3*(3), 151-165.

Petty, R.E., Wheeler, S.C., and Tormala, Z.L. (2003). Persuasion and attitude change. In T. Millon and M.J. Lerner (Eds.), *Handbook of psychology: Personality and social psychology* (vol. 5, pp. 353-382). Hoboken, NJ: John Wiley and Sons.

Reuter-Lorenz, P.A. (2002). New visions of the aging mind and brain. *Trends in cognitive sciences, 6*(9), 394-400.

Ryff, C.D., Kwan, C.M., and Singer, B.H. (2001). Personality and aging: Flourishing agendas and future challenges. In J.E. Birren and K.W. Schaie (Eds.), *Handbook of the psychology of aging* (pp. 477-499). New York: Academic Press.

Schwartz, J.E., Neale, J., Marco, C., Shiffman, S.S., and Stone, A.A. (1999). Does trait coping exist? A momentary assessment approach to the evaluation of traits. *Journal of Personality and Social Psychology, 77*(2), 360-369.

Shoda, Y., Mischel, W., and Wright, J.C. (1994). Intraindividual stability in the organization and patterning of behavior: Incorporating psychological situations into the idiographic analysis of personality. *Journal of Personality and Social Psychology, 67*(4), 674-687.

Steele, C.M., Spencer, S.J., and Aronson, J. (2002). Contending with group image: The psychology of stereotype and social identity threat. In M.P. Zanna (Ed.), *Advances in experimental social psychology* (vol. 34, pp. 379-340). San Diego: Academic Press.

Vargas, P.T., von Hippel, W., and Petty, R.E. (2004). Using partially structured attitude measures to enhance the attitude-behavior relationship. *Personality and Social Psychology Bulletin, 30*, 197-211.

Wheeler, S.C., and Petty, R.E. (2001). The effects of stereotype activation on behavior: A review of possible mechanisms. *Psychological Bulletin, 127*, 797-826.

Wilson, T.D., Lindsey, S., and Schooler, T.Y. (2000). A model of dual attitudes. *Psychological Review, 107*, 101-126.

Measurement: Aging and the Psychology of Self-Report

Norbert Schwarz
University of Michigan

INTRODUCTION

Social psychological research includes the measurement of a wide range of phenomena, from person perception and stereotyping to political attitudes and consumer preferences, and from perceptions of social change to well-being and social support. Social psychology's key contribution to measurement is not the development of particular measures for specific content domains, but basic research into the cognitive and communicative processes underlying self-reports, with implications that cut across many content domains. For comprehensive reviews of the psychology of self-reports see Schwarz (1996, 1999b); Sudman, Bradburn, and Schwarz (1996); Tourangeau, Rips, and Rasinski (2000); and the contributions in Sirken et al. (1999). As will become apparent, the cognitive changes associated with normal human aging can profoundly affect the processes underlying self-reports of opinions and behaviors, giving rise to *age-sensitive context effects* (see the contributions in Schwarz, Park, Knäuper, and Sudman, 1999). As a result, any observed age difference in self-reported attitudes and behaviors can reflect (a) a true difference, (b) a difference in the response process, or (c) an unknown mixture of both. In this paper I illustrate the problem by highlighting three age-sensitive context effects that are sufficiently pronounced to thwart meaningful cohort comparisons: question order effects, response order effects, and the effects of alternative responses.

ATTITUDE REPORTS

Social psychologists and public opinion researchers have long been aware that attitude reports are highly context dependent (for reviews see Schuman and Presser, 1981; Sudman et al., 1996). When asked to report on their opinions, respondents can rarely retrieve a ready-for-use answer from memory. Instead, they need to form an answer on the spot, drawing on information that is accessible at that point in time. This gives rise to question order and response order effects, both of which are age sensitive.

Question Order Effects Decrease with Age

Question order effects emerge when preceding questions bring information to mind that respondents may otherwise not consider in answering a subsequent question (see Sudman et al., 1996, for a discussion of the underlying processes). To reduce these effects, researchers often introduce buffer items to separate related questions, thus attenuating the accessibility of previously used information. The same logic suggests that age-related declines in memory function attenuate question order effects because they render it less likely that previously used information is still accessible. The available data support this prediction (Knäuper, Schwarz, Park, and Fritsch, 2003, unpublished manuscript; Schwarz and Knäuper, 2000).

One of the most robust question order effects in the survey literature was observed by Schuman and Presser (1981), who asked respondents if a pregnant woman should be able to obtain a legal abortion "if she is married and does not want any more children" (Question A) or "if there is a strong chance of a serious defect in the baby" (Question B). Not surprisingly, more respondents support legal abortion in response to Question B than in response to Question A. More important, support for Question A decreases when Question B is presented first: Compared to the risk of a serious birth defect, merely "not wanting any more children" appears less legitimate, reducing support for legal abortion. Secondary analyses show that this question order effect results in a difference of 19.5 percentage points for younger respondents, but decreases with age and is no longer observed for respondents aged 65 and older (Figure 1). Thus researchers arrive at different conclusions about cohort differences depending on the order in which the questions are asked. When the "no more children" question (A) is asked first, support for abortion decreases with age, suggesting that older respondents hold more conservative attitudes toward abortion. Yet no age difference can be observed when the same question is preceded by the "birth defect" question (B).

Laboratory experiments (Knäuper et al., 2003) indicate that the attenuation of question order effects among older respondents is due to age-

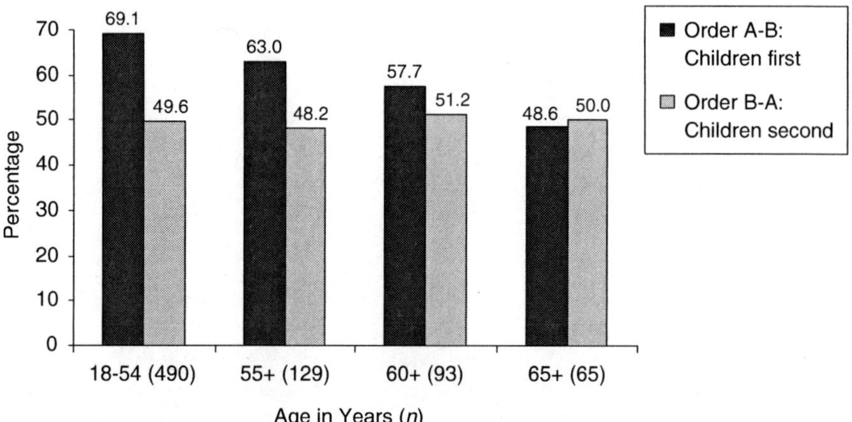

FIGURE 1 Question order effects as a function of age.
NOTE: Columns show percentages of respondents who support abortion for "a married woman who doesn't want any more children" when this question precedes (A-B) or follows (B-A) the birth defect question.

related declines in working memory capacity. Using Salthouse and Babcock's (1991) reading span test, Knäuper and colleagues (2003) found that younger respondents (age 20 to 40 years), as well as older respondents (age 60 to 100 years) with good working memory capacity, showed the familiar question order effect, whereas older respondents with poor working memory capacity did not (Figure 2), suggesting that the attenuation of question order effects among older respondents is due to age-related declines in working memory capacity. A related experiment with different questions replicated this pattern.

However, the observed attenuation of question order effects may be limited to the relatively uninvolving questions typical for public opinion surveys. In contrast, older adults' inhibition problems (Hasher and Zacks, 1988) may exaggerate question order effects when the question is of high personal relevance or emotionally involving. This possibility remains to be tested.

Response Order Effects Increase with Age

A second major source of context effects in attitude measurement is the order in which response alternatives are presented. Response order effects are most reliably obtained when a question presents several plausible response options (see Schwarz, Hippler, and Noelle-Neumann, 1992; Sudman

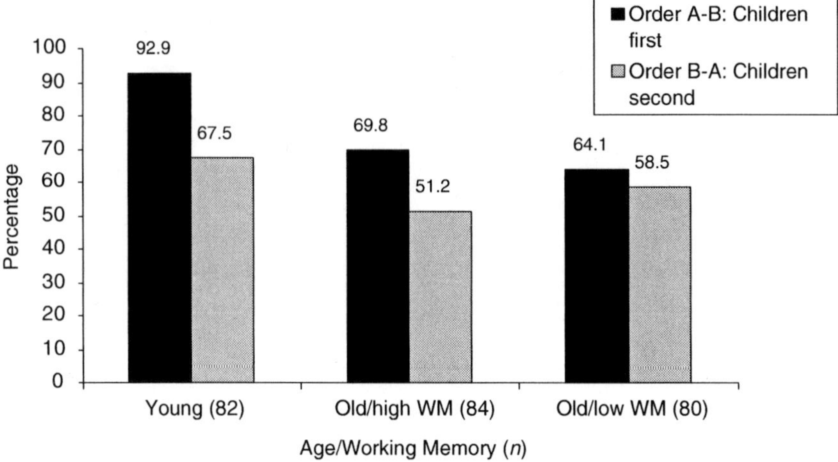

FIGURE 2 Question order effects as a function of age and working memory.
NOTE: Columns show the percentage of respondents who support abortion for "a married woman who doesn't want any more children" (question A) versus the percentage of respondents who support abortion when there is a risk of "a serious defect in the baby" (question B), when question A precedes question B (A-B) or follows it (B-A).

et al., 1996, Chapter 6, for detailed discussions). To understand the underlying processes, suppose you were asked to provide a few reasons why "divorce should be easier to get." You could easily do so, yet you could just as easily provide some reasons why "divorce should be more difficult to get." When such alternatives are juxtaposed (as in "Should divorce be easier to get or more difficult to get?"), the outcome depends on which alternative is considered first. While the researcher hopes that respondents (a) hold the question and all response alternatives in mind, (b) evaluate the implications of each alternative, and (c) finally select the one that they find most agreeable, respondents may not do so. Instead, respondents who first think about "easier" may come up with a good supporting reason and may endorse this answer without engaging in the additional steps.

Importantly, the likelihood that respondents elaborate on a given alternative depends on the order and mode in which the response options are presented (Krosnick and Alwin, 1987). When presented in writing, respondents elaborate on the implications of the response options in the order presented. In this mode, an alternative that elicits supporting thoughts is more likely to be endorsed when presented early rather than late on the list, giving rise to *primacy effects*. In contrast, when the alternatives are read to respondents, their opportunity to think about the early ones is limited by the need to listen to the later ones. In this case, they are more likely to work backward, thinking first about the last alternative read to them. When this alternative elicits supporting thoughts, it is likely to be endorsed, giving rise to *recency effects*. Thus, a given alternative is more likely to be endorsed when presented early rather than late in a visual format (primacy effect), but when presented late rather than early in an auditory format (recency effect).

On theoretical grounds, we may expect that older respondents find it more difficult to keep several response alternatives in mind, elaborating on their respective implications to select the most appropriate answer. This should be particularly true in telephone interviews, where the alternatives are read to respondents without external memory support. The available data strongly support this prediction (see Knäuper, 1999, for a comprehensive review and meta-analysis). For example, Schuman and Presser (1981) asked respondents in a telephone interview, "Should divorce in this country be easier to obtain, more difficult to obtain, or stay as it is now?" Depending on conditions, the response alternative "more difficult" was read to respondents as the second or as the last alternative. Overall, respondents were somewhat more likely to select the response alternative "more difficult" when presented last, a recency effect. However, secondary analyses reported by Knäuper (1999) indicate a dramatic age difference: As shown in Figure 3, the size of the recency effect increased with respondents' age, ranging from a nonsignificant 5 percent for age 54 and younger to 36.4 percent for age 70 and older. Thus different substantive conclusions will be drawn about the relationship of age and attitudes toward divorce, depending on the order in which the response alternatives are presented: whereas attitudes toward divorce seem to become much more conservative with age under one order condition, no reliable age differences are obtained under the other order condition.

The available data suggest that age differences in response order effects are limited to the more taxing auditory format and are not observed when all response alternatives are presented in writing and remain visible. As an example, consider a study in which younger (age 20 to 40) and older (age 65+) adults were asked, "Which of the following four cities do you find most attractive?" (Knäuper et al., 2003). Washington, DC, was presented as either the first or last choice (Table 1).

When the response alternatives were read to respondents, younger as well as older adults were more likely to choose Washington, DC, when it was presented last rather than first. Replicating the pattern of the divorce findings, this recency effect was more pronounced for older than younger respondents, with differences of 24 versus 8 percentage points. When the response options were presented in writing, however, older as well as younger respondents were more likely to choose Washington, DC, when it

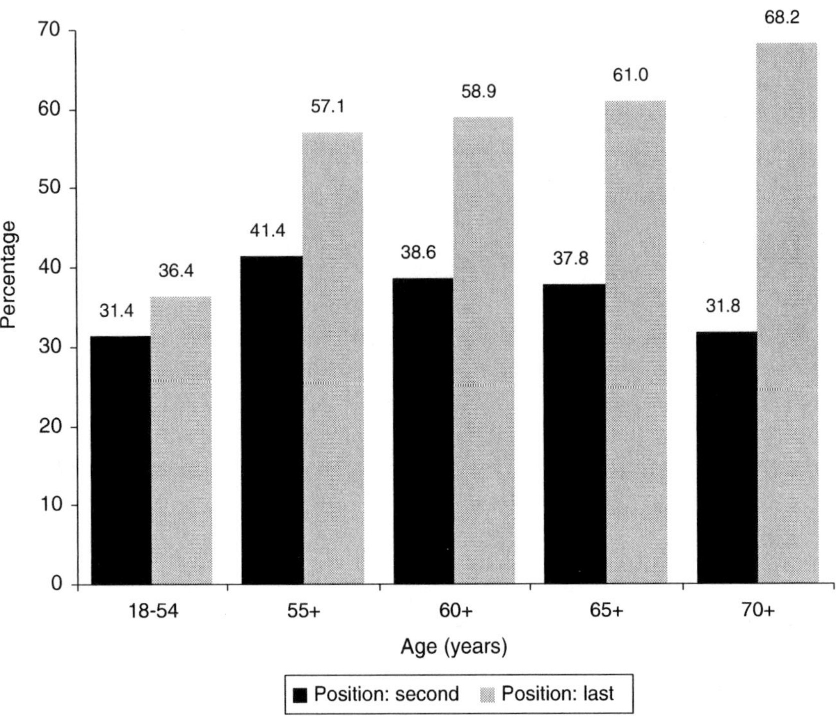

FIGURE 3 Response order effects as a function of age.
NOTE: Columns show percentage of respondents who endorse the statement that "divorce should be more difficult to get" when this alternative is presented as the second or the last of three options read during a telephone survey.

TABLE 1 Age, Mode, and Response Order Effects

	Washington, DC, Presented:		
	First (%)	Last (%)	Diff. (%)
Auditory			
Young	29	37	+8
Old	17	41	+24
Visual			
Young	36	28	–8
Old	22	13	–9

NOTE: Respondents ages 20 to 40 (young) and 65 to 90 (old) were asked, "Which of the following cities do you find most attractive?" The alternative "Washington, DC" was presented in the first or last (4th) position.

was presented first rather than last. Importantly, this primacy effect under a visual mode was of comparable size for both age groups.

Summary

In sum, the reviewed findings suggest that question order effects are likely to decrease with age, whereas response order effects are likely to increase with age. Both of these effects can be traced to age-related declines in cognitive resources. Hence, self-reports of attitudes are not only context dependent, but the size of the emerging context effects is itself age sensitive, rendering comparisons across age groups fraught with uncertainty. In addition, several studies indicate that older respondents are more likely to provide a "don't know" or "no opinion" answer (for a review see Schwarz and Knäuper, 2000). The processes underlying the latter observation are still unknown.

BEHAVIORAL FREQUENCY REPORTS

Many questions about respondents' behavior are frequency questions. Except for rare and very important behaviors, respondents are unlikely to have detailed representations of numerous individual instances of a behavior stored in memory. Rather, the details of various instances of closely related behaviors blend into one global representation (Linton, 1982; Neisser, 1986). Thus, many individual episodes become indistinguishable or irretrievable, due to interference from other similar instances (Baddeley and Hitch, 1977; Wagenaar, 1986), leading to knowledge-like representations that "lack specific time or location indicators" (Strube, 1987, p. 89). As a result, respondents usually have to resort to estimation strategies to arrive at a behavioral frequency report. See Bradburn, Rips, and Shevell (1987); Schwarz (1990); and Sudman et al. (1996) for extensive reviews, and the contributions in Schwarz and Sudman (1994) for research examples.

Subjective Theories

A particularly important estimation strategy is based on subjective theories of stability and change (see Ross, 1989, for a review). In answering retrospective questions, respondents often use their current behavior or opinion as a benchmark and invoke an implicit theory of self to assess whether their past behavior or opinion was similar to, or different from, their present behavior or opinion. Assuming, for example, that one's political beliefs become more conservative over the life span, older adults may infer that they held more liberal political attitudes as teenagers than they do now (Markus, 1986). The resulting reports of previous opinions and behaviors are correct to the extent that the implicit theory is accurate. In many domains, however, individuals assume a rather high degree of stability, resulting in underestimates of the degree of change that has occurred over time (Collins, Graham, Hansen, and Johnson, 1985; Withey, 1954), while in other domains (Ross, 1989) respondents who believe in change will detect a change even though none has occurred.

At present, little is known about whether and how subjective theories of stability and change are themselves subject to change across the life span: Which aspects of the self do people perceive as stable versus variable? And at which life stage do they expect changes to set in? Moreover, it is likely that salient life events, like retirement or the loss of a spouse, will give rise to subjective theories of profound change. If so, retrospective reports pertaining to earlier time periods may exaggerate the extent to which life was different prior to the event, conflating real change with biased reconstructions. These issues provide a promising avenue for future research.

Response Alternatives

An alternative estimation strategy draws on the frequency scale presented by the researcher (for a review see Schwarz, 1999a). In a nutshell, respondents assume that the researcher constructs a meaningful scale. Hence, values in the middle range of the scale presumably reflect the "average" or "typical" behavior, while values at the extremes of the scale correspond to the extremes of the distribution. Based on this assumption, respondents use the frequency scale as a frame of reference in estimating the frequency of their own behaviors. This results in higher frequency reports along scales with high rather than low values. For example, 37.5 percent of a sample of German respondents reported watching TV for more than 2 $^1/_2$ hours a day when given a high frequency ranging from "up to 2 $^1/_2$ hours" to "more than 4 hours" a day. In contrast, only 16.2 percent reported doing so when given a low frequency scale ranging from "up to $^1/_2$ an hour" to "more than 2 $^1/_2$ hours" (Schwarz, Hippler, Deutsch, and Strack, 1985).

Such scale-based estimation effects are more pronounced the more poorly the behavior is represented in memory (Menon, Rhagubir, and Schwarz, 1995). This suggests that the impact of response alternatives may typically be more pronounced for older than for younger respondents. The available data support this prediction, with some important qualifications. As shown in Table 2, Knäuper, Schwarz, and Park (2004) observed that older respondents were more affected by the frequency range of the response scale when asked to report on the frequency of mundane events, such as buying a birthday present. On the other hand, older respondents

TABLE 2 Impact of Response Alternatives on Behavioral Reports as a Function of Content and Respondents' Age

	Frequency Scale		
	Low (%)	High (%)	Diff. (%)
Mundane Behaviors			
Eating red meat			
Young	24	43	19
Old	19	63	44
Buying birthday presents			
Young	42	49	7
Old	46	61	15
Physical Symptoms			
Headaches			
Young	37	56	19
Old	11	10	1
Heartburn			
Young	14	33	19
Old	24	31	7

NOTE: Younger respondents are ages 29-40, older respondents 60-90. Percentage of respondents reporting eating red meat more than 10 times a month or more often; buying birthday presents 5 times a year or more often; and having headaches or heartburn twice a month or more often. Adapted from Knäuper et al. (2004). Reprinted by permission.

were less affected than younger respondents when the question pertained to the frequency of physical symptoms, which older respondents are more likely to monitor (e.g., Borchelt, Gilberg, Horgas, and Geiselmann, 1999). In combination, these findings suggest that respondents of all ages draw on the response alternatives when they need to form an estimate of how often they do something. Yet the need to estimate depends on how much attention they pay to the respective behavior, and this attention is itself age dependent.

Note that the scale format used leads to different conclusions about age-related differences in actual behavior from these reports. For example, age differences in red meat consumption (a health-relevant dietary behavior) or the purchase of birthday presents (an indicator of social integration) appear to be minor when a low frequency scale is used, but rather pronounced when a high frequency scale is used. To avoid systematic influences of response alternatives, and the age-related differences in their impact, it is advisable to ask frequency questions in open response formats that specify the relevant units of measurement. While the reports obtained under an open format are far from error free, they are at least not systematically biased by the instrument. See Schwarz (1999a) for a discussion.

CONCLUSIONS

As this review illustrates, minor changes in question wording, question format, and question order can profoundly influence the results obtained in sample surveys as well as in the psychological laboratory. Whereas researchers like to assume that respondents know what they believe and do, and can retrieve the proper information from memory, respondents usually have to compute the relevant answers on the spot, and this renders the answers highly context dependent. The underlying cognitive and communicative processes are systematic and increasingly well understood (for comprehensive reviews see Sudman et al., 1996; Tourangeau et al., 2000). Despite the general progress made, however, we know little about the impact of age-related changes in cognitive and communicative functioning on the response process; nor do we understand how age-related differences in the response process may be influenced by individuals' educational attainment and related variables. The little we do know, however, highlights that the methodological challenge is a serious one: Age-related differences in cognitive resources, memory, text comprehension, speech processing, and communication can have a profound impact on the question-answering process, resulting in *differential* context effects for older and younger respondents. As a result, any observed age differences in reported attitudes and behavior may reflect (a) a true difference, (b) a difference in the response process, or (c) an unknown mixture of both. If we want to avoid the potential misinterpretation of age-sensitive methods effects as substantive findings, we need to understand how age-related changes in cognitive and communicative functioning interact with the features of our research instruments in shaping respondents' reports. A systematic research agenda that addresses these issues is likely to advance our theoretical understanding of human cognition and communication across the life span and to improve the methodology of social research.

REFERENCES

Baddeley, A.D., and Hitch, G.J. (1977). Recency reexamined. In S. Dornic (Ed.), *Attention and performance* (vol. 6, pp. 647-667). Mahwah, NJ: Lawrence Erlbaum.

Borchelt, M., Gilberg, R., Horgas, A.L., and Geiselmann, B. (1999). On the significance of morbidity and disability in old age. In P.B. Baltes and K.U. Mayer (Eds.), *The Berlin aging study: Aging from 70 to 100* (pp. 403-429). New York: Cambridge University Press.

Bradburn, N.M., Rips, L.J., and Shevell, S.K. (1987). Answering autobiographical questions: The impact of memory and inference on surveys. *Science*, *236*, 157-161.

Collins, L.M., Graham, J.W., Hansen, W.B., and Johnson, C.A. (1985). Agreement between retrospective accounts of substance use and earlier reported substance use. *Applied Psychological Measurement*, *9*, 301-309.

Hasher, L., and Zacks, R.T. (1988). Working memory, comprehension, and aging: A review and a new view. In G.H. Bower (Ed.), *The psychology of learning and motivation* (vol. 22, pp. 193-225). San Diego: Academic Press.

Knäuper, B. (1999). The impact of age and education on response order effects in attitude measurement. *Public Opinion Quarterly, 63*, 347-370.

Knäuper, B., Schwarz, N., and Park, D.C. (2004). Frequency reports across age groups: Differential effects of frequency scales. *Journal of Official Statistics, 20*(1), 91-96.

Knäuper, B., Schwarz, N., Park, D., and Fritsch, A. (2003). *The perils of interpreting cohort differences in attitude reports: Question order effects decrease with age.* Unpublished manuscript. McGill University, Montreal, QC, Canada.

Krosnick, J.A., and Alwin, D.F. (1987). An evaluation of a cognitive theory of response order effects in survey measurement. *Public Opinion Quarterly, 51*, 201-219.

Linton, M. (1982). Transformations of memory in everyday life. In U. Neisser (Ed.), *Memory observed: Remembering in natural contexts* (pp. 77-91). San Francisco: Freeman.

Markus, G.B. (1986). Stability and change in political attitudes: Observed, recalled, and explained. *Political Behavior, 8*, 21-44.

Menon, G., Raghubir, P., and Schwarz, N. (1995). Behavioral frequency judgments: An accessibility-diagnosticity framework. *Journal of Consumer Research, 22*, 212-228.

Neisser, U. (1986). Nested structure in autobiographical memory. In D.C. Rubin (Ed.), *Autobiographical memory* (pp. 71-88). Cambridge, England: Cambridge University Press.

Ross, M. (1989). The relation of implicit theories to the construction of personal histories. *Psychological Review, 96*, 341-357.

Salthouse, T.A., and Babcock, R.L. (1991). Decomposing adult age differences in working memory. *Developmental Psychology, 27*, 763-776.

Schuman, H., and Presser, S. (1981). *Questions and answers in attitude surveys.* New York: Academic Press.

Schwarz, N. (1990). Assessing frequency reports of mundane behaviors: Contributions of cognitive psychology to questionnaire construction. In C. Hendrick and M.S. Clark (Eds.), *Research methods in personality and social psychology: Review of personality and social psychology*, (vol. 11, pp. 98-119). Thousand Oaks, CA: Sage.

Schwarz, N. (1996). *Cognition and communication: Judgmental biases, research methods and the logic of conversation.* Mahwah, NJ: Lawrence Erlbaum.

Schwarz, N. (1999a). Frequency reports of physical symptoms and health behaviors: How the questionnaire determines the results. In D.C. Park, R.W. Morrell, and K. Shifren (Eds.), *Processing medical information in aging patients: Cognitive and human factors perspectives* (pp. 93-108). Mahwah, NJ: Lawrence Erlbaum.

Schwarz, N. (1999b). Self-reports: How the questions shape the answers. *American Psychologist, 54*, 93-105.

Schwarz, N., Hippler, H.J., Deutsch, B. and Strack, F. (1985). Response categories: Effects on behavioral reports and comparative judgments. *Public Opinion Quarterly, 49*, 388-395.

Schwarz, N., Hippler, H.J., and Noelle-Neumann, E. (1992). A cognitive model of response order effects in survey measurement. In N. Schwarz and S. Sudman (Eds.), *Context effects in social and psychological research* (pp. 187-201). New York: Springer Verlag.

Schwarz, N., and Knäuper, B. (2000). Cognition, aging, and self-reports. In D. Park and N. Schwarz (Eds.), *Cognitive aging: A primer* (pp. 233-252), Philadelphia: Psychology Press.

Schwarz, N., Park, D., Knäuper, B., and Sudman, S. (1999). *Cognition, aging, and self-reports.* Philadelphia: Psychology Press.

Schwarz, N., and Sudman, S. (1994). *Autobiographical memory and the validity of retrospective reports.* New York: Springer Verlag.

Sirken, M., Hermann, D., Schechter, S., Schwarz, N., Tanur, J., and Tourangeau, R. (1999). *Cognition and survey research.* New York: Wiley.

Strube, G. (1987). Answering survey questions: The role of memory. In H.J. Hippler, N. Schwarz, and S. Sudman (Eds.), *Social information processing and survey methodology* (pp. 86-101). New York: Springer Verlag.

Sudman, S., Bradburn, N., and Schwarz, N. (1996). *Thinking about answers: The application of cognitive processes to survey methodology*. San Francisco: Jossey-Bass.

Tourangeau, R., Rips, L.J., and Rasinski, K. (2000). *The psychology of survey response.* Cambridge, England: Cambridge University Press.

Wagenaar, W.A. (1986). My memory: A study of autobiographical memory over six years. *Cognitive Psychology, 18*, 225-252.

Withey, S.B. (1954). Reliability of recall of income. *Public Opinion Quarterly, 18*, 31-34.

Optimizing Brief Assessments in Research on the Psychology of Aging: A Pragmatic Approach to Self-Report Measurement

Jon A. Krosnick
Stanford University
and

Allyson L. Holbrook
University of Illinois at Chicago
and

Penny S. Visser
University of Chicago

INTRODUCTION

In a great deal of research on the psychology of aging, as in most empirical social science, data are routinely collected from research participants via questionnaires. In the September 2004 issue of *Psychology and Aging*, for example, 16 articles appear in print, and 10 of them employed questionnaires assessing self-reports of stereotypes, confidence, depression, anxiety, social network structure, subjective well-being, positive affect, stress, and much more. And as is true of most questionnaire-based research, research on older adults often employs long batteries of questions, each intended to precisely measure a particular psychological or behavioral construct. These batteries, which have often been validated in prior research and used broadly in identical or nearly identical ways by various researchers on aging, often entail administering a dozen or more questions to measure a single construct. As is also true of most questionnaire-based research, other, nonbattery items are often in the questionnaires, routinely formatted in ad hoc ways, varying considerably from study to study and even within a single study. For example, Pruchno and Meeks' (2004) article in *Psychology and Aging* employed the Philadelphia Geriatric Center Positive and Negative Affect Scales developed by Lawton, Kleban, Dean, Rajagopal, and Parmelee (1992) as well as a mix of other questions offering rating scales with two, three, four, and five points.

The notion that social and psychological constructs can be measured precisely only by using batteries of many questionnaire items has a solid conceptual and theoretical justification. Any research participant's report of a past behavior, mood state, action tendency, hope, attitude, or goal will, of necessity, contain some random measurement error, both because of ambiguity in the memories and other internal psychological cues consulted when making the rating, and because of ambiguity in the meanings of the words used in the question and the words in the offered answer choices. As documented by the Spearman-Brown prophecy formula, the greater the number of questions asked to tap a construct, the more effectively the random measurement error in each item is cancelled out by that in the others, yielding a precise assessment of the variance shared across the items. This is why the measurement of a personality attribute, an attitude, and any other such construct is routinely accomplished by asking respondents to answer a remarkably large set of questions tapping the same thing. This practice is frustrating to some researchers, because participants can only answer a limited number of questions within the time frame of a study's data collection budget, so the more questions that tap a single construct, the fewer constructs can be gauged in a single study. The enhanced precision of assessment has routinely been preferred by researchers at the expense of breadth of construct sets and at the expense of participant fatigue in answering what may appear to be the same question over and over.

However, the above logic ignores an important fact of assessment: systematic measurement error. It has long been recognized that any measuring instrument may be biased, so error in its assessments may not all be random. And if the same bias is present in a set of questions all measuring the same construct, combining responses will not yield a canceling out of the error. Indeed, combining responses will cause the shared error to represent an increasingly prominent proportion of the variance of the final index, as the number of items combined increases and the amount of random error decreases. Thus, averaging or adding together responses to large sets of items to create indices is not the solution to all measurement problems.

Ironically, much of the shared bias in questions used to build indices is created unwittingly by the researchers themselves who seek to minimize measurement error. Even more strikingly, there appears to be a remarkably simple and practical solution to these problems that will make researchers and participants happier with the process and outcomes of their efforts. By avoiding the use of question formats that create random and systematic measurement error, researchers may be able to replace long batteries with sets of just two or three items that are well written, clear in meaning, and easy to answer, yielding psychometrics comparable to or better than those of long batteries while allowing for the measurement of a much broader array of constructs in a single questionnaire.

OPTIMIZING QUESTIONNAIRE DESIGN

Undoing the damage done in building large batteries must begin with an understanding of the principles of optimal questionnaire design. The structure, wording, and order of questions for questionnaires has traditionally been viewed as "an art, not a science," in the words of Princeton University psychologist Hadley Cantril (1951, p. vii) over five decades ago. And in his book *The Art of Asking Questions,* published the same year, Stanley Payne (1951) cautioned that "the reader will be disappointed if he expects to find here a set of definite rules or explicit directions. The art of asking questions is not likely ever to be reduced to some easy formulas" (p. xi). Thirty years later, Sudman and Bradburn (1982) agreed, saying that "no 'codified' rules for question asking exist" (p. 2). Sampling and data analysis are indeed guided by such rules that are backed by elaborate theoretical rationales. But questionnaire design has been thought of as best guided by intuition about how to script a naturally flowing conversation between a researcher and a respondent, even if that conversation is sometimes mediated by an interviewer.

Experienced questionnaire designers have followed some conventions over the years, but those conventions varied enough from individual to individual and from discipline to discipline to suggest that there are few universally accepted principles. If a questioning approach seems to work smoothly when respondents answer a questionnaire, then many researchers presume it will probably yield sufficiently useful data.

In recent years, however, it has become clear that this is an antiquated view that does not reflect the accumulation of knowledge throughout the social sciences about effective question asking. To be sure, intuition is a useful guide for designing questions, and a good questionnaire yields conversations that feel natural and comfortable to respondents. However, intuition can sometimes lead us astray, so it is useful to refine intuition with scientific evaluation. Fortunately, a large body of relevant scientific studies has now accumulated, and when taken together, their findings clearly suggest formal rules about how best to design questions to maximize the reliability and validity of measurements made by individual questions. However, this work has been scattered across the publication outlets of numerous disciplines, and this literature has not yet been comprehensively and integratively reviewed in a central place. Doing so is the goal of a forthcoming book, *The Handbook of Questionnaire Design* (Krosnick and Fabrigar, forthcoming), and we summarize some of the book's conclusions here, with a focus on optimal design of rating scales for efficient and effective brief assessments of social and psychological constructs in research on aging.

Number of Scale Points

When designing a rating scale, one must begin by specifying the number of points on the scale. As is true in Pruchno and Meeks' (2004) article in *Psychology and Aging* and in a great many social and psychological studies, rating scales vary considerably in their length, ranging from dichotomous items up to scales of 101 points (see, e.g., Robinson, Shaver, and Wrightsman, 1999). A large number of studies have compared the reliability and validity of scales of varying lengths (for a review, see Krosnick and Fabrigar, forthcoming). For bipolar scales, which have a neutral or status quo point in the middle (e.g., running from positive to negative), reliability and validity are highest for about 7 points (e.g., Matell and Jacoby, 1971). In contrast, the reliability and validity of unipolar scales, with a zero point at one end (e.g., running from no importance to very high importance), seem to be optimized at somewhat shorter lengths, approximately 5 points long (e.g., Wikman and Warneryd, 1990).

Presenting a 7-point bipolar rating scale is easy to do visually but is more challenging when an interviewer must read the seven choices aloud to a respondent, who must hold them in working memory before answering. Fortunately, research by Krosnick and Berent (1993) shows that such 7-point scales can be presented in easier ways without compromising data quality. Specifically, such scales can be presented in sequences of two questions that ask first whether the respondent is on one side of the midpoint or the other or at the midpoint (e.g., "Do you like bananas, dislike them, or neither like nor dislike them?"). Then, an appropriately worded follow-up question can ascertain how far from the midpoint the respondents are who settle on one side or the other (e.g., "Do you like bananas a lot or just a little?"). This branching approach takes less time to administer than offering the single 7-point scale all at once, and measurement reliability and validity are higher with the branching approach as well.

Scale Point Labeling

A number of studies show that data quality is better when all points on a rating scale are labeled with words than when only some are labeled thus and the others are labeled with numbers or are unlabeled (e.g., Krosnick and Berent, 1993). Furthermore, respondents are more satisfied when more rating scale points are verbally labeled (e.g., Dickinson and Zellinger, 1980). When selecting labels, researchers should strive to select ones that have meanings that divide up the continuum into approximately equal units (e.g., Klockars and Yamagishi, 1988). For example, "very good, good, and poor" is a combination that should be avoided, because the terms do not divide the continuum equally: the meaning of "good" is much closer to the meaning of "very good" than it is to the meaning of "poor" (Myers and Warner, 1968).

A very common set of rating scale labels used in questionnaires these days was initially developed by Rensis Likert (1932) and assesses the extent of agreement with an assertion: strongly agree, somewhat agree, neither agree nor disagree, somewhat disagree, strongly disagree. Yet a great deal of research shows that this response choice set is problematic because of acquiescence response bias (see, e.g., Couch and Keniston, 1960; Jackson, 1967; Schuman and Presser, 1981). Some people are inclined to agree with any assertion, regardless of its content, and content-free agreement is more common among people with limited cognitive skills, for more difficult items, and for items later in a questionnaire, when respondents are presumably more fatigued (see Krosnick, 1991). A number of studies now demonstrate how acquiescence can distort the results of substantive investigations (e.g., Jackman, 1973; Winkler, Kanouse, and Ware, 1982), and in a particularly powerful example, acquiescence undermined the scientific value of *The Authoritarian Personality*'s extensive investigation of fascism and anti-Semitism (Adorno, Frankel-Brunswick, Levinson, and Sanford, 1950).

It might seem that the damage done by acquiescence can be minimized by measuring a construct with a large set of items, half of them making assertions opposite to the other half (called "item reversals"). This approach is designed to place acquiescing respondents in the middle of the final measurement dimension but will do so only if the assertions made in the reversals are as extreme as the statements in the original items. To ensure this balance entails extensive pretesting and is therefore cumbersome to implement. Furthermore, it is difficult to write large sets of item reversals without using the word "not" or other such negations, and evaluating assertions that include negations is cognitively burdensome and error laden for respondents, thus increasing both measurement error and respondent fatigue (e.g., Eifermann, 1961; Wason, 1961). Finally, acquiescers presumably end up at the midpoint of the resulting measurement dimension, which is probably not where most belong on substantive grounds. That is, if these individuals were induced not to acquiesce and instead answered the items thoughtfully, their final index scores would presumably be more valid than placing them at the midpoint.

Most importantly, answering an agree/disagree question always involves answering a comparable rating question in one's mind first. For example, respondents asked to report their extent of agreement or disagreement with the assertion "I am not a friendly person" must first decide how friendly they are (perhaps concluding "very friendly") and then translate that conclusion into the appropriate selection in order to formulate their answer ("disagree" to the original item). It would be simpler and more direct to ask respondents how friendly they are on a rating scale ranging from "extremely friendly" to "not friendly at all." These would be called "construct-specific response options," because they explicitly state levels of the construct being measured (i.e., friendliness). In fact, every agree/disagree rating scale question implicitly requires the respondent to make a mental rating of an object along a continuous dimension representing the construct of interest, so asking about that dimension is simpler, more direct, and less burdensome. Not surprisingly, then, the reliability and validity of rating scales involving construct-specific response options are higher than those of agree/disagree rating scales (e.g., Ebel, 1982; Mirowsky and Ross, 1991; Ruch and DeGraff, 1926; Wesman, 1946). Consequently, it is best to avoid long batteries of questions in the latter format and instead to ask questions using rating scales with construct-specific response options.

Nondifferentiation

The danger of mounting systematic measurement error applies not just to agree/disagree scales but also to any long battery of questions employing the same response scale. For example, the personality construct "need to evaluate" is measured by offering respondents a series of assertions (e.g., "I form opinions about everything" and "I pay a lot of attention to whether things are good or bad") and asking them to indicate the extent to which each one describes them ("extremely characteristic," "somewhat characteristic," "uncertain," "somewhat uncharacteristic," and "extremely uncharacteristic"; Jarvis and Petty, 1996). When answering many questions using the same rating scale, a substantial number of respondents provide identical or nearly identical ratings across questions as a result of survey satisficing (Krosnick, 1991). Although these respondents could devote careful thought to the response task, retrieve relevant information from memory, and report differentiated judgments in response to the various questions, they choose to shortcut this process because they lack the cognitive skills and/or the motivation required. Instead they choose what appears to be a reasonable point on the rating scale and select that point over and over (i.e., constituting "nondifferentiation"), rather than interpreting each question carefully and answering optimally (see Krosnick, 1991; Krosnick and Alwin, 1988). Because different satisficers select different points on the rating scale, they end up at different places on the final measurement continuum built with a battery of items, and this constitutes systematic measurement error as well. For this reason, it is preferable that multiple items measuring a single construct use different sets of rating scale labels.

Order Effects

A final consideration relevant to optimizing rating scale design is the fact that people's answers to rating scale questions are sometimes influenced by the order in which the response alternatives are offered. After reading the stem of most rating scale questions, respondents are likely to begin to formulate a judgment with which to answer the question. For example, the question, "How friendly are you?" would induce respondents to generate an assessment of their level of friendliness before looking at the offered response options. As satisficing respondents read or listen to the answer choices presented, they are likely to settle for the first response option they encounter that is within their "latitude of acceptance." According to Sherif and colleagues (Sherif and Sherif, 1967; Sherif, Sherif, and Nebergall, 1965), people's judgments can be located at single points on continua, but around those points are regions on the continua that people also find acceptable representations of their beliefs. The first such acceptable response option a satisficing respondent hears is the one likely to be selected, thus inducing primacy effects in ratings, which have been observed in many studies (e.g., Belson, 1966; Carp, 1974; Chan, 1991; Mathews, 1929). To prevent this phenomenon from undetectably biasing ratings in a single direction, it is best to rotate the order of response choices across respondents and to statistically control for that rotation when analyzing the data.

However, this recommendation must be modified in light of conversational conventions about word order. Linguists Cooper and Ross (1975) outlined a series of rules for ordering words in sentences, one of which says that in pairs of positive and negative words, it is conventional to say the positive or affirmative before the negative (e.g., "plus or minus," "like or dislike," "for or against," "support or oppose"). Similarly, Guilford (1954) asserted that it is most natural and sensible to present evaluative response options on rating scales in order from positive to negative (e.g., "like a great deal" to "dislike a great deal"). Holbrook, Krosnick, Carson, and Mitchell (2000) showed that measurement validity is greater when the order of answer choices conforms to this convention.

CONCLUSION

If researchers follow all of the above guidelines in designing rating scale questions for brief assessments, reliability and validity can be maximized, systematic measurement error can be minimized, and thus the number of questions needed to measure a single construct can be reduced.

We hope that this review of research on questionnaire design is encouraging to the many scholars of aging who employ questionnaires in their work. Effective questionnaire design can be accomplished efficiently and practically in ways that minimize participant burden and maximize the breadth of constructs assessed and the accuracy of those assessments. By employing the principles of good measurement described here, researchers studying aging can move the field ahead even more successfully than they have to date.

REFERENCES

Adorno, T.W., Frankel-Brunswick, E., Levinson, D.J., and Sanford, R.N. (1950). *The authoritarian personality*. New York: Harper.

Belson, W.A. (1966). The effects of reversing the presentation order of verbal rating scales. *Journal of Advertising Research*, 6, 30-37.

Cantril, H. (1951) *Public opinion 1935-1946*. Princeton, NJ: Princeton University Press.

Carp, F.M. (1974) Position effects on interview responses. *Journal of Gerontology, 29*(5), 581-587.

Chan, J.C. (1991). Response order effects in Likert-type scales. *Educational and Psychological Measurement, 51*, 531-541.

Cooper, W.E., Ross, J.R. (1975). World order. In R.E. Grossman, L.J. San, and T.J. Vance (Eds.), *Papers from the parasession on functionalism* (pp. 63-111). Chicago: Chicago Linguistic Society.

Couch, A., and Keniston, K. (1960). Yeasayers and naysayers: Agreeing response set as a personality variable. *Journal of Abnormal Social Psychology, 60*, 151-174.

Dickinson, T.L., and Zellinger, P.M. (1980). A comparison of the behaviorally anchored rating and mixed standard scale formats. *Journal of Applied Psychology, 65*, 147-154.

Ebel, R.L. (1982). Proposed solutions to two problems of test construction. *Journal of Educational Measurement, 19*, 267-278.

Eifermann, R.R. (1961). Negation: A linguistic variable. *Acta Psychologica, 18*, 258-273.

Guilford, J.P. (1954). *Psychometric methods* (2nd ed.). New York: McGraw-Hill.

Holbrook, A.L., Krosnick, J.A., Carson, R.T., and Mitchell, R.C. (2000). Violating conversational conventions disrupts cognitive processing of attitude questions. *Journal of Experimental Social Psychology, 36*, 465-494.

Jackman, M.R. (1973). Education and prejudice or education and response-set? *American Sociological Review, 38*(June), 327-339.

Jackson, D.N. (1967). Acquiescence response styles: Problems of identification and control. In I.A. Berg (Ed.), *Response set in personality measurement*. Chicago: Aldine.

Jarvis, W.B.G., and Petty, R.E. (1996). The need to evaluate. *Journal of Personality and Social Psychology, 70*, 172-194.

Klockars, A.J., and Yamagishi, M. (1988). The influence of labels and positions in rating scales. *Journal of Educational Measurement, 25*(2), 85-96.

Krosnick, J.A. (1991). Response strategies for coping with the cognitive demands of attitude measures in surveys. *Applied Cognitive Psychology, 5*, 213-236.

Krosnick, J.A., and Alwin, D.F. (1988). A test of the form-resistant correlation hypothesis: Ratings, rankings, and the measurement of values. *Public Opinion Quarterly, 52*, 526-538.

Krosnick, J.A., and Berent, M.K. (1993) Comparisons of party identification and policy preferences: The impact of survey question format. *American Journal of Political Science, 37*(3), 941-964.

Krosnick, J.A., and Fabrigar, L.R. (Forthcoming). *Designing great questionnaires: Insights from psychology*. New York: Oxford University Press.

Lawton, M.P., Kleban, M.H., Dean, J., Rajagopal, D., and Parmelee, P.A. (1992). The factorial generality of brief positive and negative affect measures. *Journal of Gerontology: Psychological Sciences, 47*(4), P228-P237.

Likert, R. (1932). *A technique for the measurement of attitudes.* New York: McGraw-Hill.

Matell, M.S., and Jacoby, J. (1971). Is there an optimal number of alternatives for Likert scale items? Study I: Reliability and validity. *Educational and Psychological Measurement, 31*, 657-674.

Mathews, C.O. (1929). The effect of the order of printed response words on an interest questionnaire. *Journal of Educational Psychology, 20,* 128-134.

Mirowsky, J., and Ross, C.E. (1991). Eliminating defense and agreement bias from measures of the sense of control: A 2x2 index. *Social Psychology Quarterly, 55*, 217-235.

Myers, J.H., and Warner, W.G. (1968). Semantic properties of selected evaluation adjectives. *Journal of Marketing Research, 5*, 409-412.

Payne, S. (1951). *The art of asking questions.* Princeton, NJ: Princeton University Press.

Pruchno, R.A., and Meeks, S. (2004). Health-related stress, affect, and depressive symptoms experienced by caregiving mothers of adults with a developmental disability. *Psychology and Aging, 19*(3), 394-401.

Robinson, J.P., Shaver, P.R., and Wrightsman, L.S. (1999). Measures of political attitudes. In *Measures of social psychological attitudes* (vol. 2). New York: Academic Press.

Ruch, G.M., and DeGraff, M.H. (1926). Correction for chance and "guess" versus "do not guess" instructions in multiple-response tests. *Journal of Educational Psychology, 17*, 368-375.

Schuman, H., and Presser, S. (1981). *Questions and answers in attitude surveys.* New York: Academic Press.

Sherif, C.W., Sherif, M., and Nebergall, R.E. (1965). *Attitude and attitude change: The social judgment-involvement approach.* Philadelphia: W.B. Saunders.

Sherif, M., and Sherif, C.W. (1967). Attitudes as the individual's own categories: The social-judgment approach to attitude and attitude change. In C.W. Sherif and M. Sherif (Eds.), *Attitude, ego-involvement and change* (pp. 105-139). New York: Wiley.

Sudman, S., and Bradburn, N. (1982) *Asking questions: A practical guide to questionnaire design.* San Francisco: Jossey-Bass.

Wason, P.C. (1961). Responses to affirmative and negative binary statements. *British Journal of Psychology, 52*, 133-142.

Wesman, A.G. (1946). The usefulness of correctly spelled words in a spelling test. *Journal of Educational Psychology, 37*, 242-246.

Wikman, A., and Warneryd, B. (1990). Measurement errors in survey questions: Explaining response variability. *Social Indicators Research, 22*, 199-212.

Winkler, J.D., Kanouse, D.E., and Ware, J.E. (1982). Controlling for acquiescence response set in scale development. *Journal of Applied Psychology, 67*, 555-561.

Utility of Brain Imaging Methods in Research on Aging

Christine R. Hartel
National Research Council
and
Randy L. Buckner
Washington University in St. Louis

INTRODUCTION

The powerful techniques of neuroimaging have enabled the field of cognitive neuroscience to flourish, and today these techniques can be used in experiments designed to illuminate various aspects of social cognition. At the same time, the methods of social and cognitive psychology are importantly influencing experimental design in cognitive neuroscience; they have revealed that there are special measurement challenges in using neuroimaging in experiments with older adults.

The most commonly used methods of neuroimaging in cognitive studies are positron emission tomography (PET) and functional magnetic resonance imaging (fMRI) (see reviews by Buxton, 2002; Carson, Daube-Witherspoon, and Herscovitch, 1997). These two techniques measure the way the cellular functioning of the brain supports mental activities such as memory, cognition, and emotion. PET does this by measuring the changes in local blood flow that occur whenever there are changes in neural activity. Magnetic resonance imaging (MRI) measures a parallel phenomenon: the very small changes in the concentration of oxygen in blood at the sites of brain activity. The intensity of an MRI signal is proportional to the amount of oxygen carried by hemoglobin in the blood. Functional MRI (fMRI) is the use of MRI to detect what are known as blood-oxygen-level-dependent (BOLD) signals to map brain function during various activities (Ogawa et al., 1992; Kwong et al., 1992).

PET and MRI scanners, and in particular the latter, are available in virtually all hospitals today across the United States and almost all are now capable of making functional imaging measurements. There are many research centers that have scanners exclusively dedicated for research endeavors in psychology and in neuroscience. Therefore, neuroimaging resources are readily available for use as indirect measures of brain activities—including affective processes, executive function, or memory—that are not necessarily under the subject's voluntary control.

PSYCHOLOGICAL APPLICATIONS OF NEUROIMAGING

Neuroimaging methods have a temporal resolution of a few seconds. This makes it possible to ask a question such as: Are there brain areas in which activity predicts whether or not items will be remembered or forgotten? In fact, Wagner and colleagues (1998) have found that the magnitude of activity in the left prefrontal cortex and in the medial temporal cortex predicts whether or not memories will form. Such a study is important not only in relation to understanding memory but also because it illustrates how these methods can be used in experiments in social psychology. Because the methods are indirect, they might be ideal for use in experimental work in which direct questions may not (or cannot) elicit an appropriate response, although questions remain about neuroimaging methodology and measurement in the elderly population.

It is important to remember that neuroimaging techniques are based on indirect measures of blood flow response properties. There are many physical and physiological properties that change with aging and these must be assessed methodologically. For example, the vascular system changes with age and many older individuals are hypertensive. There are all sorts of small, low-level effects on the arteries during aging, and all of these changes may affect the signals that result in the neuroimage. The coupling of neural activity to the neuroimaging signal—the basic assumption of MRI use—may have different properties in young and elderly subjects (D'Esposito, Zarahn, Aguirre, and Rypma, 1999).

As an analogy, the brain imaging methods available today produce images that are much like satellite pictures of earth: they take a relatively long time to complete and provide only a survey of the activities going on. The resolution is poor relative to the brain's structural components. It would be useful to measure brain activity in a way that would show the activity of individual neurons and to observe it dynamically and across networks. But what is available is an indirect measure that provides a good cursory look at the broad regions of the brain that show activity. Even so, this measure appears to be sufficient for some of the questions being asked, especially in efforts to observe how broad pathways such as the affective systems or executive systems respond and change with age.

USES OF NEUROIMAGING IN RESEARCH ON AGING

The quality of contemporary fMRI images is also good enough that one can examine frontal cortex changes during aging. It is possible to actually reconstruct the thickness of the cortex and observe changes as people age, seeing when and where both white and gray cortical matter change. Among the many changes that occur, the ventricles enlarge and the gray matter thins. O'Sullivan and colleagues (2001) have found evidence that suggests that reduction of integrity in the white matter tracts of the brain may be an important mechanism of age-related cognitive decline. Their findings further suggest that disruption of the brain's executive functioning is a form of cerebral "disconnection" and accounts for cognitive changes in normal aging. Mikels and Reuter-Lorenz (2004) found that the corpus callosum, which interconnects the left and right cerebral hemispheres of the brain, plays an important role in resource allocation and selective attention for certain types of memory tasks, suggesting that changes in it are another cause of age-related decline. In earlier studies, Reuter-Lorenz and Stanczak (2000) had established that older adults use both hemispheres to their advantage to solve problems at lower levels of task complexity compared to young adults, but the older adults also experience impaired sensorimotor transfer between hemispheres through the corpus callosum. These studies in the functional anatomy of the aging brain use behavioral output as the end measure of brain activity.

Methodological studies are also necessary to determine whether neuroimaging in the elderly gives reliable results that can be compared to those obtained from a younger population. To illustrate with a relatively simple fMRI experiment what one type of methodological study looks like: Buckner, Snyder, Sanders, Raichle, and Morris (2000) conducted a visual flicker experiment with healthy younger and older adults and with older demented adults. Subjects were presented with the image of a large, flickering checkerboard and were asked to press a key as quickly as they could as soon as they saw it. In young adults, this resulted in a clear response in the visual cortex at the back of the brain and an equally clear motor response in the front. In both groups of older adults, the amplitude of the hemodynamic response was reduced significantly in visual cortex. The variance in regional hemodynamic response magnitude has been seen in other studies (D'Esposito et al., 1999), and differences in measured variance have been marked. Such differences mean that the main effects between groups of subjects may be difficult to interpret, since direct comparisons between groups assume the variance is similar.

Buckner and his colleagues (2000) found similar response amplitudes in the motor cortex between young and older adults, and also between nondemented and demented older adults, but because of the assumptions noted above, the results must be interpreted cautiously. Buckner et al. (2000) suggest that it is more conservative to look at group-by-region interactions, which would account for the differences in absolute response amplitude, or to look at relative change across conditions within a group rather than changes between them. These could be analyses of group-by-condition interactions or between-group parametric manipulations. The latter is particularly powerful when more than two levels of a condition are considered in each experimental group. Thus, even though various properties of the brain change with aging, and some baseline effects have to be taken into account, neuroimaging methods can be useful in these populations, but there are still measurement issues that must be attended to.

Neuroimaging techniques have also revealed that there are paradoxical differences in the ways older adults use their brains for certain kinds of memory functions. That is, in experimental memory tasks, young adults tend to use the left side of the brain for encoding and the right side for recall, while older adults recruit resources from both brain hemispheres to accomplish the task. The latter is called nonselective recruitment. Cabeza (2002) and Reuter-Lorenz (2002) have reviewed the PET and fMRI experiments that led to that generalization, and they suggest that the change observed in hemispheric asymmetry in older adults during verbal recall is not a task-specific occurrence but rather a general phenomenon of aging. Cabeza (2002), Reuter-Lorenz (2002), Buckner (2003), and others believe that this is a compensatory phenomenon. But Logan, Sanders, Snyder, Morris, and Buckner (2002) also raise the possibility that "nonselective recruitment reflects a breakdown in the appropriate selection of regions associated with controlled task performance," citing the work of O'Sullivan et al. (2001) on cortical "disconnection" described above. Logan, Sanders, Snyder, Morris, and Buckner (2002) suggest that age-related changes in white matter integrity may cause nonselective recruitment that in turn leads to the processing difficulties so common in an elderly population.

Furthermore, in memory tasks, older adults, unlike younger ones, do not recruit the frontal areas of the brain that are the sites of the control processes needed for memory; this is called underrecruitment. The phenomena of nonselective recruitment and underrecruitment are paradoxical and seem to be due not to context or other effects but simply to differences in how the systems are recruited by younger and older adults. Researchers are really just beginning to understand how these work, both neuroanatomically and functionally.

However, under certain conditions, older adults can recruit the same executive areas of the brain and at the same level of intensity as younger adults. In fact, under a different set of conditions, the brains of younger adults can be made to look much like those of older adults in their recruitment strategies. This is a very important measurement issue, and is, in a sense, like that described by Schwarz (this volume) with respect to surveys: results depend on the context in which you ask the question, and differences between younger and older adults can appear or disappear depending on the context. Such effects apply in many different experimental situations and must be taken into account in designing properly controlled experiments.

For example, Logan and colleagues (2002) have looked at memory formation in younger and older adults under several conditions. Under one condition, subjects were asked to memorize (intentional encoding) words (verbal stimuli) and faces (nonverbal stimuli) and told that they would be tested on these later while in the MRI scanner. This type of memory encoding is actually rather difficult because one must initiate strategies for memorization by oneself. In this situation, there are large differences between older and younger adults in the recruitment of the frontal regions (especially the left hemisphere) that are part of the brain's executive system to encode memories. One might conclude that during aging the brain is actually losing some of its physical properties because of atrophy in these areas and that executive resources simply disappear with aging. But this turns out not to be true.

Under a different experimental condition (for words only), environmental support for memory encoding was provided by giving subjects an effective strategy for memorization by using meaning-based (semantic) elaboration. Under this condition, the memory of older adults was improved but not fully to that of younger adults, while the left frontal activity performance was nearly the same in both groups. However, the lack of selectivity in recruiting various brain areas was not reversed by semantic elaboration techniques in the elderly, suggesting a true and permanent decline in functioning with age. When both groups learned words "accidentally" (shallow incidental encoding), left frontal activity and memory in younger adults decreased to levels seen in older adults. In these experiments, care was taken to ensure that baseline differences in hemodynamic response properties that might be observed in between-population comparisons were controlled for. Baseline differences could result from internal physiological properties of individuals or from external properties of the analysis, like misregistration. Thus it seems clear that context effects are among the most salient, even at the neural level, in exploring the differences between younger and older adults.

Efforts to determine causal mechanisms for these phenomena are under way in many laboratories, but our understanding is still very limited. It is important to note that nonimaging methods can also provide important data for understanding causal mechanisms. For example, older people are not unaware of their memory deficits, and sometimes if asked to perform in a memory experiment they demur, asking to do some other task. By changing the nature of the experiment slightly, this problem can be overcome. For example, one can take advantage of the fact that people accidentally memorize things (incidental encoding) during an experiment that does not appear to be a memory test: participants may be shown a series of words, asked to complete an unrelated task, and then given another task that uses the original series of words without reference to the fact that it is the same list of words seen earlier. Neuroimages can be obtained during each phase of the experiment, taking advantage of the fact that participants will have unintentionally remembered some of the words and forgotten others.

CONCLUSION

The convergence of data from experiments using techniques like these that were developed in other sciences, and the use of the data, methods, and techniques of other sciences generally, will both improve scientists' understanding and also constrain what can be learned from the current level of neuroimage resolution. While the resolution of PET and fMRI images is not of the quality desired to carry out all the types of experiments needed to explore the brain phenomena of aging, the quality of images we have is still remarkable. And the promise of these techniques—and their successors—is enormous for all fields of research involving brain function and the aging population.

REFERENCES

Buckner, R.L. (2003). Functional-anatomic correlates of control processes in memory. *Journal of Neuroscience, 23*, 3999-4004.

Buckner, R.L., and Logan, J.M. (2002). Frontal contributions to episodic memory encoding in the young and elderly. In A.E. Parker, E.L. Wilding, and T. Bussey (Eds.), *The cognitive neuroscience of memory encoding and retrieval.* Philadelphia: Psychology Press.

Buckner, R.L., Snyder, A.Z., Sanders, A.L., Raichle, M.E., and Morris, J.C. (2000). Functional brain imaging of young, nondemented, and demented older adults. *Journal of Cognitive Neuroscience, 12*(Suppl. 2), 24-34.

Buxton, R.B. (2002). *Introduction to functional magnetic resonance imaging: Principles and techniques.* New York: Cambridge University Press.

Cabeza, R. (2002). Hemispheric asymmetry reduction in older adults: The HAROLD model. *Psychology and Aging, 17*, 85-100.

Carson, R.E., Daube-Witherspoon, M.E., and Herscovitch, P. (1997). *Quantitative functional brain imaging with positron emission tomography.* San Diego: Academic Press.

D'Esposito, M., Zarahn, E., Aguirre, G.K. and Rypma, B. (1999). The effects of normal aging on the coupling of neural activity to the BOLD hemodynamic response. *NeuroImage, 10*, 6-14.

Head, D., Snyder, A.Z., Girton, L.E., Morris, J.C., and Buckner, R.L. (2004). Frontal-hippocampal double dissociation between normal aging and Alzheimer's disease. *Cerebral Cortex, 14*, 410-423.

Kwong, K.K., Belliveau, J.W., Chesler, D., Goldberg, I.E., Weiskoff, R.J., Poncelet, B.P., Kennedy, D.N., Hoppel, B.E., Cohen, J.S., Turner, R., Cheng, H., Brady, T.J., and Rosen, B.R. (1992). Dynamic magnetic resonance imaging of human brain activity during primary sensory simulation. *Proceedings of the National Academy of Sciences, 89*, 5675-5679.

Logan, J.M., Sanders, A.L., Snyder, A.Z., Morris, J.C., and Buckner, R.L. (2002). Underrecruitment and nonselective recruitment: Dissociable neural mechanisms associated with aging. *Neuron, 33*(5), 827-840.

Mikels, J.A., and Reuter-Lorenz, P.A. (2004). Neural gate keeping: The role of interhemispheric interactions in resource allocation and selective filtering. *Neuropsychology, 18*, 328-339.

Ogawa, S., Tank, D.W., Menon, R., Ellermann, J.M., Kim, S.-G., Merkle, H., and Ugurbil, K. (1992). Intrinsic signal changes accompanying sensory stimulation: Functional brain mapping with magnetic resonance. *Proceedings of the National Academy of Sciences, 89*, 5951-5955.

O'Sullivan, M., Jones, D.K., Summers, P.E., Morris, R.G., Williams, S.C.R., and Markus, H.S. (2001). Evidence for cortical "disconnection" as a mechanism of age-related cognitive decline. *Neurology, 57*, 632-638.

Reuter-Lorenz, P. (2002). New visions of the aging mind and brain. *Trends in Cognitive Science, 6*, 394-400.

Reuter-Lorenz, P.A., and Stanczak, L. (2000). Differential effects of aging on the functions of the corpus callosum. *Developmental Neuropsychology, 18*, 113-137.

Wagner, A.D., Schacter, D.L., Rotte, M., Koutstaal, W., Maril, A., Dale, A.M., Rosen, B.R., and Buckner, R.L. (1998). Building memories: Remembering and forgetting of verbal experiences as predicted by brain activity. *Science, 281*, 1188-1191.

Research Infrastructure

Committee on Aging Frontiers in Social Psychology, Personality, and Adult Developmental Psychology

As stated in our recommendation in Chapter 1, the committee strongly supports the development of integrated interdisciplinary grants that will take the best conceptual and measurement work from social, personality, and adult development psychology and link it with comparable work from other disciplines, such as economics, biostatistics, neurosciences, demography, health psychology, geriatric medicine, behavioral economics, social neuroscience, psychoneuroimmunology, and engineering, in order to address important social and health problems of relevance to the mission of the National Institute on Aging (NIA).

Currently, the Behavioral and Social Research Program at NIA offers a variety of research funding mechanisms, including traditional individual research grants, small business innovation research grants, training and conference grants, research program projects, and grants for research centers, including exploratory, center core, specialized centers, and comprehensive centers. However, stimulation of interdisciplinary work might involve not only innovative variations of current mechanisms, but also new mechanisms, innovative use of review resources, and partnerships among government agencies, foundations, and professional societies.

In order to facilitate collaboration between disciplines, funding mechanisms need to provide for sustained contact between disciplines and mutual education in the approaches of each discipline. For example, short-term salary support for researchers of different disciplines would enable those in one field to learn enough about the other field in order to plan an interdisciplinary research project. Another new mechanism might be a "paired K award" (perhaps called KK awards, after the K awards from the

National Institutes of Health [NIH][1]), in which two scientists from the same or neighboring institutions jointly apply for career development awards that specify continued collaboration over the life of the award. Similarly, there might be senior KK awards that are career awards for collaborative leadership.

Flexibility in the use of K awards for academic faculty could also stimulate interdisciplinary training and development. For example, the award might provide summer salary rather than a percentage of the academic year salary, or a research costs category for a faculty member. This type of customization to fit the needs of academic faculty would be parallel in intent to customizing physician-scientist K awards to meet the structure of the career paths of physician-scientists.

We encourage interdisciplinary center grants designed to facilitate collaboration. These grants could be modeled, for example, on the R24 infrastructure grants given by the Office of Behavioral and Social Sciences Research and other NIH entities to support research in mind-body medicine[2] or on the grants for transdisciplinary centers given by the National Institute on Drug Abuse, in which the first phase of the award provides funds for meeting and talking in order to generate new ideas. Center grants could also require setting aside funds for a certain number of cross-disciplinary pilot projects to be funded within the center.

In addition, small grants could be given for holding technical assistance workshops or other training events that would teach about one discipline and would take place the day before the professional meeting of another discipline. Another possibility for NIA is to give grants to develop and hold short courses (e.g., 1 or 2 weeks) on methodology. There are several models for successful short courses on technical topics. NIA support of the costs of developing and offering such courses could substantially promote dissemination of new ideas and methodological developments across fields.

We suggest consideration by NIH of encouraging nonprofit organizations or even universities to apply for NIA funding to administer a small

---

[1]K02 awards allow early to mid-career investigators—who have received prior funding—to develop skills and collaborations to become leaders in their research fields; K07 awards allow senior investigators to develop an area of aging research at a university or other research institution. There are also many other types of K awards. See http://grants2.nih.gov/training/careerdevelopmentawards.htm (accessed December 2005).

[2]A central goal of this program is to facilitate interdisciplinary collaboration and innovation in mind-body and health research while providing essential and cost-effective core services in support of the development, conduct, and translation into practice of mind-body and health research based in centers or comparable administrative units. See http://obssr.od.nih.gov/RFA_PAs/MindBody/MBFY04/Start.htm#infrastructure%20initiatives (accessed December 2005).

grants program to promote specific aspects of interdisciplinary work. A very successful model of such a program is the "small grants in behavioral economics" program run by the Russell Sage Foundation (for details, see http://www.russellsage.org/programs/other/behavioral/smallgrants/, accessed October 13, 2005). This program supports junior faculty who are pursuing new, small-scale research projects and also serves as a mechanism for faculty to fund diverse graduate student projects. Both of these types of projects are very difficult to fund with traditional funding mechanisms and yet can contribute significantly to interdisciplinary research. Another model is the program sponsored by the Retirement Research Foundation, which funded an autonomy initiative that entailed both awarding a number of small grants and bringing grantees together to create greater synergy.

There are precedents for NIH to fund scientific or professional organizations or universities to build momentum in an area of study through training grants. For example, StartMH Program of the National Institute of Mental Health, administered by the University of California-San Diego, partners students at all levels with faculty mentors across the country for a summer-long research apprenticeship, and holds one workshop for all participants.

Since it is difficult for the NIH to administer small grants, it might be useful to use the model of professional organizations for training grants. For example, the American Psychological Association administers training grants that support students at universities across the United States, while also providing opportunities for networking among those students. The grants funded under such a program might be very small (e.g., less than $10,000) with a very minimal application process (e.g., a 1-3 page proposal conveyed by email), a very rapid review (e.g., 1-2 weeks), and minimal requirements for a final report.

A new type of training grant could be made by NIA to centers in social, personality, and adult development psychology for predoctoral and postdoctoral trainees to partner with demography centers at the same or a nearby university for interdisciplinary training.

Because the evaluation of interdisciplinary work is so difficult, the Center for Scientific Review of the NIH could establish a special peer review group devoted to grants of this type. It would be relatively easy for NIH or National Science Foundation to evaluate any of these alternative mechanisms for facilitating interdisciplinary work after a 5-year trial period and then decide whether or not it should be continued.

The topics we recommend for a focused research program on aging for the NIA can benefit enormously from the kind support envisioned by the committee's recommendation on infrastructure. With flexibility to cross disciplines, foster small-scale efforts, and encourage innovative ways to approaching the exciting questions in aging research, we believe major strides in understanding certain key aspects of aging can be realized in a short time. The promise of those strides is a better quality of life for the nation's older adults, as well as better contributions from them to the nation's well-being.

Appendix

Biographical Sketches of Committee Members and Contributors

Laura L. Carstensen (*Chair*) is professor of psychology at Stanford University, where she is also chair of the Psychology Department. She has published extensively about emotional, cognitive, and motivational changes with age, and has formulated socioemotional selectivity theory. She is a Fellow of the American Psychological Society, the American Psychological Association, and the Gerontological Society of America. Dr. Carstensen received the Kalish Award for Innovative Research from the Gerontological Society in 1993 and was selected as a Guggenheim Fellow in 2003.

Fredda Blanchard-Fields is a professor in the School of Psychology at the Georgia Institute of Technology in Atlanta. She was associate chair of the School from 1996-2002 and was chair of the National Institutes of Health study section, Social Psychology, Personality, and Interpersonal Processes. She is currently associate editor for *Psychology and Aging*. Her research focuses on adult development and aging in the areas of social cognition, cognitive change, attributional processes, and everyday problem solving.

Randy L. Buckner is interested in discovering the brain systems that support human memory and how these systems are disrupted by Alzheimer's disease. In addition to being an Investigator at the Howard Hughes Medical Institute, he is associate professor of psychology at Washington University in St. Louis. Dr. Buckner is also professor of psychology at Harvard University, where he is affiliated with the Center for Brain Science and faculty of the Athinoula A. Martinos Center for Biomedical Imaging at Massachusetts General Hospital/Harvard Medical School. Dr. Buckner received his B.A.

degree in psychology and his M.A. and Ph.D. degrees in psychology and neuroscience from Washington University. Dr. Buckner has published over 100 articles and book chapters and has received the Young Investigator Awards from the Organization of Human Brain Mapping and the Cognitive Neuroscience Society.

Margaret Gatz is professor in the Department of Psychology at the University of Southern California. She is also a foreign adjunct professor with the Department of Medical Epidemiology at the Karolinska Institute in Stockholm. Her research interests encompass age-related change in depressive symptoms, risk and protective factors for Alzheimer's disease, successfulness of coping mechanisms of the aged, and evaluation of the effects of interventions. Dr. Gatz is past chair of the behavioral sciences section of the Gerontological Society of America and a former Zenith Fellow of the Alzheimer's Association. She served on the advisory committee for the Minority Aging Network in Psychology and hosted two of its summer institutes. She received her Ph.D. in clinical psychology from Duke University, completed her clinical psychology internship at West Virginia University Medical Center, and was a postdoctoral fellow at Duke University's Center for the Study of Aging and Human Development.

Christine R. Hartel is the director of the Center for Studies of Behavior and Development at the National Research Council, where she also directs the Board on Behavioral, Cognitive, and Sensory Sciences. She is the study director for the Committee on Aging Frontiers in Social Psychology, Personality, and Adult Developmental Psychology. Previously, she served as associate executive director for science at the American Psychological Association and as deputy director for basic research at the National Institute on Drug Abuse. As a research psychologist at the U.S. Army Research Institute for the Behavioral and Social Sciences, Dr. Hartel earned the Army's highest civilian award for technical excellence. She is a Fellow of the American Psychological Association. She has a Ph.D. in biopsychology from the University of Chicago.

Todd F. Heatherton is the Champion International Professor of Psychological and Brain Sciences at Dartmouth College. After 4 years on the faculty at Harvard University, in 1994 he joined the faculty at Dartmouth College, where he is the Director of the Center for Social Brain Sciences and an affiliate of the Center for Cognitive Neuroscience. His research examines processes related to self, particular self-regulation, self-esteem, and self-referential processing. He has been on the executive committees of several professional societies. He is associate editor of the *Journal of Cognitive Neuroscience,* and on the editorial boards of *Psychological Science, Journal* *of Abnormal Psychology, Journal of Personality and Social Psychology, Journal of Personality,* and *Review of General Psychology.* His books include: *The Social Psychology of Stigma* (2000), *Can Personality Change?* (1994), and, with Michael Gazzaniga, *Psychological Science: The Mind, Brain, and Behavior* (2003). He received the Petra Shattuck Award for Teaching Excellence from the Harvard Extension School in 1994, the McLane Fellowship from Dartmouth College in 1997, and the Friedman Family Fellowship from Dartmouth College in 2001. He received his Ph.D. in psychology from the University of Toronto.

Allyson L. Holbrook is assistant professor at the University of Illinois at Chicago in public administration, the Survey Research Laboratory, and the Psychology Department. Dr. Holbrook teaches courses primarily in methodology and statistics and conducts research on survey methodology, particularly the role that social and psychological processes play in the task of answering survey questions, and on attitudes and persuasion, and the role attitude strength plays in moderating the impact of attitudes on thoughts and behaviors. She received her Ph.D. from Ohio State University.

Jon A. Krosnick is the Frederic O. Glover Professor in Humanities and Social Sciences and professor of communication, political science, and (by courtesy) psychology, at Stanford University. Dr. Krosnick received his B.A. degree in psychology from Harvard University and M.A. and Ph.D. degrees in social psychology from the University of Michigan. Prior to joining the Stanford faculty in 2004, Dr. Krosnick was professor of psychology and political science at Ohio State University, where he co-directed the Summer Institute in Political Psychology. He has taught courses on survey methodology around the world at universities, for corporations, and for government agencies. He has provided expert testimony in court and has served as an on-air election-night television commentator. Dr. Krosnick has served as a consultant to such organizations as Pfizer Pharmaceuticals, the Office of Social Research at CBS, the News Division of ABC, the National Institutes of Health, Home Box Office, NASA, the U.S. Bureau of the Census, and the Urban Institute.

George Loewenstein is professor of Economics and Psychology at Carnegie Mellon University. He received his Ph.D. from Yale University in 1985 and since then has held academic positions at the University of Chicago and Carnegie Mellon University, and fellowships at the Center for Advanced Study in the Behavioral Sciences, the Institute for Advanced Study in Princeton, the Russell Sage Foundation, and the Institute for Advanced Study in Berlin. His research focuses on applications of psychology to economics, and his specific interests include decision making over time, bargaining and negotiations, psychology and health, law and economics, the psychology of adaptation, the role of emotion in decision making, the psychology of curiosity, conflict of interest, and "out of control" behaviors such as impulsive violent crime and drug addiction.

Mara Mather is associate professor of psychology at the University of California, Santa Cruz. She is a cognitive psychologist whose research interests focus on aging, memory, emotion, and decision making. She completed her undergraduate degree at Stanford University and her Ph.D. at Princeton University. Dr. Mather has been examining how changes in emotional processing across the life span affect cognitive processes, such as attention, memory, and decision making. Dr. Mather also investigates how people remember and misremember past decisions.

Denise C. Park is professor in the Department of Psychology at the University of Illinois and a faculty member in the Biological Intelligence Group at the Beckman Institute. She directs the Center for Healthy Minds, an NIA-supported Roybal Center. Her fields of professional interest are the cognitive neuroscience of aging; culture, cognition, and aging; and the impact of social/cognitive interventions in minimizing neurobiological changes that occur with age. Dr. Park received the Distinguished Contribution Award to the Psychology of Aging from the American Psychological Association in 2003. She is a Fellow of the American Association for the Advancement of Science, a member of the Board of Directors of the American Psychological Society, past chair of the Board of Scientific Affairs of the American Psychological Association, and past president of the Division of Adult Development and Aging of the APA.

Lawrence A. Pervin received his Ph.D. from Harvard University in 1962. He was professor of psychology at Rutgers University from 1971-2004 and is currently professor emeritus. He is the editor of *The Handbook of Personality: Theory and Research* (1st edition, 1990; 2nd edition, 1999), as well as author of *Current Controversies and Issues in Personality* (1st edition, 1978; 2nd edition, 1984; 3rd edition, 2001). Dr. Pervin also wrote the personality textbook *Personality: Theory and Research*, now in its ninth edition, and several of his books have been translated into eight foreign languages.

Richard E. Petty received his B.A. from the University of Virginia in 1973, and his Ph.D. in social psychology from Ohio State University in 1977. He began his career as assistant professor of psychology at the University of Missouri, where he was named the Frederick A. Middlebush Professor in 1985. He returned to Ohio State in 1987 as professor and director of the

Social Psychology Doctoral Program. In 1998, he was named Distinguished University Professor. Dr. Petty's research focuses broadly on the situational and individual difference factors responsible for changes in beliefs, attitudes, and behaviors. This work has resulted in 7 books and over 200 journal articles and chapters. Dr. Petty has received several honors for his work including the Distinguished Scientific Contribution Awards from the Society for Personality and Social Psychology (2001) and the Society for Consumer Psychology (2000). Dr. Petty served as associate editor of the *Personality and Social Psychology Bulletin* for two years, and later became the journal's editor from 1988-1991. He has also served as associate editor for the journal, *Emotion,* and has served on the editorial boards of 10 other journals. Dr. Petty has served as a consultant and panelist for various federal agencies such as the National Institute on Drug Abuse, the National Science Foundation, the National Cancer Institute, and also for the National Academy of Sciences.

Jennifer A. Richeson is associate professor of psychology and a faculty fellow at the Institute for Policy Research at Northwestern University. She received her B.S. in psychology at Brown University and her Ph.D. at Harvard University in social psychology. Dr. Richeson's research focuses on prejudice, stereotyping, and intergroup relations. Her work generally concerns the ways in which social group memberships such as race and gender affect the way people think, feel, and behave during intergroup interactions. She is currently working on three primary lines of research: the dynamics and consequences of interracial contact; detecting and controlling racial bias; and racial categorization and identity. Through the development of these research streams, Dr. Richeson hopes to contribute to a better understanding of intergroup relations, as well as to elucidate pitfalls in current approaches to prejudice reduction.

Alexander J. Rothman received his Ph.D. in psychology from Yale University and is currently associate professor in the Department of Psychology at the University of Minnesota. Dr. Rothman's primary program of research concerns the application of social psychological theory to illness prevention and health promotion and is comprised of a synthesis of basic research on how people process and respond to health information with the development and evaluation of theory-based interventions to promote healthy behavior. In his most recent work, Dr. Rothman has focused on how the relation between people's health beliefs and health behavior unfolds over time. In particular, he has begun to delineate the different decision processes that guide the initiation and maintenance of long-term self-regulatory behavior. In recognition of his work, Dr. Rothman received the 2002 Distinguished Scientific Award for Early Career Contribution to

Psychology in the area of Health Psychology from the American Psychological Association.

Norbert Schwarz is professor of psychology at the University of Michigan, professor of marketing at the University of Michigan Business School, and research professor in the Survey Research Center and the Research Center for Group Dynamics at Michigan's Institute for Social Research. He received a Ph.D. in sociology and psychology from the University of Mannheim, Germany, in 1980. Prior to joining the University of Michigan in 1993, he taught psychology at the University of Heidelberg, Germany (1981-1992), and served as Scientific Director of ZUMA, a social science research center in Mannheim (1987-1992). Dr. Schwarz's interests focus on human judgment and cognition, including the interplay of feeling and thinking, the socially situated nature of cognition, and the implications of basic cognitive and communicative processes for public opinion and social science research. He is a fellow of the American Academy of Arts and Sciences, the American Psychological Society, and the Society for Personality and Social Psychology.

J. Nicole Shelton is assistant professor of psychology at Princeton University. She received her Ph.D. from the University of Virginia in 1998. Her research focuses on interracial interaction, prejudice, and ethnic identity. She explores how interpersonal concerns about issues of prejudice (i.e., concerns with appearing prejudiced and concerns with being rejected) influence the dynamics of intergroup contact. Additionally, she has been exploring personality and situational factors that influence the development and maintenance of cross-racial friendships. She is also studying issues related to targets' detection of and responses to prejudice and discrimination, and the personal and social costs of confronting, or not confronting, perpetrators of prejudice.

Ilene C. Siegler is professor of medical psychology in the Department of Psychiatry and Behavioral Sciences, Department of Psychology: Social and Health Sciences, Duke University, and adjunct professor of epidemiology at the University of North Carolina School of Public Health. She is a developmental psychologist and behavioral epidemiologist whose research is at the intersection of the psychology of adult development and aging and behavioral medicine. Her research involves the understanding of behavioral factors in chronic disease. She is the director of the UNC Alumni Heart Study, a former member of the National Advisory Council of the National Institute on Aging, past president of Division 20 (Adult Development and Aging) of the American Psychological Association, and former associate editor of *Health Psychology*.

Penny S. Visser is associate professor of psychology at the University of Chicago. She earned her undergraduate degree at Grand Valley State University, and her M.A. and Ph.D. from Ohio State University. Dr. Visser was an assistant professor at Princeton University from 1998 through 2001, with a joint appointment in the Psychology Department and the Woodrow Wilson School of Public and International Affairs. She joined the faculty at the University of Chicago in 2001. Dr. Visser is primarily interested in attitudes: how they influence the way we process information, how they motivate and guide our behavior, how they are influenced by the social context in which we hold them, and how we maintain them in the face of persuasive appeals.

Linda J. Waite is the Lucy Flower Professor of Sociology and director of the Center on Aging at the University of Chicago, where she also co-directs the Alfred P. Sloan Center on Parents, Children and Work. She is past president of the Population Association of America and a member of the Advisory Committee to the Director of NIH. Her research focuses on the family, from the youngest to the oldest ages. She is author, with Frances Goldscheider, of *New Families, No Families?: The Transformation of the American Home* (University of California Press, 1991) and, with Maggie Gallagher, of *The Case for Marriage: Why Married People are Happier, Healthier and Better Off Financially* (Doubleday, 2000). One current project examines the role of the social context in the etiology of loneliness and stress, and their impact on health and well-being at older ages. Another project focuses on the relationship between social networks, intimacy, physical health, emotional well-being, and cognitive function at older ages.

Keith E. Whitfield is associate professor in the Department of Biobehavioral Health at Pennsylvania State University. His current research focuses on individual differences in aging in African Americans. Dr. Whitfield has written about health disparities and minority aging, conceptual and methodological issues involving individual differences and aging in African Americans, and the effects of race and health on cognition. His current projects include a study of the impact of health and personality on cognitive functioning and a study of health and psychosocial factors in older African American twins. He served on the National Academies' Committee on Future Directions for Cognitive Research on Aging.

Index

A

AARP. *See* American Association of Retired Persons
Ability to change, without any form of professional assistance, 37
Abortion, 220
Accommodation, 187
Action
  attitudes guiding, 46
  consequences of, 137
  likelihood of taking, 134n
Activity restriction, 26
Adaptation, 24
Addictive behaviors, 42, 153
Adult developmental psychology, recent developments in, 12
Adulthood, 20
Advance directives, 34
Affect, role in self-regulation, 43
Affective disorders, major, 23
Affective forecasting, 62–63
Affective heuristics, 3
Affective neural systems, 60–61
Age, protective factor in etiology of mental health disorders, 29
Age differences in self-regulation, 38–39
Age discrimination, consequences of, 87
Age distribution by population, 10–11
Age identity and self-concept, 86–87
Age-related decline, beliefs about, 80
Age stigma from the perceiver's perspective, 175–186
  attitudes and stereotypes, 175–180
  behavior toward older adults, 180–184
  emerging themes and directions for future research, 184–186
Age stigma from the perspective of older adults, 186–197
  consequences of exposure to ageist stereotypes, 190–191
  coping with a negative age identity, 191–196
  emerging themes and directions for future research, 196–197
  identity and self-concept, 186–188
  implications of self-stereotyping, 189
Ageism, 4
  consequences of, 197
  coping in the face of, 198
  multiple dynamics of, 198
Ageist views, of patients in a medical setting, 82
Aging
  influences on course of, 24
  and prefrontal decline, 151–152
  uneasiness about, 9

Aging and social engagement, 69–72
  mental stimulation and cognitive aging, 71–72
  neurocognitive function and cognition, 70–71
Aging societies, future of, 13
Agreeableness, 22
Alcoholism, 37, 42, 58
Alzheimer's disease, 68, 75, 77
America
  the "aging of," 1
  well-being of, 250
American Association of Retired Persons (AARP), 163–164
American Psychological Association, 249
Amygdala, 70, 148
Anger, and risk aversion, 152
Anti-Semitism, 235
Antonucci, Toni, 25
Art of Asking Questions, The, 233
Attenuation, of question order effects, 220–221
Attitude change processes, thoughtful or automatic, 47–49
Attitude reports, 220–225
  negative, 24
  question order effects decreasing with aging, 220–221
  response order effects increasing with age, 221–225
  strong and positive, 24
Attitudes, 175–180
  automatic, 52
  guiding people's decisions and actions, 46
  implicit or unconscious, 179–180
  toward different older adult subtypes, 176
  toward the future, 60
Attitudes toward body image, racial and ethnic differences in, 32
Authoritarian Personality, The, 235
Automatic attitudes, 52
Automatic biases, challenging, 90
Automatic evaluations, 85

B

Bandura, Albert, 23
Beatles, 9
Behavior. *See also* Addictive behaviors
  genetic explanations for, 21
  importance of context in maintaining, 41
  key to all aging scenarios, 13
  neuroscience studying its relation to the brain, 37
  prediction of, 210
Behavior-based research, 3
Behavior change, sustaining, 134–138
Behavior toward older adults, 180–184
  interventions, 183–184
  patronizing *versus* accommodating speech, 181–183
Behavioral and Social Research Program, 2, 11, 16, 247
Behavioral forecasting measures, 62
Behavioral frequency reports, 225–227
  response alternatives, 226–227
  subjective theories, 225–226
Behavioral observations, 83–84
Behavioral practices, 5
Behavioral science, recent developments in, 12
Beliefs, 21
  about age-related decline, 80
  about aging, 89
  about memory loss, 30
  acquired, 23
  self-efficacy, 44
Binge eating, 42
Blood-oxygen-level-dependent (BOLD) signals, 240
Body image, racial and ethnic differences in attitudes toward, 32
BOLD. *See* Blood-oxygen-level-dependent signals
Boomer generation, 9
Brain imaging methods, 241

C

Cantril, Hadley, 233
Capabilities for deciding, 56–59
  individual, 56–58
  meta-awareness, 58–59
Caregiving, 12, 26
Cellular senescence, 21
Center for Scientific Review, 249

Change. *See also* Ability to change; Life change
external sources of, 36
initiating and maintaining, 39–41, 50–51
involving novelty, 41
measurement of over time, 17
need for, 34
older people's unique motives for, 35
readiness to make, 122–139
Changing implicit and explicit attitudes, 51–52
Choices
intertemporal, 60
made earlier in life, consequences of, 55
"tyranny" of, 54
Cognitive deficits, age-related, 82
Cognitive function
documented declines in, 88
engagement as augmenting, 77
preserving good, 68
Cognitive impairments, 138
Cognitive neuroscience, 39
of aging, 146
Cognitive science, recent developments in, 12
Cognitive tests, 73
Cognitive training, 71
Cognitive value, fostering, 71
Collaboration between theory and practice, enhancing, 138–139
Committee on Aging Frontiers in Social Psychology, Personality, and Adult Developmental Psychology, 2, 13–14, 58
charge and approach, 11–13
Communication, patronizing forms of, 82
Communication strategies that motivate behavior change, 125–134
message framing, 130–134
message tailoring, 127–130
Competence stereotypes, 177–178
forgetfulness, 177–178
mental incompetence, 178
Compliance, with medical regimens, 47
Confidence, 161, 164, 188
Conscientiousness, 23
Consequences
of actions, 137
of age discrimination, 87
of ageism, 197
of choices made earlier in life, 55
considering, 49
of exposure to ageist stereotypes, 190–191
introduction of new, 49
Context effects, age-sensitive, 219, 228
Continuum-based framework, 124
Control, over the environment, 44
Coping, 43
with distress, 23
in the face of ageism, 198
with traumatic events, 28
Coping with a negative age identity, 191–196
primary compensatory strategies, 192–194
secondary compensatory strategies, 194–196
Cortical "disconnection," 243
Cross-disciplinary research, 37
Cross-racial studies, 78
Cross-sectional studies, 12, 24–25
Cultural and ethnic factors, role of, 78–79
Cultural effects, 1, 5, 15, 21
recommendation regarding, 15

D

Deciding whether to decide, 155–158
Decision avoidance, 156–157
Decision-making processes
emotion, and older adults' decisions, 58
long-range planning and, 59–61
meta-awareness of one's own, 59
at older ages, 3
Decisions
attitudes guiding, 46
medical, 155
memories of past, 147
types most often regretted, 65
"Delay discounting," 154
Deliberative forms of thinking, 48
Deliberative neural systems, 60–61
Deliberative processes, 3, 52
Dementia, 12
defining, 70–71
delaying the onset of, 79
educational level and, 31
physiology of, 242–243
Depressed performance, 88

Depression
and cognitive and neural function, 74
predicting, 189
Detection behaviors, 131
Developmental diathesis-stress model, 21
Diets, 21, 35, 129
failing at, 42
nutritious, 13
Differences in people's readiness to change, 122–139
Disambiguation, of stereotypes, 183, 186
Discrimination
age, consequences of, 87
stress from being the target of, 87
Disease onset, engagement as delaying, 77
Disidentification, 194–195
Disinhibition, 42
Dissatisfaction, post-change, 51
Distress
coping, 23
emotional, 52
Diversity, developing a psychology of, 4–5, 15–16
Dorsolateral prefrontal cortex, 149–151
Driving ability, 58
link to independence, 59
Drug cards, increasingly complicated, 55
Drug regimens. *See* Medical regimens

E

Economy, of an aging workforce, 11
Educational level, and dementia, 31
Elderspeak, 182–183
Eliot, Andrew, 129
Emotion
attention to, 57
in the decision process, 58
effectiveness of regulation of, 146
intraindividual variability in the experience of, 213
and older adults' decisions, 147–149
regulation of, 156
Emotional distress, 52
Emotional factors in attitudes and decision making, 49–50
Emotional processes and self-regulation, 42–43. *See also* Self-regulation
Emotional responses, to options, 66
Emotional solidarity, between parents and adult children, 25
Emotional well-being, 27–29
End-of-life care, 65–66
Engagement
as augmenting cognitive function or delaying disease onset, 77
most effective types of, 77
Environments
control over, 44
exposure to different types of, 23
mastery of, 28
natural, change in, 37
stable cues in, 41
Escapist strategies, 42
Ethnicity issues, 1, 5, 15, 21
recommendation regarding, 15
Exercising regularly, 13, 21, 35, 73–74, 121
Expectations
acquired, 23
of aging, 81
becoming self-fulfilling prophecies, 181
studying, 51
Experience
increasing complexity of, 214
learning from, 63
openness to, 22
Experience sampling, 212–214
Explicit stereotypes, 81–83
Extraversion, 23

F

Family
receiving care from, 32
relationships of self to, 61
Fascism, 235
Fear, and risk aversion, 152
"Feared" selves, 188
Feature-based strategies, 159–160
Five-factor model of traits, 22
Flexibility. *See also* Neural plasticity
fMRI. *See* Functional magnetic resonance imaging
Forgetfulness, 177–178
Formal treatment, ability to change without any form of, 37
Free to Choose, 54
Friedman, Milton, 54
Functional magnetic resonance imaging (fMRI), 58, 214–215, 240, 242, 245
Funding mechanisms, 6
Future, attitudes toward, 60

Future feelings, ability to predict, 62
Future research needed, 13–15
emerging themes and directions for, 184–186, 196–197

G

Gage, Phineas, 149, 151
Gain-framed appeals, 130–131, 133
Gambling games, 153–154
studies using, 150
Gender, race, and socioeconomic status, 31–33
Gender differences, 5, 15, 21, 180
recommendation regarding, 15
Genetic explanations, for behavior, 21
Gerontology, 12, 198
Glucocorticoid dysregulation, 74
Grants
R24 infrastructure, 17
for transdisciplinary centers, 17, 248
Great Depression, "birth dearth" during, 9
Growth, personal, 24, 28

H

Handbook of Questionnaire Design, The, 233
Health, subjective perceptions of, 38
Health interventions, costly and degrading, 66
"Healthy mind," maintaining, 4
Healthy People 2010, 90, 134
Healthy regimens, in everyday life, 13
Heterogeneity, of America's older population, 15
Heuristics. *See* Affective heuristics
High-risk situations, 44
Hippocampal structures
loss of neurons in, 74
neurogenesis in, 73
"Hoped-for" selves, 188
5-HTT (serotonin transporter) gene, 21
Human genome project, 21
Hypertension, 151

I

IAT. *See* Implicit Association Test
Identity, and self-concept, 186–188
Illness, recovery from, 23
Implicit Association Test (IAT), 52, 84, 179, 211
Implicit attitudes and stereotypes, 179–180
activation of, 83–85
gender differences in, 180
Implicit constructs and processes, 83
Impression management, 193
Impulsivity, 154
Incidental encoding, 244–245
Incontinence, 193
Individual adjustments, 24
Individual beliefs and attitudes, 43–44
Individual differences, 23
role of, 78
Individuals, 56–58
Inertia, overcoming, 35
Information about health
more effective presentation of, 36, 126
reduced seeking of, 158–159
Initiation and maintenance of change, 39–41, 50–51, 121–144
Interactional perspective, on personality, 23
Interdisciplinary research, 5–6, 14, 16, 198, 248
Intergenerational interactions, 181
dynamics of, 184
Internalized stereotypes, effects of, 88–89
Intertemporal choice, normative models of, 60
Interventions, 183–184. *See also* Health interventions
to change ageist attitudes, 89–90
culturally appropriate, programmatic, 79
strategies for, 138–139
Intraindividual variability, in emotional experience, 213
Intuitive modes of thinking, 48
Isolation, 12

J

Journal of Cognitive Neuroscience, 214

K

K awards, 247–248
flexibility in, 248
Kahn, Robert, 25

L

Late-life outcomes, 1
Learning from experience, 63
Leisure activities, mentally engaging, 68–69
Life change, successful, 44
Life experiences, accumulating, 24, 33
Life-prolonging medical care, 32
Life-span approach, 12, 14, 19–21, 24, 63
Likert, Rensis, 235
Long-term care institutions, 73
Long-term relationships, loss of, 26–27
Longer life expectancies, impact on societies, 1
Loss-framed appeals, 130–131, 133

M

Magnetic resonance imaging (MRI), 240, 244
Magnetoencephalogram (MEG), 214
Major theory building, 13
Marijuana use, 58
Marital satisfaction, 26
"Matthew effect," 20
Measurement of implicit constructs, 210–212
  introduction, 219
Measurement of psychological mechanisms, 15, 17, 58, 209–216
  experience sampling, 212–214
  measuring implicit constructs, 210–212
  social neuroscience, 214–216
Medical care, life-prolonging, 32
Medical decisions, 155
Medical regimens, compliance with, 47, 59, 121
Medical setting, ageist views of patients in, 82
Medicare, increasingly complicated, 55
Medications, adherence in taking, 35, 37, 40
Memories, of past decisions, 147
Memory bias, 165–166
Memory enhancement effect, and self-reference, 215
Memory loss
  beliefs about, 30
  meta-awareness of, 59, 244
Mental capabilities, significant declines in, 56
Mental health issues, 20, 29
Mental incompetence, 178
Mental stimulation, and cognitive aging, 71–72
Mental vitality, ability to maintain, 68
Message framing, 130–134
Message tailoring, 40, 48–49, 126–130
  defined, 127n
Meta-awareness, 58–59
Methodology, issues of, 17
Mischel, Walter, 60
Models, of behavior change, 128
Mortality, 121
  predictors of, 38
Motivation, and health, 44
Motivation and behavioral change, 2–3, 34–53
  developing methods for, 139
  persuasion and attitude change, 45–52
  recommendation regarding, 14
Motivation and self-regulation, 36–45
  age differences in self-regulation, 38–39
  the avoidance of novelty, 41–42
  emotional processes and self-regulation, 42–43
  individual beliefs and attitudes, 43–44
  initiating or maintaining change, 39–41
  social facilitation and barriers to change, 44–45
MRI. *See* Magnetic resonance imaging
Multilevel factors, 5, 14, 16
Multiparty decision making, 61–66
  affective forecasting, 62–63
  regrets, 64–65
  risk aversion, 63–64
Multiple categories of identity, 85–86

N

National Health Interview Survey, 29
National Institute of Mental Health, StartMH Program, 249
National Institute on Aging (NIA), 2, 5, 13–17, 247–248
  Behavioral and Social Research Program, 2, 11, 16, 247
National Institutes of Health (NIH), 17, 248–249
  Center for Scientific Review, 249
  Office of Behavioral and Social Sciences Research, 248

National Institute on Drug Abuse, 248
National Research Council, 2
National Science Foundation, 249
Natural environments, change in, 37
Negative affect, 152
Negative emotional experiences, 128, 147, 160
Negative pictures, memory for, 148
Negative stereotypes, 176
Neural plasticity, role in social tasks, 216
Neural substrates of decision making, 149–151
Neural systems, types of, 60
Neurocognitive function and cognition, 70–71
Neurogenesis, 73
Neuroimaging, 152, 243
Neuron loss, 151
Neuroscience
  cognitive, 39
  methods of, 58
  recent gains in, 37, 39
Neuroticism, 23
New consequences, introduction of, 49
NIA. *See* National Institute on Aging
NIH. *See* National Institutes of Health
Nondifferentiation, 236
Novelty, the avoidance of, 41–42

O

Obesity, effectiveness of programs to reduce, 32
Office of Behavioral and Social Sciences Research, 248
Older adult subtypes, attitudes toward different, 176
Older adults
  affective heuristics for, 3
  behavior toward, 180–184
  coping with traumatic events, 28
  defined, 11n, 185–187, 189
  differential treatment of, 4
  emotional self-control in, 28
  growing diversity of, 15
  growth in, 20
  identifying problems of, 12
  impulse control in, 38–39
  and the Internet, 76
  predicting lower satisfaction in the future, 27
  reported distance between actual and ideal selves, 24
  self-satisfaction among, 43
  societies top-heavy with, 9
  solving interpersonal problems, 29
  spending more time alone, 25
Older adults' decisions, prefrontal cortex and, 149–164
Optimism-pessimism, dimension of, 23
Optimizing questionnaire design, 233–237
  nondifferentiation, 236
  number of scale points, 234
  order effects, 237
  scale point labeling, 234–236
Orbitofrontal cortex, 149–150
Order effects, 237
Overconfidence, 161

P

Paradox of Choice, The, 54
Park, Denise C., 254
Passivity, 40
Patronizing forms of communication, 82
  versus accommodating speech, 181–183
Payne, Stanley, 233
Performance deficits, age-related, 88
Personal growth, 24, 28
Personality, and self-concept, 22–24
Personality studies, 213
  interactional or transactional perspective on, 23
  recent developments in, 12
  stability and, 22
Perspectives, changing, 24
Persuasion and attitude change, 45–52
  attitude change processes, thoughtful or automatic, 47–49
  changing implicit and explicit attitudes, 51–52
  emotional factors in attitudes and decision making, 49–50
  initiation and maintenance of change, 50–51
  knowledge about, 53
PET. *See* Positron emission tomography
Philadelphia Geriatric Center Positive and Negative Affect Scales, 231
Physical activity. *See* Exercising regularly
Plasticity. *See* Neural plasticity
Positive affect, 149

Positive emotional experiences, 128
Positive social identity, maintaining, 194
Positive stereotypes, 82, 184–185
Positivity effect, 30–31
Positron emission tomography (PET), 214, 240, 245
Prediction, 210
  of depression, 189
  of future feelings, 62
  of mortality, 38
  of self-esteem, 189
Prefrontal cortex and older adults' decisions, 149–165
  aging and prefrontal decline, 151–152
  deciding whether to decide, 155–158
  neural substrates of decision making, 149–151
  repeated decisions, 161–162
  risky decisions, 152–155
  seeking information, 158–161
  susceptibility to scams, 162–164
Prejudice
  negotiating, 197
  reducing, 183
Prevention behaviors, 131
Primacy effects, 222–223
Primary compensatory strategies, 192–194
  self-presentation theory, 192–193
  socioemotional selectivity theory, 193–194
Priming measure, 52, 84, 211
Problem-solving, 156–157
  social, 57
Procrastination, 34–35
Professional assistance, ability to change without any form of, 37
Prospect theory, framing postulate of, 130
Psychological applications of neuroimaging, 241
Psychological disengagement, 194
Psychological processes, 5
Psychological transformation of events, 63
Psychology
  of diversity, developing, 4–5, 15–16
  role in understanding motivation for change, 35
Psychology and Aging, 231, 234
Psychopathologies, 23
  age not increasing risk of, 29
Psychotherapy, efficacy of, 41
Purpose in life, 28

Q

Question order effects, decreasing with aging, 220–221
Question wording, format, and order, 228

R

R24 infrastructure grants, 17
Race effects, 1, 5, 15, 21
  on health, 31
  recommendation regarding, 15
"Rational" processes, 66
Readiness to make change, 122
Reasoned action, theory of, 123
Recency effects, 223
Recommendations, 2, 5–6, 14, 16
Recovery from illness, 23
Regret, 64–66
  anticipated, 64
Relationships. *See also* Social networks
  positive, 28
  of self to the family, 61
Repeated decisions, 161–162
Report structure, 18
Research infrastructure, 5–6, 247–250
  developing, 6
  supporting, 16–17
Research topics, 3–4
  motivation and behavioral change, 3
  opportunities lost: stereotypes of self and by others, 4
  social engagement and cognition, 4
  socioemotional influences on decision making, 3–4
Resilience, 24
Response alternatives, 226–227
Response order effects, increasing with age, 221–225
Retirement "decisions," 21
Retirement Research Foundation, 249
Retirement savings, 55–56
Review process, innovative use of, 6
Reward anticipation, 215
Risk aversion, 63–64, 66, 152
Risk tolerance, 152
Risky decisions, 152–155. *See also* High-risk situations
Russell Sage Foundation, 249

S

Satisfaction, 136–137. *See also* Dissatisfaction; Self-satisfaction
 marital, 26
 studying, 51
Scale points
 labeling, 234–236
 number of, 234
Scams, susceptibility to, 162–164
Schwartz, Barry, 54
Screening behaviors, 132
Secondary compensatory strategies, 194–196
 disidentification, 194–195
 psychological disengagement, 194
 social comparison, 195–196
Seeking information, 158–161
 reduced, 158–159
Selection, 20
Self, views of, 24
Self-acceptance, 28
Self-concept, 198
 changing with age, 24
Self-confidence, 145–146
Self-control, maintaining, 66–67
Self-efficacy, 128
 beliefs about, 44
Self-esteem
 not changing with age, 24
 predicting, 189
Self-fulfilling prophecies, expectations becoming, 181
Self-knowledge, 20
Self-persuasion, 128
Self-presentation theory, 192–193
Self-questioning, 47
Self-regulation, 35
 and aging, 39, 50
 role of affect in, 43
 skills in, 20, 214
 strategies for, 137
Self-Regulatory Model of Illness Behavior, 135
Self-report scales, 62
Self-reports, 84, 209
 of constructs or processes, 83
Self-satisfaction, among older adults, 43
Self-stereotypes, 198
 implications of, 189
Senescence, cellular, 21
Senior citizen community settings, 73
Shifting standards framework, 86
Smoking, 13, 42, 127
Social class effects, 15
Social cognition, 29–31, 214
Social cognitive approach, 85
Social cognitive theory, 135
Social comparison, 195–196
Social concepts, 21
"Social convoys," 25
Social downgrading, 195
Social engagement, 72–76
 technology training as engagement, 75–76
 underlying mechanisms, 73–75
Social facilitation, and barriers to change, 44–45
Social identity, maintaining a positive, 194
Social networks, 1
 composition of, 25
 over time, 25
 size of, 27
 strong and lasting, 13
Social neurosciences, 214–216
 recent developments in, 12
 transforming our understanding of behavior, 14
Social pressure, 162
Social problem solving, 57
Social psychology, 32, 81, 83, 86–87, 89
 recent developments in, 12
Social relations, 20, 25–27
Social Security system, 56
 proposed changes in, 55
Social support, 44–45
Social tasks, role of neural plasticity in, 216
Sociocultural perspective, 83
Socioeconomic status, 21, 31
 recommendation regarding, 15
Socioemotional selectivity theory (SST), 42, 128, 148, 193–194
Spearman-Brown prophecy formula, 232
SST. *See* Socioemotional selectivity theory
Stable environmental cues, 41
Stable personality traits, 23
Stage-based framework, 124
StartMH Program, 249
Status quo, acceptance of, 34
"Stereotype threat" theory, 88, 190
Stereotypes, 175–180. *See also* Self-stereotypes
 activation of, 83

- age identity and self-concept, 86–87
- competence, 177–178
- disambiguation of, 183, 186
- effects of internalized, 88–89
- explicit, 81–83
- impact on self and others, 2, 4, 16, 30, 80–91
- implicit or unconscious, 179–180
- interventions to change ageist attitudes, 89–90
- multiple categories of identity, 85–86
- negative, 81–83
- positive, 82, 184–185
- recommendation regarding, 14

Stigma-related stress, 191
Stimulation, most effective types and combinations of, 79
Strains of later life, 26
Stress
- from being the target of discrimination, 87
- and cognitive and neural function, 74
- stigma-related, 191

Stressful life events, 21, 23
Subjective perceptions of health, 38
Subjective theories, 225–226
Subjective well-being, 23
Sustaining behavior change, 134–138

T

Tailoring. *See* Message tailoring
Taxonomies of traits, 22
Technology
- training in as engagement, 75–76
- using to tailor messages, 128

Telomere shortening, 21
Temperamental inheritance, 23
Thematic apperception tests, 83
Thinking continuum, 47–48
Thoughts about thoughts, 47
Trade-offs, 160
Training designs, 72
Transactional perspective, on personality, 23
Transdisciplinary centers, grants for, 17, 248
Transformation of events psychologically, 63
Traumatic events, coping with, 28
Treatment, ability to change without any formal, 37
"Tyranny of choice," 54

U

Unconscious attitudes and stereotypes, 179–180
- gender differences in, 180

Underconfidence, 161
Underlying mechanisms of behavior, 73–75
- investigating, 3

Understanding. *See* Meta-awareness
University of California-San Diego, 249
"Use it or lose it" argument, 74

V

Vacations, retrieving memories about, 61
Validity checking, 47

W

Well-being
- conceptualizing, 28
- emotional, 27–29
- of the nation, 250
- subjective, 23

Widowhood, 26–27
Wisdom, 24
Workshops, extended, 6